21·32

# Prescribing Scenarios at a Glance

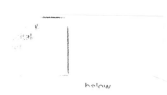

This title is also available as an e-book.
For more details, please see
www.wiley.com/buy/9781118570869
or scan this QR code:

# Prescribing Scenarios at a Glance

**Emma Baker** PhD FRCP

Professor of Clinical Pharmacology
St George's, University of London
Consultant Physician
St George's Healthcare NHS Trust, London


**Daniel Burrage** BSc(Hons) MBBS MRCP FHEA

Academic Clinical Fellow
St George's, University of London
Specialty Registrar (ST3) in Clinical Pharmacology, General Medicine and
Stroke Medicine
St George's Healthcare NHS Trust, London


**Dagan Lonsdale** BSc(Hons) MBBS MRCP FHEA

Academic Clinical Fellow
St George's, University of London
Specialty Registrar (ST3) in Clinical Pharmacology, General Medicine and
Intensive Care Medicine
St George's Healthcare NHS Trust, London


**Andrew Hitchings** BSc(Hons) MBBS MRCP FHEA

Clinical Research Fellow
St George's, University of London
Specialty Registrar (ST7) in Clinical Pharmacology, General Medicine and
Intensive Care Medicine
St George's Healthcare NHS Trust, London

**WILEY** Blackwell

This edition first published 2014 © John Wiley & Sons, Ltd.

*Registered Office*

John Wiley & Sons Ltd, The Atrium, Southern Gate, Chichester, West Sussex, PO19 8SQ, UK

*Editorial Offices*

350 Main Street, Malden, MA 02148-5020, USA

9600 Garsington Road, Oxford, OX4 2DQ, UK

The Atrium, Southern Gate, Chichester, West Sussex, PO19 8SQ, UK

For details of our global editorial offices, for customer services, and for information about how to apply for permission to reuse the copyright material in this book please see our website at www.wiley.com/wiley-blackwell.

The right of Emma Baker, Daniel Burrage, Dagan Lonsdale and Andrew Hitchings to be identified as the authors of this work has been asserted in accordance with the UK Copyright, Designs and Patents Act 1988.

Wiley also publishes its books in a variety of electronic formats. Some content that appears in print may not be available in electronic books.

Designations used by companies to distinguish their products are often claimed as trademarks. All brand names and product names used in this book are trade names, service marks, trademarks or registered trademarks of their respective owners. The publisher is not associated with any product or vendor mentioned in this book. The simulated prescribing chart, variable rate IV insulin infusion chart and discharge prescription are reproduced with permission from St George's, University of London.

SKU: 978EWTLP26358

*Library of Congress Cataloging-in-Publication Data*

Baker, Emma, author.
  Prescribing scenarios at a glance / Emma Baker, Daniel Burrage, Dagan Lonsdale, Andrew Hitchings.
       p. ; cm. – (At a glance)
  Includes bibliographical references and index.
    ISBN 978-1-118-57086-9 (pbk.)
  I. Burrage, Daniel, author.  II. Lonsdale, Dagan, author.  III. Hitchings, Andrew, author.  IV. Title.  V. Series: At a glance series (Oxford, England).
    [DNLM:  1.  Drug Therapy–Case Reports.   2.  Pharmaceutical Preparations–Case Reports. WB 330]
  RM300
  615.1–dc23
                               2014000049

A catalogue record for this book is available from the British Library.

Cover image: Reproduced from iStock © joyfnp
Cover design by Meaden Creative

Set in 9/11.5 pt Time New RomanMTStd by Toppan Best-set Premedia Limited
Printed and bound in Malaysia by Vivar Printing Sdn Bhd

1  2014

# Contents

*Please note that the prepared drug charts can be found in the accompanying workbook.*

## Section 3: Routine inpatient review

# Acknowledgements

We are indebted to Dr Katie Pearson, Specialist Trainee in Paediatrics, Penninsula Deanery for her contribution as lead author for paediatric cases 21–23. These cases arose from a survey she performed, which found that over half of foundation doctors were required to prescribe for children, with analgesia, antibiotics and fluids being the most common prescriptions.

We are grateful to Dr Natasha Patel, Consultant in Acute Medicine and Diabetes, for her comments on insulin prescribing in Case 42.

# Dedication

This book is dedicated to our families for their support and patience over the many months of late evenings and lost weekends that they've had to endure in the course of its preparation!

# List of abbreviations

| | | | |
|---|---|---|---|
| ABCDE | approach to the critically unwell patient: airway; breathing; circulation; disability; exposure | FDA | Food and Drug Administration |
| Abdo | abdomen (examination) | FFP | fresh frozen plasma |
| ACE | angiotensin converting enzyme | FP10 | NHS prescription forms used in the community |
| ACR | albumin : creatinine ratio | FH | family history |
| ACS | acute coronary syndrome | FT4 | free thyroxine (concentration) |
| Adj Ca$^{2+}$ | adjusted calcium concentration | GABA | gamma-aminobutyric acid |
| ADP | adenosine diphosphate | GGT | gamma glutamyl transferase |
| ADR | adverse drug reaction | GI | gastrointestinal |
| AKI | acute kidney injury | Gluc | glucose (concentration) |
| ALP | alkaline phosphatase | GP | general practitioner |
| ALT | alanine transaminase | GRACE | Global Registry of Acute Coronary Events |
| APTT | activated partial thromboplastin time | GSL | general sales list (medicines) |
| ARB | angiotensin receptor blocker | GTN | glyceryl trinitrate |
| ARF | acute renal failure | H | histamine |
| BBB | blood–brain barrier | Hb | haemoglobin (concentration) |
| BD | (bis die) twice daily | HbA$_{1c}$ | glycated haemoglobin |
| BE | base excess | HCO$_3^-$ | bicarbonate ion (concentration) |
| Bil | bilirubin (concentration) | HIV | human immunodeficiency virus |
| BMI | body mass index | HPC | history of presenting complaint |
| BNF | British National Formulary | HR | heart rate |
| BNFc | BNF for Children | 5HT | serotonin |
| BNP | brain natriuretic peptide | Ig | immunoglobulin |
| BP | blood pressure | IM | intramuscular |
| Ca$^{2+}$ | calcium ion (concentration) | INH | inhaled |
| CBG | capillary blood glucose | INN | international non-proprietary name |
| CIWA-Ar | Clinical Institute Withdrawal Assessment for Alcohol Scale, revised | INR | international normalised ratio |
| CKD | chronic kidney disease | IV | intravenous |
| CLO | Campylobacter-like organism (test) | JVP | jugular venous pressure |
| CMV | cytomegalovirus | K$^+$ | potassium ion (concentration) |
| COPD | chronic obstructive pulmonary disease | kg | kilogram |
| CPAP | continuous positive airway pressure | kPa | kilopascals |
| Creat | creatinine (concentration) | LMWH | low molecular weight heparin |
| CRP | C-reactive protein | MC&S | microscopy, culture and sensitivity |
| CSCI | continuous subcutaneous insulin infusion | MCV | mean corpuscular volume |
| CT | computed tomography | MHRA | Medicines and Healthcare products Regulatory Agency |
| CTPA | computed tomography pulmonary angiogram | MI | myocardial infarction |
| CTZ | chemoreceptor trigger zone | mmHg | millimetres of mercury |
| CURB-65 | pneumonia severity score (confusion, urea, respiratory rate, blood pressure, age) | MR or m/r | modified release |
| | | MRSA | meticillin resistant *Staphylococcus aureus* |
| CVS | cardiovascular system | MSS | musculoskeletal system |
| CXR | chest X-ray | Na$^+$ | sodium ion (concentration) |
| D | dopamine | NAC | *N*-acetylcysteine |
| DH | drug history | NAPQI | *N*-acetyl-*p*-benzoquinone imine |
| DXA | dual-energy X-ray absorptiometry | NEB | nebulised |
| EBV | Epstein–Barr virus | Neut | neutrophil (count) |
| ECG | electrocardiogram | NG | nasogastric (tube) |
| eGFR | estimated glomerular filtration rate | NICE | National Institute for Health and Care Excellence |
| eMC | electronic Medicines Compendium | NKDA | no known drug allergies |
| EMA | European Medicines Agency | NMDA | *N*-methyl-D-aspartate |
| Eos | eosinophil (count) | NOAC | novel oral anticoagulant |
| EPO | erythropoietin | NPH | neutral protamine Hagedorn (refers to intermediate-acting insulin) |
| ESR | erythrocyte sedimentation rate | NRT | nicotine replacement therapy |
| FBC | full blood count | NS | nervous system |

| | | | | |
|---|---|---|---|---|
| NSAID | non-steroidal anti-inflammatory drug | | RS | respiratory system |
| NSF | National Service Framework | | SC | subcutaneous |
| NSTEMI | non-ST elevation myocardial infarction | | SH | social history |
| Obs | observations | | SIGN | Scottish Intercollegiate Guidelines Network |
| OD | (*omni die*) every day | | SPC | Summary of Product Characteristics |
| OM | (*omni mane*) every morning | | $SpO_2$ | oxygen saturations |
| ON | (*omni nocte*) every night | | STEMI | ST elevation myocardial infarction |
| $PaO_2$ | partial pressure of oxygen | | T | temperature |
| $PaCO_2$ | partial pressure of carbon dioxide | | TDM | therapeutic drug monitoring |
| PC | presenting complaint | | TDS | (*ter die sumendum*) to be taken three times daily |
| PCC | prothrombin complex concentrate | | TIA | transient ischaemic attack |
| PE | pulmonary embolism | | TRALI | transfusion-associated lung injury |
| PEFR | peak expiratory flow rate | | TRH | thyrotropin releasing hormone |
| PEG | percutaneous endoscopic gastrostomy | | Trop | troponin |
| PIL | patient information leaflet | | TSH | thyroid stimulating hormone |
| Plt | platelet (count) | | TTA | to take away |
| PMH | past medical history | | TTO | to take out |
| $PO_4^{2-}$ | phosphate ion (concentration) | | UFH | unfractionated heparin |
| PoM | prescription only medicines | | Ur | urea (concentration) |
| PPI | proton pump inhibitor | | USS KUB | ultrasound scan of kidneys, ureters and bladder |
| PR | per rectum | | Vit | vitamin |
| PRN | (*pro re nata*) as required | | VRIII | variable rate intravenous insulin infusion |
| PT | prothrombin time | | VTE | venous thromboembolic/ism |
| PV | per vagina | | WCC | white (blood) cell count |
| QDS | (*quater die sumendum*) to be taken four times daily | | WHO | World Health Organization |
| RR | respiratory rate | | % w/w | percentage weight/weight |

# How to use your textbook

## Features contained within your textbook

Each case comprises a prescribing scenario and a prepared drug chart, contained in the accompanying workbook, on which to write your answer.

These are accompanied by full explanations and completed drug charts.

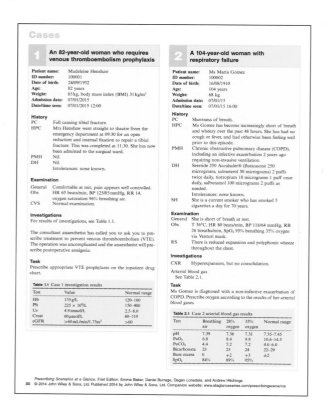

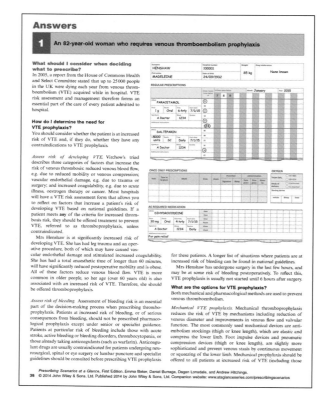

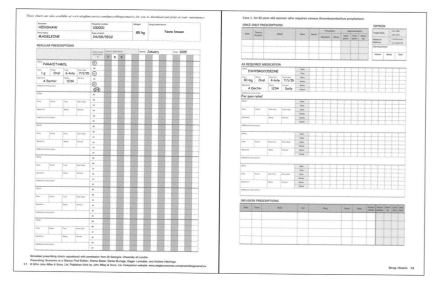

 **The website icon** indicates that you can find accompanying resources on the book's companion website.

## The anytime, anywhere textbook

### Wiley E-Text

Your book is also available to purchase as a **Wiley E-Text: Powered by VitalSource** version – a digital, interactive version of this book which you own as soon as you download it.

Your Wiley E-Text allows you to:

**Search:** Save time by finding terms and topics instantly in your book, your notes, even your whole library (once you've downloaded more textbooks)

**Note and Highlight:** Colour code, highlight and make digital notes right in the text so you can find them quickly and easily

**Organize:** Keep books, notes and class materials organized in folders inside the application

**Share:** Exchange notes and highlights with friends, classmates and study groups

**Upgrade:** Your textbook can be transferred when you need to change or upgrade computers

**Link:** Link directly from the page of your interactive textbook to all of the material contained on the companion website

The Wiley E-Text version will also allow you to copy and paste any photograph or illustration into assignments, presentations and your own notes.

**To access your** Wiley E-Text:

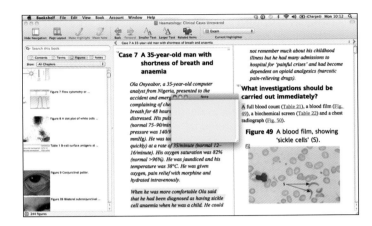

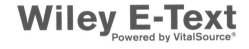

- Visit **www.vitalsource.com/software/bookshelf/downloads** to download the Bookshelf application to your computer, laptop, tablet or mobile device.
- Open the Bookshelf application on your computer and register for an account.
- Follow the registration process.

### The VitalSource Bookshelf can now be used to view your Wiley E-Text on iOS, Android and Kindle Fire!

- **For iOS:** Visit the app store to download the VitalSource Bookshelf: **http://bit.ly/17ib3XS**
- **For Android:** Visit the Google Play Market to download the VitalSource Bookshelf: **http://bit.ly/ZMEGvo**
- **For Kindle Fire, Kindle Fire 2 or Kindle Fire HD:** Simply install the VitalSource Bookshelf onto your Fire (see how at **http://bit.ly/11BVFn9**). You can now sign in with the email address and password you used when you created your VitalSource Bookshelf Account.

Full E-Text support for mobile devices is available at: **http://support.vitalsource.com**

## CourseSmart

**CourseSmart** gives you instant access (via computer or mobile device) to this Wiley-Blackwell e-book and its extra electronic functionality, at 40% off the recommended retail print price. See all the benefits at: **www.coursesmart.com/students**

**Instructors . . . receive your own digital desk copies!**

**CourseSmart** also offers instructors an immediate, efficient, and environmentally friendly way to review this book for your course.

For more information visit **www.coursesmart.com/instructors**.

With CourseSmart, you can create lecture notes quickly with copy and paste, and share pages and notes with your students. Access your **CourseSmart** digital book from your computer or mobile device instantly for evaluation, class preparation, and as a teaching tool in the classroom.

Simply sign in at **http://instructors.coursesmart.com/bookshelf** to download your Bookshelf and get started. To request your desk copy, hit 'Request Online Copy' on your search results or book product page.

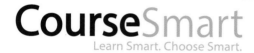

We hope you enjoy using your new book. Good luck with your studies!

# About the companion website

Don't forget to visit the companion website for this book:

 **www.ataglanceseries.com/prescribingscenarios**

There you will find:
- Refill drug charts for each scenario in the book for you to download and print
- Additional useful charts for you to download and print

Scan this QR code to visit the companion website:

# Introduction: Practical prescribing scenarios

## Purpose of the book

A prescription is a written order from a suitably qualified health-care professional that authorises the dispensing or administration of a medicine for a patient. Prescribing is an essential skill, central to the practice of medicine, and has many component parts. Deciding what to prescribe requires you to have up-to-date knowledge of diagnosis, pharmacology and therapeutics, backed up by use of appropriate reference material and underpinned by good clinical and consultation skills. Writing the prescription requires you to apply this knowledge, with clear communication and consideration of the implications of the prescription for the patient, healthcare system and society.

The right to prescribe is controlled by legislation. In the UK, prior to 1992, only doctors, dentists and veterinary surgeons could write prescriptions. Prescribing training for these practitioners is therefore included in their undergraduate courses, with supervised prescribing early in postgraduate training required prior to professional registration. Subsequent legislation widened prescribing rights to allow nurses, pharmacists and optometrists, and soon radiographers, podiatrists and chiropodists, to be independent prescribers. These 'non-medical prescribers' are required to be experienced practitioners, to complete an accredited postgraduate prescribing course and to register this qualification on their professional register.

Whether you are learning prescribing at undergraduate or postgraduate level, you will require considerable practice to attain competence. The aim of this book is to allow you to practise making treatment decisions and writing realistic prescriptions for a wide range of simulated patients, to develop skills that will translate readily into clinical practice. This book is designed around the types and levels of tasks expected of a foundation doctor, but should also be useful for other healthcare professionals training to prescribe.

## How to use this book

### Contents

The book comprises an introductory chapter, which gives an overview of prescribing skills, and 50 simulated patients requiring treatment. For each patient there is a clinical scenario, a prepared chart for you to write the prescription and suggested answers including a model completed chart and an explanation of the prescription. The scenarios, model charts and explanations are presented consecutively in the main book. The prepared charts are provided in a separate workbook in patient order so that you can use them alongside the clinical information and compare them easily with the model answers.

### Cases

The cases are organised by clinical setting, and have been chosen as situations likely to be encountered by foundation doctors. The three settings are: the acute take; on call in the hospital; and routine or specialty inpatient review. Each case requires you to perform a task at the level expected of a foundation doctor. Within each setting, the cases have been organised by approximate level of complexity, using the scheme shown in Box I.1. This is given as

---

### Box I.1 Complexity of cases

**Issues considered:**
- Several medicines to prescribe or review where interactions/adverse drug reactions may be important/complex
- A difficult patient with contraindications/special circumstances
- Lateral thinking required, e.g. considering prophylaxis against venous thromboembolism where not specifically asked to do so
- Complicated prescription, dose calculations, infusions

**Level allocated:**
1 No issues, single medicine, following protocol or guidelines, straightforward patient
2 One issue
3 Two issues
4 Three or more issues

---

a rough guide to allow you to work through more straightforward cases, before tackling more complex patients.

### Working through the cases

We recommend that you first read the clinical information, work out what you think should be done, then write the prescription(s) required before reading the model answer. Completion of the prepared charts is a very important part of the process. For example, knowing that you need to prescribe 'an angiotensin converting enzyme (ACE) inhibitor' is very different from choosing between the dozen or so ACE inhibitors available, then selecting a dose and frequency of administration and committing this to paper. When completing the prescriptions you should refer to a paper or online (https://www.evidence.nhs.uk/formulary/bnf/current) version of the British National Formulary (BNF), which provides up-to-date information about the use of medicines licensed for prescription in the UK. In the clinical situation you will also use local and national guidelines to support your practice. For an example of local guidelines, you could refer to the St George's *Guidelines for the Management of Common Medical Emergencies and for the Use of Antimicrobial Drugs*, which is freely available online (www.greybook.sgul.ac.uk) or as an iPhone/iPad app (https://itunes.apple.com/gb/app/greymobile/id566912801?mt=8). In the model answer we have provided references and links to appropriate national guidelines as further reading. As antibiotic prescribing is a particularly difficult area we have provided suggested antibiotic guidelines in Appendix 1 to support your prescribing as you work through the cases.

### Model answers

Medicine is very complex and there is seldom one single correct solution to any clinical problem. Two patients with similar clinical presentations may end up with very different prescriptions, depending on the underlying characteristics of the patient (comorbidities, other therapies, allergies, special circumstances and treatment preferences), prescriber (experience, specialty, knowledge, perspective and preferences) and the consultation process (concordance).

*Prescribing Scenarios at a Glance*, First Edition. Emma Baker, Daniel Burrage, Dagan Lonsdale, and Andrew Hitchings.

Guidelines provide support for treatment decisions but do not cover all eventualities and there are often areas of uncertainty.

When writing our model prescriptions we have followed BNF guidance and national guidelines where available. However, each answer should be considered as one way of managing the patient described, rather than the single correct way. The answers are tailored to that patient and, although wider management considerations may be discussed, they are not intended to provide a guideline on the management of the condition more generally. Where uncertainty exists we have tried to reflect this in the discussion. Our explanations are set out in two parts: what to consider when deciding what to prescribe; and how to write the prescription. Both parts are essential to the development of prescribing skills. The multiple skills required to be a competent prescriber are emphasised by the blueprint for the proposed national Prescribing Safety Assessment which includes: writing a new prescription; reviewing existing prescriptions; planning management; providing information; identifying and avoiding adverse drug reactions; monitoring drug treatment; dose calculations; and data interpretation (www.prescribe.ac.uk/psa/?page_id=23).

### Disclaimer
The cases in this book are designed to reflect real life, with their own reports of symptoms and concerns. However, they and their identities are entirely fictitious and any similarity to real patients, alive or dead, is coincidental.

## The prescribing process
The World Health Organization provides a 6-step guide to the process of rational prescribing (http://apps.who.int/medicinedocs/en/d/Jwhozip23e/):
1. Define the patient's problem
2. Specify the therapeutic objective
3. Choose a drug for the condition and verify suitability for the individual
4. Write the prescription
5. Give the patient information and warnings
6. Monitor the treatment.

Throughout this book we will consider these 6 steps in two main stages: how to decide what to prescribe (steps 1–3); and how to write the prescription (step 4), with discussion of patient information and monitoring as appropriate.

### How to decide what to prescribe
#### The tools
Good prescribing decisions require expertise in sourcing and using reliable up-to-date reference material to support personal knowledge, clinical skills and experience. The main reference material you need is contained in formularies and guidelines.

#### Formularies
A formulary is a list of prescribable medicines that includes details to support their prescription. Formularies can be international, national, local or personal. The World Health Organization issues a list of medicines to guide countries in making essential medicines available to their citizens. National formularies list medicines approved for prescription within that country.

The British National Formulary (BNF) lists all drugs licensed for prescription in the UK. It is an independent publication, produced by an editorial team of experienced pharmacists, supported by expert clinical advisers, and overseen by a committee representing national bodies including the Royal Pharmaceutical Society, Medicines and Healthcare products Regulatory Agency (MHRA) and UK health departments. It brings together validated guidance on best practice and drug information. The electronic version (available at https://www.evidence.nhs.uk/formulary/bnf/current) is updated monthly and a printed edition is currently produced every 6 months.

The BNF is divided into chapters, by body system (e.g. cardiovascular, respiratory) or aspect of medical care (e.g. infection, malignant disease). Each chapter is subdivided into sections (e.g. cardiovascular sections include diuretics, anti-arrhythmic drugs and drugs for hypertension and heart failure), which provide prescribing notes and information about relevant drugs, grouped according to their pharmacology and therapeutic effects. For individual drugs, the BNF describes indications, safety considerations and potential side effects, provides practical information including dosage and route of administration, and lists preparations available with their prices. The BNF is a valuable resource to support prescribing in the UK and you should become experienced in its use.

Local formularies developed by hospitals or primary care trusts usually contain a subset of medicines from the national formulary approved for prescribing in that locality. Local formularies can improve medicines safety, e.g. by limiting the availability of different preparations of a single drug, reducing dosing errors. They can also reduce cost, e.g. by selecting the cheapest drug within a class or by limiting drug stocks in hospital pharmacies to prevent waste. Local formularies are usually published electronically or on paper, or you can find out what medicines are available in your hospital by asking your pharmacy.

Personal formularies are lists of drugs that an individual becomes familiar with, usually by prescribing them regularly. You can use this book to develop your personal formulary as you practise writing prescriptions for drugs in situations commonly encountered by F1 doctors. Experience in the use of a well-defined subset of drugs allows you to care for patients more effectively and to practise more efficiently.

#### Guidelines
Clinical guidelines are recommendations on the appropriate treatment and care of people with specific diseases and conditions. They are usually based on the best available evidence and are designed to support and raise the general standard of clinical practice, without replacing the knowledge and expertise of individual practitioners.

In the UK, guidelines for care of patients in the NHS are produced by the National Institute for Health and Care Excellence (NICE). The Scottish Medicines Consortium (SMC) and Scottish Intercollegiate Guidelines Network (SIGN) undertakes similar work for the NHS in Scotland. NICE guidelines are produced by groups that include healthcare professionals, patient and carer representatives, and technical advisers. NICE issues two main types of guidance of relevance to prescribing:
1 *Clinical guidelines* are recommendations on the management of a condition based on the assessment of the best available evidence. They are advisory.
2 *Technology appraisals* are recommendations on how technologies (such as medicines) should be used in the NHS. A positive

recommendation in a NICE technology appraisal mandates that the technology be made available for all NHS patients in whom it is indicated. This approach aims to eliminate local variations in treatment, sometimes referred to as a 'postcode lottery'.

NICE guidelines are easy to access online (www.nice.org.uk). Quick reference guides and patient pathways can help you to make timely decisions about patient care, whereas full guidance provides a comprehensive summary of the evidence. Other national guidelines, including those from the Royal Colleges or specialty bodies, also provide helpful information, although the process used to produce them is sometimes less transparent. Where guidance from such bodies bears the NICE accredited mark, it means that the process has been assessed by NICE and deemed to be of high quality.

Primary or secondary care organisations or individual practitioners may produce bespoke guidelines for local use. These are often based on national guidance but have the purpose of defining local practice (e.g. antibiotic use according to local sensitivities), bringing together sets of guidance for easy access (e.g. guidelines for common medical emergencies) or directing specialty care (e.g. management of haematological malignancies). When starting a new job, you should find out what the local guidelines are for management of patients under your care and make sure you consult these.

### Approach to the patient

The first two steps in rational prescribing are to define the patient's problem and specify the therapeutic objective. In addition, each patient contact provides an opportunity to review existing treatment and ensure that measures to prevent complications, deterioration or recurrence of the clinical problem have been implemented. The extent to which each aspect of care is prioritised will depend on the clinical setting and illness severity. In this section, we consider how you should approach patients seen on the acute take, on call in the hospital, and at routine or specialty inpatient review.

#### Acute take

Many patients presenting to the hospital as an emergency on the 'acute take' are critically unwell. You should therefore prioritise identification and treatment of life-threatening abnormalities, using an ABCDE approach (Resuscitation Council (UK) www.resus.org.uk/pages/alsabcde.htm).

**A** – Check that the airway is patent. Use airway manoeuvres, suction, or oral, nasal, laryngeal or tracheal airways to open the airway as needed.

**B** – Ensure that the patient is breathing sufficiently to achieve adequate oxygenation and ventilation. Prescribe high flow oxygen as needed to correct hypoxia.

**C** – Check circulation. Does the patient have an adequate blood pressure for perfusion of essential organs? Secure adequate intravenous (IV) access as appropriate and prescribe IV fluids as needed to treat hypotension/shock.

**D** – Disability. In patients with reduced conscious level, ensure hypoxia and hypotension have been corrected. Consider drug causes and administer an antagonist if appropriate (e.g. naloxone for opioid overdose). Measure blood glucose and administer intravenous glucose to correct hypoglycaemia if appropriate.

**E** – Exposure. Look for and address external sources of critical illness, such as an infusion that may be precipitating an anaphylactic reaction. Once priorities to sustain life have been addressed, other treatment priorities include symptom relief; treatment of the primary diagnosis; review of existing treatment; and prevention of complications, deterioration or recurrence.

As a foundation doctor you should always call for senior help when managing patients with critical illness. After initial assessment and treatment, it is essential that you monitor and review patients carefully. You should assess the effects of treatment to make sure there has been clinical improvement or, if not, to identify the need for further measures. On-going care for patients with critical illness is less well represented than initial treatment in this book, but is extremely important.

#### On call in the hospital

Outside normal working hours, medical care in hospitals is provided by on-call staff. The on-call team is usually too small to provide routine review of all inpatients, so a handover system is used to identify patients who need review or change in treatment. The on-call team is also called by ward staff to see patients who deteriorate acutely or develop new care needs.

Inpatients who deteriorate acutely should be assessed and managed using the ABCDE approach in a similar manner to those presenting acutely. In other situations, clinical assessment or handover instructions should identify the therapeutic objective.

Although time may be limited on call, prescribing in this situation still requires a quick review of existing medication. You should determine whether the patient's medication could account for new symptoms, or whether it may be complicated by new diagnoses (cautions and contraindications) or treatments (drug–drug interactions). It is particularly important to check that 'dangerous' existing medications, such as warfarin, insulin or gentamicin, are being correctly monitored and prescribed.

#### Routine or specialty inpatient review

When you review hospital inpatients on a routine ward round, there are several prescribing-related aspects to consider.

1 *Presenting problem.* You should check that the presenting problem/diagnosis has been treated effectively with control of symptoms. You should enquire about side effects of new treatments and check that drugs have been prescribed correctly (e.g. that antibiotics have a review date and indications).

2 *Prior complaints.* You should check that existing medicines for long-term conditions have been prescribed as appropriate and consider potential interactions between new and existing medicines. You should keep long-term conditions under review and make sure that any new treatment does not cause them to deteriorate.

3 *Prophylaxis.* You should check that measures to prevent complications, deterioration or recurrence have been taken, e.g. low molecular weight heparin to prevent venous thromboembolism, statins for secondary prevention of ischaemic heart disease.

4 *Discharge planning.* You should review routes of administration of treatment and make changes (e.g. intravenous to oral, nebulised to inhaled) when appropriate. You should stop any treatment that is no longer required, e.g. aspirin if cardiovascular disease has been ruled out, and plan review dates for other medicines as appropriate. You should prepare a provisional

discharge prescription as soon as possible to allow for efficient patient discharge when the time comes.

## Deciding what to prescribe

When you prescribe a medicine you need to weigh up likely benefits (efficacy), potential harm (safety), other side effects and inconvenience (tolerability) and share these considerations with the patient through consultation. Where other factors are balanced, cost may also be a consideration. In this section we review these steps, illustrating them with the processes involved in prescribing an ACE inhibitor for a patient with hypertension.

### Efficacy

You need to consider: how the medicine works; whether it is indicated for the problem you are trying to treat; and its place in therapy, relative to other medicines available for the same indication.

*Mechanism of action.* A good understanding of pharmacology helps you to prescribe rationally.

Example: Angiotensin converting enzyme (ACE) inhibitors prevent conversion of angiotensin I to angiotensin II. As angiotensin II acts as a vasoconstrictor and (via aldosterone) stimulates sodium and water retention, reduction in angiotensin II production lowers blood pressure. ACE inhibitors alone do not lower blood pressure effectively in people who have low-renin hypertension, where the renin–angiotensin system is suppressed (most commonly in elderly patients and those of African descent).

*Indications.* Clinical trials are performed to establish indications for medicines. Evidence from these trials is presented to regulatory bodies such as the MHRA, the European Medicines Agency (EMA) and the US Food and Drug Administration (FDA). If the medicine is found to be of sufficient safety, quality and efficacy, these agencies issue a marketing authorisation (licence), which allows it to be prescribed and sold. The licensed indications for medicines in Europe are listed in their Summary of Product Characteristics (SPC). The SPC is a document provided to inform healthcare professionals about the nature and use of the medicine. For products licensed in the UK, the SPC can be obtained online from the electronic Medicines Compendium (eMC, http://www.medicines.org.uk/emc/). The BNF also lists licensed indications for medicines, and additionally may state unlicensed but widely accepted indications. The use of medicines in unlicensed indications is permitted, but this places some additional responsibilities on the prescriber (detailed in guidance from the General Medical Council provided at http://www.gmc-uk.org/guidance/ethical_guidance/14327.asp) and is usually outside the remit of a foundation doctor.

Example: Licensed indications for ACE inhibitors listed in the BNF include hypertension, heart failure, diabetic nephropathy, prophylaxis of cardiovascular events.

*Place in therapy.* Where more than one medicine is licensed for an indication, treatment guidelines and pathways, developed from clinical trial evidence, are used to define their relative place in therapy. NICE provides national guidance in many clinical areas for the UK.

Example: Other drugs that are licensed for the treatment of hypertension include calcium-channel blockers, angiotensin II receptor blockers, thiazide diuretics, alpha- and beta-adrenoceptor blockers. NICE guidance describes the relative place of these different treatments in therapy and states, for example, that ACE inhibitors are a first-line treatment for hypertension in people aged <55 years who are not of black African or Caribbean origin.

### Safety

You need to consider the risks associated with prescribing the medicine: adverse drug reactions (side effects); risk of interactions of new medicines with existing treatment (drug–drug interactions) or underlying disease (cautions and contraindications); and whether patients have increased susceptibility to harm from the drug (special circumstances).

*Adverse drug reactions.* All drugs have adverse effects. There are various systems for the classification of adverse drug reactions, one of which defines them according to whether they are dose-related (augmented, type A), idiosyncratic (bizarre, type B), continued use (type C), delayed onset (type D) or end of dose (type E) effects (see Case 33). When choosing a drug, you should check whether your patient has known intolerance of or is allergic to any medication, and avoid drugs known to cause adverse reactions. You should be able to counsel your patient on the most likely or potentially serious side effects of treatment, monitor for and recognise adverse drug reactions if they occur. Drug side effects are listed for drugs and classes in the BNF, in the SPC, and on the patient information leaflet (PIL) included with all medicines in the UK (these are also available from the eMC at http://www.medicines.org.uk/emc/). Serious adverse drug reactions need to be reported to the MHRA using the Yellow Card Scheme.

Example: Common side effects of ACE inhibitors include first-dose hypotension, cough, hyperkalaemia and renal impairment. Allergic reactions and angioedema are rare and potentially life-threatening idiosyncratic reactions.

*Drug–drug interactions.* Where more than one drug is taken, there is potential for drug–drug interactions. These interactions may be pharmacokinetic, where one drug alters the absorption distribution, metabolism or excretion of another, or pharmacodynamic, where drugs with similar or opposite actions augment or cancel each other's effects. Some interactions have therapeutic benefit; others increase the risk of harm. Before prescribing a new medicine, it is important to take a thorough medical history to identify existing prescribed medicines, drugs purchased by the patient (over the counter), any complementary or herbal remedies and illicit drug use. It is good practice to consult Appendix 1 of the BNF to check for potential interactions between proposed and existing medicines.

Example: Pharmacokinetic interaction: ACE inhibitors reduce lithium excretion, which increases the risk of lithium toxicity. Pharmacodynamic interactions: the hypotensive effect of ACE inhibitors is enhanced by other drugs that lower blood pressure, including diuretics, calcium-channel blockers, alpha- and beta-adrenoceptor blockers. This may be of therapeutic benefit, e.g. where combination treatment is required for hypertension, or harmful, e.g. where diuresis in heart failure is limited by hypotension. There is an increased risk of hyperkalaemia in patients taking ACE inhibitors with potassium-sparing diuretics or potassium salts.

*Cautions and contraindications.* Where patients have more than one problem or diagnosis, drugs used to treat one condition can exacerbate the other(s). When prescribing, it is important to identify other conditions (comorbidities) and check whether these require caution with, or are contraindications to, your planned treatment. 'Caution' is a general term which can be difficult to interpret even for experienced doctors, as specific guidance on what 'being cautious' actually constitutes is rarely provided. The BNF lists cautions and contraindications under individual drugs or classes.

Example: Caution should be used when prescribing ACE inhibitors for patients taking concurrent diuretic therapy, as they are at increased risk of first-dose hypotension. Caution in this situation could include: starting ACE inhibitor treatment at the lowest dose; taking extra care to ensure that the patient is aware of the possible first-dose effect; and omitting the dose of diuretic that precedes the first dose of ACE inhibitor. ACE inhibitors are contraindicated, so should not be used, in patients with known hypersensitivity, because of the risk of a life-threatening allergic reaction.

*Tolerability.* Taking a medicine invariably causes some inconvenience for the patient, whether because of a troublesome but non-serious adverse effect, or simply because of the bother of having to take medicine doses. Such issues can seem trivial to the prescriber but may be of great important to the patient, and may result in non-adherence. The better you know your patient, and the more you discuss and prioritise the issues important to them, the greater the chances of maintaining a productive therapeutic relationship.

Example: The various ACE inhibitors available have different half-lives in the body, which influences how frequently they need to be taken. Prescribing a product that needs only to be taken once a day (e.g. ramipril, lisinopril) may cause less inconvenience to the patient and promote better adherence than prescribing captopril, an older drug that needs to be taken two or three times daily.

*Special circumstances.* Pharmacokinetics (handling of drugs by the body) and pharmacodynamics (response of the body to drugs) are altered in people with renal or hepatic impairment, those who are pregnant or breast feeding, and the very young (neonate) or elderly. You should therefore be very cautious when prescribing for people with these 'special circumstances', minimising the use of medicines and using drugs with well-established safety profiles at low doses. It is important to recognise these conditions, e.g. by testing renal or hepatic function and considering possible pregnancy in all women of child-bearing age, before starting treatment.

Example: ACE inhibitors should not be used during pregnancy, as they may have adverse effects on the fetus, including impaired blood pressure control and renal function. They are not recommended during breast feeding, as they can cause hypotension in the infant. As many ACE inhibitors are pro-drugs (require hepatic metabolism for activation), their action may be unpredictable in patients with hepatic impairment and requires close monitoring. Hyperkalaemia and other side effects of ACE inhibitors are more common in people with renal impairment, in whom dose reduction may be required.

*Costs*
You need to consider the cost of medicines both to the individual and NHS and minimise this where possible.

*Individual patients.* In England, patients are required to pay a fixed charge for primary care prescriptions, which is £8.05 per item from April 2014. Many patients are exempt from this fee, including young (<16 years or 16–18 years old in full-time education), pregnant or older (≥60 years) people, people with medical exemption for chronic disease (e.g. diabetes mellitus, epilepsy) and those with low income. Where patients are taking multiple medicines, a 3- or 12-month pre-payment certificate can reduce costs. Despite this, some patients will not be able to afford prescription charges and therefore will not take prescribed medicines. You should consider checking this when writing outpatient prescriptions.

*NHS.* The cost of prescribed medicines to the NHS in England is around £13 billion each year, with primary care accounting for two-thirds and hospitals for one-third of the total spend. Where safety and efficacy of two drugs are equal, cost should be taken into consideration when choosing between them. Prescribing a drug by its generic name allows dispensing of cheaper non-branded versions of drugs, which can also reduce costs.

Example: Depending on the dose, generic ramipril is 5–10 times cheaper than Tritace®, a proprietary (branded) form of ramipril. In England in 2011, there were approximately 22.5 million prescriptions for ramipril. If these had all been written as Tritace®, rather than as generic ramipril, this would have increased the national annual cost of providing ramipril by approximately £175 million.

**Monitoring and follow up**
Selecting a medicine and writing a prescription is only part of the prescribing process. You need to consider how treatment should be monitored and how the patient should be followed up. Planning a stop date for a medicine is just as important as starting treatment. Without this forethought, patients can accumulate medicines that are no longer indicated, increasing the risk of harm.

*Monitoring*

Treatment should be monitored both to see if it has worked and to make sure that it is safe. Methods of monitoring include:

- History, e.g. of improvement in symptoms or of side effects
- Examination, e.g. measurement of blood pressure, peak flow rate
- Blood tests to measure response, e.g. international normalised ratio (INR) for warfarin, or adverse effects, e.g. hepatic function for methotrexate
- Measurement of plasma concentration of drugs with a narrow therapeutic index (see Cases 26 and 41).

It is important to act on the outcome of monitoring. If treatment is not fully effective, you may need to increase the dosage, add a second medicine or stop treatment and change to an alternative. If adverse effects develop, you may need to reduce the dosage or change the treatment.

---

Example: An ACE inhibitor is being prescribed to treat hypertension. Efficacy should therefore be monitored by measurement of blood pressure to ensure control. If blood pressure is not reduced to target, you could increase the dosage of ACE inhibitor, or add a calcium channel blocker to treatment.

Important side effects of ACE inhibitors are renal impairment and hyperkalaemia. You should measure renal function before and 2 weeks after starting an ACE inhibitor or changing the dosage. You should also measure serum potassium, particularly in patients at high risk of hyperkalaemia, e.g. those with pre-existing renal impairment or taking spironolactone (aldosterone antagonist). You should stop the ACE inhibitor and change to an alternative drug if significant new renal impairment or hyperkalaemia develops on treatment (see Case 46).

Patients should be advised that ACE inhibitors are a long-term treatment to control blood pressure. They should therefore collect repeat prescriptions and not stop the drug without consultation with their healthcare professional.

---

## How to write the prescription
### The tools
The form on which a prescription is written depends on the healthcare setting in which you see the patient and the extent to which your organisation has adopted IT. Many hospitals and other institutions still use paper-based drug charts for prescription of medicines to be taken by the patient during their stay. There is no one standard drug chart, so these can vary widely between organisations. Paper drug charts are gradually being superseded by electronic prescribing, with different systems being adopted by different organisations. In the community, prescribing material is more harmonised, with universal use of the FP10 prescribing form. Most GP practices use electronic prescribing, although FP10 prescriptions can still be written by hand. Other forms of prescription you may use include paper or electronic prescribing of discharge ('to take out' (TTO)) medicines and hospital prescriptions for outpatient dispensing by hospital pharmacies.

### Paper and electronic prescribing
Prescribing on paper requires you select your medicine, dose and frequency from experience, the BNF and/or guidelines and write these down by hand. Potential advantages are that this can be done by any trained prescriber with a pen. Potential disadvantages include errors in dispensing and administration arising from illegible handwriting, lack of embedded decision-making support (e.g. you have to remember to check for potential interactions drug by drug), having to rewrite drug charts when they are full and limitations around data collection for audit.

Electronic prescribing requires you to select your medicine, dose and frequency from a drop-down menu on a computer screen. Advantages are that this is always legible, that decision support can be embedded with alarms and alerts for prescribing errors and that data collection is automated, making audit and monitoring easier. Although electronic prescribing systems are commonly implemented for safety reasons, they may generate just as many errors as paper prescribing. For example, errors can easily be made when selecting drugs or doses from drop-down menus, e.g. picking cyclophosphamide (a cytotoxic drug) instead of cyclizine (an anti-emetic). Alerts and alarms are often overridden. Use of electronic prescribing systems requires training, which may preclude prescribing by temporary staff, sufficient hardware and good IT support, as it is potentially disastrous if the system goes down.

Whatever the system used, a prescription is a form of communication between prescriber, dispenser and administrator that results in a patient taking a medicine. Writing the prescription is therefore just the start of this communication process. You need to ensure that your medicine order is handed over to the pharmacist, to ensure it is dispensed, and to the patient, nurse or carer to ensure that it is taken or administered. The more clarity and accuracy you can bring to the prescribing process, the more likely it is that it will result in a favourable outcome.

### Writing a legal prescription
In the UK, the Medicines Act 1968 and the Council Directive 2001/83/EC provides the main statutory framework governing the control of medicines for human use. There are three main classes of medicines:

1 Prescription only medicines (PoM) that can only be obtained from a pharmacist with a prescription from an approved practitioner
2 Pharmacy only medicines that can only be purchased under supervision of a registered pharmacist
3 General sales list (GSL) medicines that can be bought from any outlet without a prescription or supervision by a pharmacist.

The Medicines Act 1968 defined practitioners that can prescribe (doctors, dentists and veterinary surgeons) and administer medicines. Subsequent legislation has widened prescribing rights to allow nurses, pharmacists and optometrists, and soon radiographers, podiatrists and chiropodists, to be independent prescribers.

When writing a prescription, the legal requirements are that it should be written in indelible ink and signed in ink by the prescriber. It should contain the address and professional status of the prescriber, the date, and the name, address and age (if under 12) of the person for whom the treatment is prescribed.

### Components of a prescription
When writing a prescription you should include the following information.

## Box I.2 Appropriate use of proprietary (brand) names in prescribing

- Drugs without approved non-proprietary names. This applies to many compound preparations (e.g. Adcal-D3®), but not all (e.g. co-amoxiclav and co-codamol are approved compound names)
- Drugs where bioavailability and/or dosage differs significantly between different brands of the same drug. This is often the case for modified-release (m/r) preparations, e.g. oral morphine (Oramorph® or MST Continus®), diltiazem m/r (Adizem-SR®, Tildiem LA®).
- Drugs with a narrow therapeutic index (e.g. phenytoin, carbamazepine, theophylline)
- Drugs with a specific administration device (e.g. inhalers Seretide® 250 Evohaler, Spiriva® HandiHaler®, insulin Novomix® 30 FlexPen®)

*The patient.* You should write the name and date of birth of the patient at the top of the prescription. On hospital inpatient charts you need to include the patient's hospital identification (ID) number and ward. On outpatient prescriptions, write the patient's address. When adding to an existing prescription, e.g. on a hospital drug chart, you should always check these details to make sure that you are prescribing for the correct patient.

*The prescriber.* You need to identify yourself with your name and contact details. In hospital, your contact information is likely to be a bleep or extension number. In the community it is likely to be a practice address and telephone number. Good practice is for this identifying information to be additional to your signature to ensure that it is legible. Do not forget that you are responsible for all prescriptions bearing your signature.

*The medicine.* You should usually prescribe medicines using their international non-proprietary name (INN, also called the 'generic' or 'non-brand' name). There are exceptions to this, shown in Box I.2. In the BNF, proprietary (branded) drug names are denoted by an initial capital and a registered (®) symbol (e.g. Microgynon 30®), whereas generic names have an initial lower case letter (e.g. ethinylestradiol). We observe the same convention in this book. You are not expected to reproduce this in prescriptions, where best practice is to write all drug names in capital letters.

*Administration.* You need to include sufficient information on the prescription for the patient to take the medicine. This should include dose, frequency and timing of administration as well as instructions on when to start and stop the drug.

*Dispensing.* You should state the formulation of the medicine and include dispensing information, such as the number of tablets to be dispensed or days of treatment required.

### Practical considerations

*Dose and dosage.* A dose is a specified quantity of a medicine taken at a single time point. Dosage describes the treatment regimen, specifying amount, number and frequency of doses to be taken over a specified time period. In practice, the terms are often used interchangeably.

The BNF gives the dosage of individual drugs recommended for their licensed indications. For many drugs, a range of dosages are described and it can be difficult for you to select a starting dose. Local guidelines or advice from specialists and colleagues can help. Some general considerations apply:

*For chronic conditions* treatment is often started at a low dosage and titrated up depending on side effects and/or response. For example, in the treatment of heart failure, the starting dose of the ACE inhibitor ramipril is 1.25 mg, given once daily. The patient is monitored for side effects, such as hypotension and renal impairment. As long as these do not develop, the daily dose is increased to a maximum of 10 mg for optimal treatment of heart failure.

*For acute conditions* treatment is often started at a high dose and weaned down as the patient recovers. For example, you may prescribe the beta-2 agonist salbutamol at a dose of 5 mg for administration via a nebuliser for optimal bronchodilation during an acute asthma attack, but will reduce the dosage to 200 micrograms (two puffs) by inhaler to minimise side effects as the asthma comes under control.

The starting dose of many drugs is determined by individual patient characteristics. The most common influential characteristic is body weight, with drugs such as the anticoagulant heparin and the antibiotic gentamicin being dosed in units or milligrams of drug per kilogram of body weight, respectively. Special circumstances such as renal or hepatic impairment, pregnancy or the extremes of age also require adjustment of dosage. For example, in a patient with renal impairment, the dosage of gentamicin (which is both excreted by the kidney and is nephrotoxic) should be reduced. Drug doses for children are listed in the BNF for Children (BNFc). For the very elderly, a 'start low and go slow' approach to dosage selection is recommended.

It is important that the number relating to the prescribed dose is written clearly to reduce the risk of dispensing and administration errors. The use of decimal points should be avoided where possible: write 7 mg not 7.0 mg; avoid quantities less than one by changing the units (e.g. 700 mg not 0.7 g, 700 micrograms not 0.7 mg); where unavoidable use a zero before the decimal place (e.g. 0.7 mg not .7 mg).

*Units.* Drugs are usually dosed by mass, units, number of tablets, volume or molecular weight. It is important to indicate the unit of dose clearly to minimise the risk of life-threatening errors when dispensing and administering drugs.

Acceptable abbreviations are as follow:
- Mass: milligrams (mg), grams (g)
- Number: tablets (tab(s))
- Volume: millilitres (mL), litres (L). A capital 'L' is preferred to a lower case 'l' to reduce the risk of confusion with the number '1'
- Molecular weight: millimoles (mmol), moles (mol)

All other units should be written out in full e.g. 'micrograms', 'nanograms', 'units', 'puffs'. The Ť symbol should not be used to denote the number of tablets; instead write, for example, '1 tab'.

*Frequency and timing.* You should specify the frequency of administration and the interval between doses. Drugs are usually taken one or more times each day, but dosing frequency can range from continuous (e.g. heparin infusion for urgent anticoagulation) to

**Table I.1** Terminology used to convey dosage frequency

| Abbreviation | In full (Latin) | Meaning | Preferred instruction |
|---|---|---|---|
| **BD** | *bis die* | twice daily | **12-hrly** or **twice daily** |
| **OD** | *omni die* | every day | **daily** |
| **OM** | *omni mane* | every morning | **daily** |
| **ON** | *omni nocte* | every night | **nightly** |
| **PRN*** | *pro re nata* | as required* | **as required*** |
| **QDS** | *quater die sumendum* | to be taken four times daily | **6-hrly** or **4 times daily** (as appropriate) |
| **TDS** | *ter die sumendum* | to be taken three times daily | **8-hrly** or **3 times daily** (as appropriate) |

*For as required prescriptions you should state a minimum dosage interval (e.g. paracetamol 1 g 6-hrly) or maximum daily dose (e.g. paracetamol max 4 g/day)

**Table I.2** Acceptable prescribing abbreviations for route of administration

| Abbreviation | Route of administration |
|---|---|
| IM | Intramuscular |
| INH | Inhaled |
| IV | Intravenous |
| NEB | Nebulised |
| NG/PEG | By enteral tube (NG, nasogastric; PEG, percutaneous endoscopic gastrostomy) |
| ORAL | Oral (PO is discouraged) |
| PR | Rectal |
| PV | Vaginal |
| SC | Subcutaneous |

monthly (e.g. depot antipsychotic injections) or annual (e.g. bisphosphonate infusions for osteoporosis) administration. Drugs with similar frequency of administration may require different time intervals between doses. For example, twice-daily salmeterol, a long-acting beta-2 adrenoceptor agonist, is taken at 12-hourly intervals for consistent bronchodilatation in patients with airways disease. By contrast, twice-daily isosorbide mononitrate for angina is best taken asymmetrically, e.g. at 8am and 2pm, to provide a nitrate-free interval in the night and prevent the development of tolerance. Some drugs are prescribed to be taken as needed by the patient, without a pre-specified regimen. For these you should state a minimum dosage interval (e.g. paracetamol 1 g 6-hrly as required) or maximum daily dose (e.g. paracetamol max 4 g/day).

It can be difficult to convey complex information about frequency and timing on a prescription. Abbreviations in common practice are shown in Table I.1. The use of English without abbreviations is preferred to Latin where possible to increase the clarity of prescriptions.

*Starting and stopping.* For some prescriptions, specific instructions are required on when to start the medicine. For patients with critical illness in hospital, treatment (e.g. antibiotics for meningitis) should start immediately. This should be indicated clearly by the timing of the prescription and through prompt handover to staff administering the medicine. Some medicines should not be started immediately. For example, taking the first dose of the first course of a combined oral contraceptive pill may be best deferred until the beginning of the next menstrual cycle.

Stopping medicines also requires clear instruction. Some medicines are prescribed as a course, e.g. 5 days of flucloxacillin for mild cellulitis, whereas others are continued indefinitely for long-term conditions, e.g. metformin for diabetes mellitus.

*Administration.* Most patients take their own medicines. Help with administration is required where administration is technical or complex (e.g. nursing administration of intravenous drugs), or where the patient cannot do it themselves (e.g. caregiver support for patients with impaired memory, cognition or physical function).

*Route.* Most drugs are taken by mouth and absorbed in the intestine. This enteral administration has the advantages of being easy and acceptable for patients and is generally an effective means of delivering medicines. Alternative routes are required when patients are vomiting, have impaired enteral absorption or for drugs with no or poor bioavailability when taken by mouth (e.g. heparin, insulin, gentamicin).

Parenteral administration is where medicines are given by routes other than via the intestine for an effect at a different site. Examples of parenteral drug administration include injection (intravenous, e.g. antibiotics; intramuscular, e.g. analgesia; subcutaneous, e.g. insulin), inhalation (e.g. nasal desmopression for diabetes insipidus, nebulised salbutamol as additive treatment in management of hyperkalaemia) or transdermal delivery (e.g. nicotine replacement for smoking cessation). Parenteral delivery can allow administration of drugs where the oral route is not possible or more rapidly and at higher concentrations (intravenous) than oral administration in an emergency situation. Disadvantages include route-specific adverse effects, such as infection complicating injections or local irritation complicating nasal or transdermal delivery.

Topical administration delivers medicines directly to their site of action. Examples include inhalers for airways disease, ointments for skin disease or pessaries for vaginal complaints. Advantages include reduction in systemic side effects. Disadvantages include difficulty with administration and need for frequent administration if medicines are cleared rapidly from their site of action.

Some acceptable abbreviations for routes of administration for use when prescribing are given in Table I.2.

*Formulation.* A drug is a substance that changes a biological system by interacting with it. It becomes a medicine when it is presented in a form intended for restoring or preserving health. Drugs are often mixed with other substances (excipients) to allow delivery or control onset or duration of action, or simply to make it practical for administration (e.g. as a suitably sized tablet). Different formulations of a single drug may be prepared that have different pharmacokinetics.

## REGULAR PRESCRIPTIONS

| | | | | Circle / enter times below ↓ | ↘ Enter dates below | | Month: | | Year: | |
|---|---|---|---|---|---|---|---|---|---|---|
| **DRUG** | | | | 06 | | | | | | |
| | | | | 08 | | | | | | |
| Dose | Route | Freq | Start date | | | | | | | |
| | | | | 12 | | | | | | |
| Signature | | Bleep | Review | 16 | | | | | | |
| | | | | 18 | | | | | | |
| Additional instructions | | | | 22 | | | | | | |

**Figure I.1** Regular prescriptions.

Example: The drug nifedipine is a calcium channel blocker that causes arterial dilatation. Adalat® is a brand of medicine taken three times a day for the treatment of hypertension that contains nifedipine and excipients (glycerol, purified water, saccharin sodium, peppermint oil and macrogol 400) in a gelatin capsule coloured with sunset yellow (E110). The utility of Adalat® for the treatment of hypertension is limited by its rapid onset and short duration of action. Other nifedipine formulations have therefore been developed, including Adalat® Retard, a modified-release tablet for twice-daily administration and Adalat® LA, a film coated tablet for once-daily administration.

You may need to specify the formulation of a drug when prescribing, particularly where modified-release or long-acting preparations are required.

*Special instructions.* Where medicines require specific instructions for their administration, you should include these in the prescription. For example, some medicines should be taken after food (e.g. non-steroidal anti-inflammatory drugs (NSAIDs)), whereas others require an empty stomach (e.g. bisphosphonates). Medicines may require the patient to avoid alcohol (e.g. the antibiotic metronidazole) or take care when driving or using heavy machinery (e.g. sedatives).

### Writing a prescription

Although the components of a prescription are similar in all situations, the process of writing the prescription will differ between clinical situations, depending on the prescribing form used. In this book we have focused on writing inpatient prescriptions.

*Prescribing on an inpatient drug (prescription) chart.* Although the layout of hospital drug charts is not standardised, they usually contain sections for prescribing regular, as required and once only medicines, as well as infusions and oxygen. Throughout this book we use an example chart for prescribing for simulated hospital inpatients, containing all these sections. It differs from real inpatient prescription charts in having space for fewer prescriptions than would usually be the case. When moving to a new hospital, you should familiarise yourself with the layout of the local chart.

*Drug intolerances.* Drug intolerances should be clearly documented so that the patient does not receive medicines that are known to cause allergic reactions or other adverse effects. You should write both the culprit drug and the reaction caused in this section (e.g. penicillin – rash).

*Regular prescriptions.* All drugs to be taken regularly should be prescribed in this section. Space is provided to indicate the name of the drug, dose, route and frequency of administration, start and stop (review) dates (Figure I.1). The prescription should be signed and the prescriber identified by bleep number. Nursing staff will review prescriptions in this section of the chart at regular intervals and administer doses at their prescribed times, unless there is a compelling reason not to (when, ideally, a numerical coding system should be used to record the reason for non-administration).

Important instructions about the administration of the medicine should be written in the additional information box. This may relate to timing (e.g. with food) or method (e.g. drive nebulised treatment with oxygen or air) of drug delivery. When prescribing antibiotics you should always ensure that the indication is given and that the duration of treatment is specified. This allows good antibiotic stewardship to minimise the development of antibiotic resistance and side effects.

You should indicate the timing of drug administration by circling these times as appropriate. If a drug needs to be administered at an unusual time (e.g. 2am), this should be indicated in the time column and handed over to the nursing staff so that the medicine dose is not missed. When a drug has been given, the nurse will indicate this with their initials in the appropriate box for the date and time of administration.

*As required medication.* This section is used for prescribing medicines that are administered only when needed, usually for symptom relief. Examples include analgesics, anti-emetics, laxatives and bronchodilators. These drugs are not administered automatically, but if a patient has a symptom that may be treated by an as required prescription, the nurse can administer it (within the terms of the prescription) without needing to seek further authorisation from the prescriber. When prescribing as required medication, make sure you do not duplicate regular medication inappropriately (e.g. do not prescribe as required paracetamol and regular co-codamol (paracetamol and codeine)). Also ensure you have

## INFUSION PRESCRIPTIONS

| Date | Time | Fluid | Vol | Drug | Dose | Rate | Doctor initials | Nurse initials | Batch no | Start time | Stop time |
|------|------|-------|-----|------|------|------|-----------------|----------------|----------|------------|-----------|
| 7/1/15 | 08:00 | 0.9% SODIUM CHLORIDE | 1 L | POTASSIUM CHLORIDE | 20 mmol | 8 hours | AD | | | | |

**Figure I.2** Example prescription for intravenous fluid and electrolyte replacement.

## INFUSION PRESCRIPTIONS

| Date | Time | Fluid | Vol | Drug | Dose | Rate | Doctor initials | Nurse initials | Batch no | Start time | Stop time |
|------|------|-------|-----|------|------|------|-----------------|----------------|----------|------------|-----------|
| 7/1/15 | 08:00 | 0.9% SODIUM CHLORIDE | 40 mL | GLYCERYL TRINITRATE | 50 mg in 10 mL | See below | AD | | | | |
| Start at 1 mL/hr. Increase by 0.5 mL/hr every 15 min, ensuring systolic BP >100 mmHg until chest pain controlled | | | | | | | | | | | |

**Figure I.3** Example prescription of an intravenous glyceryl trinitrate (GTN) infusion.

indicated a maximum frequency of administration or total daily dose as needed.

*Once only prescriptions.* This section can be used to prescribe an initial dose of a drug, where delay in administration would be detrimental (e.g. first dose of an antibiotic for severe infection). It can also be used where only a single dose is required (e.g. oral fluconazole for vaginal candidiasis) or when it is preferable not to administer further doses without a reassessment by a doctor (e.g. when prescribing a sleeping tablet such as a temazapam for a patient with a changing clinical condition).

*Infusions.* The purpose of this section is the prescription of intravenous infusions, which may be for fluid and electrolyte replacement or for continuous administration of a drug. Subcutaneous infusions should also be prescribed in this section, with the route of administration being clearly indicated.

• *Intravenous fluids.* The nature and volume of the fluid should be clearly indicated, with the nature and amount of any additive required indicated in the drug and dose boxes. An example fluid and electrolyte prescription is shown in Figure I.2. The date and time that the fluid infusion is to commence should be clearly indicated. The fluid can be prescribed to be given over a time period (e.g. 8 hours) or at an infusion rate (e.g. 125 mL/hour).

When prescribing fluids, you should use the names specified in the BNF and/or on product labelling (Table I.3). These may describe the composition of the fluid (e.g. 0.9% sodium chloride), or be a recognised eponymous (e.g. Hartmann's solution) or brand (e.g. Gelofusine®) name. The base composition of a fluid is usually described as percentage weight/weight (% w/w), which indicates the number of grams of solute per 100 grams of water. For example, 0.9% sodium chloride contains 0.9 g sodium chloride in 100 g water (equivalent to 100 mL). Additives are usually described in terms of mass. In the example (Figure I.2), potassium chloride 20 mmol is specified as an additive. You should be aware that in practice 0.9% sodium chloride with potassium chloride 20 mmol is supplied ready-made.

**Table I.3** Acceptable, discouraged and unacceptable names for intravenous fluids

| Acceptable | Discouraged | Unacceptable |
|------------|-------------|--------------|
| 0.9% sodium chloride | 0.9% NaCl | Normal saline |
| 5% glucose | 0.9% saline | N. saline |
| Compound sodium lactate | Physiological saline | |
| Hartmann's solution | Dextrose | |
| Gelofusine® | | |
| Volplex® | | |

• *Intravenous drugs.* There is often confusion over when a drug should be prescribed in this section. Where drugs require intermittent intravenous administration (e.g. 4-hourly penicillin for *Streptococcus pneumoniae* infection) they should be written in the regular prescriptions section, even if in practice they are infused (e.g. benzylpenicillin may be administered in 100 mL of 5% glucose over 30–60 min). However, drugs with a short half-life that require continuous intravenous administration – in which the rate of infusion is a fundamental determinant of their clinical effect – are written in the infusion section. Examples include intravenous glyceryl trinitrate (GTN) for unstable angina, intravenous heparin for anticoagulation and intravenous insulin for diabetic ketoacidosis.

Prescription of intravenous drug infusions requires choice of a suitable intravenous fluid vehicle. Appendix 6 of the BNF lists drugs that are given by intravenous infusion, with compatible fluids. Drug infusions can be given in small fluid volumes (up to 50 mL) via a syringe driver (e.g. GTN) or larger volumes (up to 1 L) via a flow regulator (e.g. aminophylline, acetylcysteine). Drugs should ideally be diluted to concentrations that allow easy conversion between required dosing (e.g. micrograms per minute) and flow rate (e.g. mL per hour). For example, if the required starting dose of GTN is 10 micrograms per minute (600 micrograms per hour) and GTN is diluted in sodium chloride to a concentration of 1 mg/mL (Figure I.3), it is relatively easy to calculate the required infusion rate of 0.6 mL/hour. The rate of infusion for some drugs where adjustment is required is usually prescribed as a range. In practice, GTN infusions are usually commenced at 1 mL (1000 micrograms) per hour and increased until chest pain is controlled. At the same time blood pressure is monitored and the infusion rate slowed if hypotension develops (Figure I.3).

In practice, hospital infusion protocols, ready-made drug solutions and pre-programmed 'smart' infusion pumps simplify prescription and administration of drug infusions and reduce the risk of error.

*Oxygen.* Oxygen is supplied as a medical gas from cylinders, concentrators or larger storage containers. Delivery devices are used to mix oxygen at different flow rates with air, to deliver increased inspired oxygen concentrations to the patient.

The administration of oxygen should always be supported by a written prescription, except in emergencies when it may initially be administered without prescription. When prescribing oxygen you should set a target concentration for oxygen saturations (Figure I.4). This should be 94–98% for most patients, but 88–92% for people with chronic type 2 respiratory failure (see Case 2). Oxygen should usually be prescribed on a 'continuous' basis, because this prescription allows for the possibility that the concentration of supplemental oxygen may be down-titrated to air, if the patient's oxygen saturation remains within target. The 'as required' prescription is usually reserved, for example, for people who desaturate

during physiotherapy. The starting device will depend on the severity of hypoxia and underlying illness. Non-rebreather devices (typically those with reservoir bags) that deliver inspired oxygen concentrations of up to 90% should be used for patients with critical illness. For most patients with less severe illness, nasal cannulae are preferred. These deliver relatively low concentrations of oxygen (25–39% depending on flow rate) somewhat unpredictably, but are comfortable for the patient, allowing them to talk and eat. Venturi devices deliver a consistent oxygen concentration (specified on the device) and are particularly useful for patients with chronic type 2 respiratory failure, in whom inspired oxygen concentrations need to be carefully controlled.

*Additional charts.* Drugs that require intensive monitoring and regular dose adjustment may have separate charts for their prescription, additional to the standard drug chart. For example, an insulin chart records blood glucose measurements and daily insulin requirements (see Case 42) and a warfarin chart records the INR and daily prescribed warfarin dose. When you prescribe drugs on additional charts, it is important that you record their existence on the standard chart so that they are not overlooked by the person administering treatment. One way of doing this is to write up the drug in the regular prescriptions section, referring to the additional chart for dose (Figure I.5).

*Modifying inpatient prescriptions.* Any changes in prescription on an inpatient chart should be indicated clearly, usually by stopping the medicine and rewriting it clearly on a new line. This is important both to make sure that the patient gets the correct medicine and to allow a clear audit trail of prescribing. When medicines are stopped, this should be indicated with a line that does not obscure the underlying prescription. The date, responsible doctor and contact details should be clearly indicated (Figure I.6). Remember that stopping a medicine is an active decision, which you should take responsibility for in the same way as when you start a medicine.

*Prescribing discharge medicines.* The transition of a patient between hospital and home requires provision of a 7–14 day supply of medicines and clear communication to allow the GP to continue

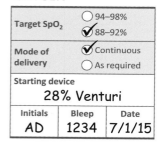

**Figure I.4** Oxygen prescribing.

| | Circle / enter times below ↓ | ↘ Enter dates below | | | | | Month: | | | Year: | | |
|---|---|---|---|---|---|---|---|---|---|---|---|---|
| DRUG  WARFARIN | 06 | | | | | | | | | | | |
| | 08 | | | | | | | | | | | |
| Dose See chart | Route ORAL | Freq Daily | Start date 7/1/15 | 12 | | | | | | | | | | | |
| Signature A Doctor | Bleep 1234 | Review | 16 | | | | | | | | | | | | |
| Additional instructions See warfarin chart for daily dose | (18) | | | | | | | | | | | |
| | 22 | | | | | | | | | | | |

**Figure I.5** Prescribing drugs needing additional charts.

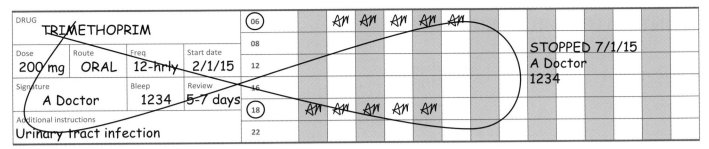

**Figure I.6** Stopping medicines.

medicines as required in the community. This is usually achieved by preparing a discharge prescription, which is now electronic in most hospitals (see Case 45). You will often hear discharge prescriptions being referred to by the abbreviations TTA or TTO, which are derived from their traditional names (to take away or to take out).

*Controlled drugs.* These are drugs associated with a risk of misuse and dependence, where manufacture, supply and possession are controlled by law. The drugs with the most potential to cause harm if misused are subject to particular control relating to prescription, safe custody and the need to keep registers. These include strong opioids such as morphine, diamorphine and pethidine.

The law requires that prescriptions for controlled drugs contain indelible information that specifies the prescriber, the patient and the exact quantity of drug to be dispensed to reduce the risk of misuse. An example is shown in Figure I.7 and referred to in brackets below. You should include the prescriber's address and signature, the name and address of the patient and the date of the prescription. The prescription should specify the form and strength of the preparation (e.g. MST Continus 30 mg tablets), the total quantity of the preparation or number of dosage units to be supplied in both words and figures (e.g. supply twenty eight (28) tablets) and the dose of drug to be taken (e.g. take one tablet twice daily). If all this information is not supplied, the pharmacist is not legally allowed to dispense the drug. A prescription for controlled drugs is valid for up to 28 days and should not usually supply drugs for more than 30 days (14 days supplied in the example).

## Dose calculations

When prescribing medicines you may be required to make calculations to determine the required dose. It is useful to practice these to minimise errors when prescribing for patients. In clinical practice, back up from pharmacy, local guidelines and pre-programmed 'smart' infusion pumps helps to reduce the risk of error.

### Dosing by body weight

It is relatively common for drugs to require dosing by body weight (the term 'mass' is technically more precise, but when referring to patients we use 'weight' for consistency with common usage). For such drugs, the BNF states the dose required per kilogram of body weight. You therefore need to multiply the recommended dose by the patient's body weight to determine the total dose.

> Example: A 70-kg man requires dalteparin (low molecular weight heparin) for unstable coronary artery disease. The recommended dalteparin dose for this indication is 120 units/kg every 12 hours. His required dose therefore is $120 \times 70 = 8400$ units 12-hrly.

When performing this relatively straightforward task, make sure you read the prescribing instructions carefully to minimise the risk of error. For example, for unstable coronary disease, the maximum recommended dose of dalteparin is 10 000 units twice daily. Therefore anyone heavier than 83 kg should receive this ceiling dosage, rather than a higher calculated dosage. The calculated dose may also need to be administered twice daily – as in this example – or may be a total daily dosage to be given in two divided doses. Finally, make sure the weight on which you are basing your calculation is accurate. Using an estimated weight is highly unreliable and usually negates the value of a weight-based dose calculation.

### Converting doses between common units

The most common dosing unit used is mass. Drugs may be prescribed in grams (g), milligrams (mg) and micrograms (micrograms). The conversion factors are: 1 g = 1000 mg, 1 mg = 1000 micrograms. For volume, 1 L = 1000 mL.

> Example: A patient requires digoxin 0.125 mg to be prescribed. It is preferable in prescribing to avoid unnecessary use of a decimal point. As 1 mg = 1000 micrograms, the digoxin dose can be converted from mg to micrograms by multiplying by 1000, i.e. $0.125 \times 1000 = 125$ micrograms, which can now be prescribed without the decimal point. Make sure you write micrograms out in full for clarity.

### Converting doses between concentrations expressed as percentage and mass

Some medicines, including ointments, eye, nose and ear drops are expressed as % w/w, which indicates the number of grams of drug

## CONTROLLED DRUG PRESCRIPTION

| Surname | Hospital number | Date of admission | Ward |
|---|---|---|---|
| PATIENT | 123456 | 05/01/2015 | RESPIRATORY |

| First name | Date of birth | Date of discharge | Consultant |
|---|---|---|---|
| ANY | 07/01/50 | 07/01/2015 | BAKER |

| Address | Drug intolerances | General practitioner name and address |
|---|---|---|
| 76 ANY STREET ANYTOWN AT1 2BC | NIL KNOWN | DR G DOCTOR ANYSTREET ANYTOWN |

**Drug**
MST CONTINUS

**Formulation (tablets/liquid etc)**
TABLETS

**Dose**
30 MG (ONE TABLET) TWICE DAILY

**Quantity to be supplied (numbers)**
28 TABLETS

**Quantity to be supplied (words)**
TWENTY EIGHT TABLETS

| Print name | Grade | Bleep | Signature | Date |
|---|---|---|---|---|
| A DOCTOR | SpR | 1234 | A Doctor | 07/01/2015 |

**Figure I.7** Example discharge prescription for a controlled drug.

per 100 g of diluent, e.g. 0.5% hydrocortisone ointment contains 0.5 g hydrocortisone in 100 g ointment. The total amount of drug administered can be determined by multiplying the % w/w by the volume administered divided by 100.

---

Example: A patient treated with 0.5% hydrocortisone ointment uses a 30-g tube. The total hydrocortisone dose contained in this is $0.5 \times (30/100) = 0.15$ g (or 150 mg without the decimal point).

---

### Calculations for drug infusions

This is probably the most complex calculation task in medicine as it may require conversions between drug concentration, expressed in mass/volume (e.g. mg/mL), required dosage, expressed in mass (e.g. mg) or mass/time (e.g. micrograms/minute), and infusion rates, expressed in volume/time (e.g. mL/hr). You may also need to convert mass between grams, milligrams and micrograms, volume between mL and L and time between seconds, minutes and hours.

Example: A patient on the coronary care unit requires treatment with dobutamine (an inotrope) for cardiogenic shock. He weighs 84 kg. The hospital formulary states that dobutamine 250 mg should be diluted with 5% glucose to a total volume of 50 mL, then infused at an initial rate of 5 micrograms/kg/min. What initial rate (in mL/hr) should be set on the infusion pump?

We first need to know the concentration of the dobutamine in the prepared solution:

$$250 \text{ mg} \div 50 \text{ mL} = 5 \text{ mg/mL}.$$

We then need to work out the required initial infusion rate for this patient and convert it into mg/hr:

$$5 \text{ micrograms/kg/min} \times 84 \text{ kg} = 420 \text{ micrograms/min}$$

$$420 \text{ micrograms/min} \times 60 \text{ min/hr} = 25\,200 \text{ micrograms/hr}$$
$$= 25.2 \text{ mg/hr}.$$

Finally, we need to take account of the concentration of dobutamine in the solution to work out the rate to set on the infusion pump:

$$25 \text{ mg/hr} \div 5 \text{ mg/mL} = 5 \text{ mL/hr}.$$

## Minimising medication errors

Approximately 10% of prescriptions contain errors and 10% of prescribing errors have potential to cause serious or life-threatening harm to the patient. Errors can occur at any part of the treatment process, from making the diagnosis and treatment decision to administering the medication and monitoring its effects. It is inevitable that you will make some errors when prescribing. However, it is both your responsibility and the responsibility of the system in which you work to minimise the number and severity of these errors and, most importantly, their impact on patients.

### Types of error and their prevention

Errors can arise in the process of formulating a plan ('thinking errors'), or in executing it ('doing errors'):

Thinking errors are termed *mistakes*. These most commonly occur when dealing with unfamiliar tasks that require the application of knowledge or judgement. Mistakes are therefore best prevented by improving your knowledge (both of the individual patient, and of the disease and its treatment). This may be supplemented by the correct applications of rules. Such rules may be informal (e.g. 'when prescribing a regular opioid always consider prescribing a laxative') or formal (e.g. a protocol for the management of a particular condition in your hospital).

Doing errors may be *slips* or *lapses*. Slips are where a component of the plan is executed incorrectly (e.g. when intending to prescribe the antibiotic azithromycin, the immunosuppressive drug azathioprine is accidently prescribed). Lapses are where a component of the plan is incorrectly omitted (e.g. forgetting to check a patient's allergy status before prescribing a drug). Slips and lapses occur most commonly when dealing with familiar tasks, particularly when there are other sources of distraction. They are best prevented by *checking*. Provided your underlying plan is sound (e.g. you know the correct drug should be azithromycin, not azathioprine, and you know to check the patient's allergies), there is a high chance of identifying your error when you double check what you have done.

As well as considering the measures you can take individually, remember that your prescribing will take place within a system that should have multiple checks and balances to identify errors and reduce the risk of harm to the patient. These may include a pharmacist checking your prescribing on a post-take ward round and senior nurses checking that drugs have been prescribed and prepared correctly before administration. Harm is most likely to happen when all of these checks go wrong at once (e.g. the pharmacist is off sick on the first day in charge for a new nurse).

The purpose of this book is to provide an opportunity for you to practise prescribing on simulated patients without the risk of causing harm. We hope this will allow you to improve your knowledge, decision-making and practical prescribing skills towards good prescribing practice and minimising error when you start to prescribe for real.

# Section 1: The acute take

# Cases

## 1 An 82-year-old woman who requires venous thromboembolism prophylaxis

| | |
|---|---|
| **Patient name:** | Madeleine Henshaw |
| **ID number:** | 100001 |
| **Date of birth:** | 24/09/1932 |
| **Age:** | 82 years |
| **Weight:** | 85 kg, body mass index (BMI) 31 kg/m$^2$ |
| **Admission date:** | 07/01/2015 |
| **Date/time seen:** | 07/01/2015 12:00 |

### History

| | |
|---|---|
| PC | Fall causing tibial fracture. |
| HPC | Mrs Henshaw went straight to theatre from the emergency department at 09:30 for an open reduction and internal fixation to repair a tibial fracture. This was completed at 11:30. She has now been admitted to the surgical ward. |
| PMH | Nil. |
| DH | Nil. |
| | Intolerances: none known. |

### Examination

| | |
|---|---|
| General | Comfortable at rest, pain appears well controlled. |
| Obs | HR 65 beats/min, BP 125/85 mmHg, RR 14, oxygen saturation 96% breathing air. |
| CVS | Normal examination. |

### Investigations

For results of investigations, see Table 1.1.

The consultant anaesthetist has called you to ask you to prescribe treatment to prevent venous thromboembolism (VTE). The operation was uncomplicated and the anaesthetist will prescribe postoperative analgesia.

### Task

Prescribe appropriate VTE prophylaxis on the inpatient drug chart.

**Table 1.1** Case 1 investigation results

| Test | Value | Normal range |
|---|---|---|
| Hb | 135 g/L | 120–160 |
| Plt | 225 × 10$^9$/L | 150–400 |
| Ur | 4.9 mmol/L | 2.5–8.0 |
| Creat | 60 μmol/L | 60–110 |
| eGFR | >60 mL/min/1.73m$^2$ | >60 |

## 2 A 104-year-old woman with respiratory failure

| | |
|---|---|
| **Patient name:** | Ms Maria Gomez |
| **ID number:** | 100002 |
| **Date of birth:** | 16/08/1910 |
| **Age:** | 104 years |
| **Weight:** | 68 kg |
| **Admission date:** | 07/01/15 |
| **Date/time seen:** | 07/01/15 16:00 |

### History

| | |
|---|---|
| PC | Shortness of breath. |
| HPC | Ms Gomez has become increasingly short of breath and wheezy over the past 48 hours. She has had no cough or fever, and had otherwise been feeling well prior to this episode. |
| PMH | Chronic obstructive pulmonary disease (COPD), including an infective exacerbation 2 years ago requiring non-invasive ventilation. |
| DH | Seretide 250 Accuhaler® (fluticasone 250 micrograms, salmeterol 50 micrograms) 2 puffs twice daily, tiotropium 18 micrograms 1 puff once daily, salbutamol 100 micrograms 2 puffs as needed. |
| | Intolerances: none known. |
| SH | She is a current smoker who has smoked 5 cigarettes a day for 70 years. |

### Examination

| | |
|---|---|
| General | She is short of breath at rest. |
| Obs | T 36°C, HR 80 beats/min, BP 118/64 mmHg, RR 26 breaths/min, SpO$_2$ 95% breathing 35% oxygen via Venturi mask. |
| RS | There is reduced expansion and polyphonic wheeze throughout the chest. |

### Investigations

| | |
|---|---|
| CXR | Hyperexpansion, but no consolidation. |

Arterial blood gas
  See Table 2.1.

### Task

Ms Gomez is diagnosed with a non-infective exacerbation of COPD. Prescribe oxygen according to the results of her arterial blood gases.

**Table 2.1** Case 2 arterial blood gas results

| Test | Breathing air | 28% oxygen | 35% oxygen | Normal range |
|---|---|---|---|---|
| pH | 7.39 | 7.36 | 7.31 | 7.35–7.45 |
| PaO$_2$ | 6.8 | 8.4 | 9.8 | 10.6–14.5 kPa |
| PaCO$_2$ | 4.4 | 5.2 | 7.2 | 4.0–6.0 kPa |
| Bicarbonate | 23 | 23 | 24 | 22–29 mmol/L |
| Base excess | 0 | +2 | +3 | ±2 mmol/L |
| SpO$_2$ | 84% | 89% | 95% | |

*Prescribing Scenarios at a Glance*, First Edition. Emma Baker, Daniel Burrage, Dagan Lonsdale, and Andrew Hitchings.
© 2014 John Wiley & Sons, Ltd. Published 2014 by John Wiley & Sons, Ltd. Companion website: www.ataglanceseries.com/prescribingscenarios

## 3   A 64-year-old man with severe acute abdominal pain

| | |
|---|---|
| **Patient name:** | Eoghan O'Connor |
| **ID number:** | 100003 |
| **Date of birth:** | 18/10/1950 |
| **Age:** | 64 years |
| **Weight:** | 73 kg |
| **Admission date:** | 07/01/2015 |
| **Date/time seen:** | 07/01/2015 18:10 |

### History

PC   Severe abdominal pain.

HPC   Mr O'Connor has had left lower quadrant pain, fevers and malaise for the past 2 days. His abdominal pain has increased markedly and become more generalised over the past few hours and he now rates it as 10/10 in severity.

PMH   Diverticular disease with one previous episode of uncomplicated diverticulitis.

DH   Cod liver oil 1 capsule daily.
Intolerances: none known.

SH   Smokes 1–2 cigarettes per day and drinks about 30 units of alcohol per week. He works as a security guard and is usually fit and active.

### Examination

General   He looks unwell and is clearly distressed by severe pain from his abdomen.

Obs   T 38.1°C, HR 118 beats/min, BP 116/72 mmHg, RR 28 breaths/min, SpO$_2$ 97% breathing oxygen 10 L/min via a facemask.

Systems   Cardiorespiratory examination is normal. On abdominal examination, he has generalised rebound tenderness and guarding consistent with peritonitis.

### Investigations

Baseline investigations are not yet available.

Your registrar has seen him and made a provisional diagnosis of acute abdomen due to diverticular perforation. She is arranging for him to be transferred urgently from the emergency department to the operating theatre for a laparotomy, and has asked you to 'deal with analgesia'. She has asked the nurses to keep Mr O'Connor 'nil by mouth'.

### Task

Prescribe acute analgesia for immediate administration (all other aspects of his management are being appropriately addressed by colleagues).

## 4   A 55-year-old woman with atrial fibrillation

| | |
|---|---|
| **Patient name:** | Edna Sullivan |
| **ID number:** | 100004 |
| **Date of birth:** | 26/12/1959 |
| **Age:** | 55 years |
| **Weight:** | 78 kg |
| **Admission date:** | 07/01/2015 |
| **Date/time seen:** | 07/01/2015 15:00 |

### History

PC   Palpitations.

HPC   Edna Sullivan has been referred to the emergency department by her GP with palpitations for the past 3 days. She has had no chest pain, is not short of breath and has been otherwise feeling well.

PMH   Hypertension and hypercholesterolaemia.

DH   Amlodipine 5 mg daily and simvastatin 40 mg daily.
Intolerances: none known.

SH   She is a retired head teacher who lives independently with her husband. She has never smoked. She drinks 8 units of alcohol per week.

### Examination

Obs   T 36.5°C, HR 162 beats/min, BP 138/82 mmHg, RR 18 breaths/min, SpO$_2$ 96% breathing room air.

CVS   She has an irregularly irregular pulse. Her jugular venous pressure (JVP) is not raised, and she has normal heart sounds. There is no peripheral oedema.

RS   Normal.

### Investigations

For results of investigations, see Table 4.1.

A diagnosis of atrial fibrillation is made.

### Task

Prescribe appropriate initial treatment for the management of Mrs Sullivan's atrial fibrillation.

**Table 4.1** Case 4 investigation results

| Test | Value | Normal range |
|---|---|---|
| Na$^+$ | 140 mmol/L | 135–145 |
| K$^+$ | 4.6 mmol/L | 3.5–4.7 |
| Ur | 6.1 mmol/L | 2.5–8.0 |
| Creat | 68 μmol/L | 60–110 |
| Adj Ca$^{2+}$ | 2.42 mmol/L | 2.20–2.50 |
| Mg$^{2+}$ | 1.0 mmol/L | 0.7–1.0 |
| FT4 | 16 pmol/L | 10–23 |
| TSH | 3.0 mU/L | 0.4–5.0 |
| ECG | Rate 160 beats/min, no visible p-waves, irregular rhythm, no other abnormalities | |
| CXR | Normal | |

## 5 A 32-year-old man with community-acquired pneumonia

**Patient name:** Dragos Hasdeu
**ID number:** 100005
**Date of birth:** 17/09/1982
**Age:** 32 years
**Weight:** 85 kg
**Admission date:** 07/01/2015
**Date/time seen:** 07/01/2015 10:00

### History
**PC** Dragos Hasdeu presented to the emergency department with left-sided chest pain and shortness of breath.

**HPC** The pain has come on gradually over 2 days. He initially thought it was a strained muscle, but now has a sharp left-sided chest pain on breathing or coughing. He normally has unlimited exercise tolerance. However, as the pain has got worse he has felt breathless walking short distances. He feels feverish and shivery and has developed a cough productive of brown sputum. He is able to eat and drink.

**PMH** He is usually fit and well with no previous significant illness.

**DH** None.
Intolerances: none known.

**SH** He works on a building site and lives in a flat with two friends. He smokes 15 roll up cigarettes per day and drinks alcohol at the weekends.

### Examination
**General** He is in obvious discomfort on breathing.
**Obs** T 38.5°C, HR 102 beats/min, BP 112/86 mmHg, RR 32 breaths/min, SpO$_2$ 93% breathing air.
**RS** His left lung base is dull to percussion. On auscultation there are crackles and bronchial breathing at the left lung base.

### Investigations
For results of investigations see Table 5.1.

### Task
A diagnosis of community-acquired pneumonia is made. Prescribe appropriate admission medication.

**Table 5.1** Case 5 investigation results

| Test | Value | Normal range |
|------|-------|--------------|
| Hb | 146 g/L | 130–180 |
| WCC | 19.4 × 10⁹/L | 4.0–11.0 |
| Neut | 15.2 × 10⁹/L | 1.7–8.0 |
| Plt | 178 × 10⁹/L | 150–400 |
| Na⁺ | 144 mmol/L | 135–145 |
| K⁺ | 4.1 mmol/L | 3.5–4.7 |
| Ur | 9.6 mmol/L | 2.5–8.0 |
| Creat | 72 μmol/L | 60–110 |
| CRP | 284 mg/L | <10 |
| CXR | Left lower lobe consolidation | |

## 6 A 45-year-old woman with status epilepticus

**Patient name:** Helen Yarwood
**ID number:** 100006
**Date of birth:** 03/12/1969
**Age:** 45 years
**Weight:** 69 kg
**Admission date:** 07/01/2015
**Date/time seen:** 07/01/2015 02:00

### History
**PC** Helen Yarwood was brought into the emergency department by ambulance with repeated tonic–clonic seizures. You are called to see her because she is having a further seizure, which has lasted 9 minutes so far.

**HPC** Collateral history is available from her son who heard Mrs Yarwood fall out of bed. He found her having a seizure and called the ambulance. She had two further seizures in the ambulance and has not fully recovered consciousness in between.

**PMH** Mrs Yarwood has had epilepsy since her mid-teens. She usually has 1–2 seizures per year, each lasting around 3–5 minutes.

**DH** Carbamazepine 600 mg twice daily.
Intolerances: none known.

**SH** Mrs Yarwood lives with her son and daughter and is usually independent. She is a non-smoker and does not drink alcohol. She eats well and is not underweight.

### Examination
**General** She is on her left side and is undergoing a tonic–clonic seizure. The trolley has rails which have been raised and padded. She has a nasal airway and intravenous cannula *in situ*. There are no contusions.

**Obs** T 36.4°C, HR 110 beats/min, BP 138/84 mmHg, SpO$_2$ 92% breathing oxygen via non-rebreathe mask at 15 L/minute. Capillary blood glucose 5.9 mmol/L.

### Investigations
Blood tests sent on admission, including full blood count, renal and hepatic function and electrolytes were all normal apart from:

Carbamazepine 1 mg/L 4–12 mg/L

A diagnosis of status epilepticus is made.

### Task
Prescribe appropriate medication on the drug chart provided.

# A 27-year-old woman with suspected bacterial meningitis

| | |
|---|---|
| **Patient name:** | Florence Menzes |
| **ID number:** | 100007 |
| **Date of birth:** | 01/02/1987 |
| **Age:** | 27 years |
| **Weight:** | 65 kg |
| **Admission date:** | 07/01/2015 |
| **Date/time seen:** | 07/01/2015 23:00 |

## History

PC    Florence Menzes is seen in the emergency department complaining of a severe headache.

HPC    A generalised headache has come on over the past 8 hours, gradually increasing in severity. It is now so bad that it is painful for her to move and the light is hurting her eyes. She feels hot and cold and has vomited twice. There is no history of head injury or ear or sinus disease.

PMH    No previous hospital admissions, no recent illness.

DH    Microgynon 30 ® (ethinyloestradiol 30 micrograms, levonorgestrel 150 micrograms).
Intolerances: none known.

SH    Mrs Menzes lives with her husband. She is a non-smoker who drinks 6 units of alcohol per week. Her last foreign travel was 5 years ago. She does not have any contacts that are unwell.

## Examination

General    She looks unwell and in pain. She is shading her eyes from the light.

Obs    T 38.2°C, HR 98 beats/min, BP 138/82 mmHg, RR 14 breaths/min, SpO$_2$ 100% breathing room air.

NS    Glasgow Coma Scale 15/15, severe neck stiffness, positive Kernig's sign.
No focal neurological abnormalities.
Photophobia but no abnormalities on fundoscopy.

Skin    No rash.

## Investigations

For results of investigations, see Tables 7.1 and 7.2.

Computed tomography (CT) brain scan – no abnormality, no evidence of raised intracranial pressure.

Blood cultures, a blood sample for molecular studies and a throat swab have also been taken.

## Task

A presumptive diagnosis of bacterial meningitis is made. Prescribe appropriate admission medication.

**Table 7.1** Case 7 investigation results

| Test | Value | Normal range |
|---|---|---|
| Hb | 134 g/L | 120–160 |
| WCC | 20.4 × 10$^9$/L | 4.0–11.0 × 10$^9$ |
| Neut | 18.2 × 10$^9$/L | 1.7–8.0 × 10$^9$ |
| Plt | 433 × 10$^9$/L | 150–400 × 10$^9$ |
| Na$^+$ | 141 mmol/L | 135–145 |
| K$^+$ | 4.0 mmol/L | 3.5–4.7 |
| Ur | 6.0 mmol/L | 2.5–8.0 |
| Creat | 76 μmol/L | 60–110 |
| Gluc (random) | 5.6 mmol/L | 3.9–7.8 |
| CRP | 125 mg/L | <10 |
| PT | 14 sec | 11–16 |
| INR | 0.9 | 0.8–1.1 |
| APTT ratio | 1.06 | 0.85–1.15 |

**Table 7.2** Case 7 cerebrospinal fluid investigation results

| Test | Result | Normal range |
|---|---|---|
| Appearance | Turbid | |
| Protein | 1.2 g/L | 0.2–0.4 |
| Glucose | 1.6 mmol/L | 2/3 to 1/2 blood glucose |
| Polymorphs | 244/mm$^3$ | Nil |
| Organisms | No organisms seen on Gram-stain | |

## 8 A 31-year-old woman with paracetamol overdose

**Patient name:** Eleanor Briggs
**ID number:** 100008
**Date of birth:** 04/04/1983
**Age:** 31 years
**Weight:** 65 kg
**Admission date:** 07/01/2015
**Date/time seen:** 07/01/2015 14:00

### History

PC     Paracetamol overdose.

HPC    Eleanor Briggs took 28 paracetamol 500-mg tablets 6 hours ago. She ingested all the tablets over the course of a few minutes. She had intended to hurt herself, but now regrets this. She did not take any other medicines, recreational drugs or alcohol. At present, she has no symptoms.

PMH    None.

DH     None.
          Intolerances: none known.

SH     She drinks alcohol socially, consuming about 14 units per week. She does not smoke cigarettes or take any other drugs.

### Examination

General   She looks anxious but well.

Obs      T 36.8°C, HR 90 beats/min, BP 124/85 mmHg, RR 18 breaths/min, SpO$_2$ 99% breathing air.

Systems   Normal. In particular, she is not icteric and her abdomen is soft, with no hepatomegaly or right upper quadrant tenderness.

### Investigations

For results of investigations see Table 8.1.

### Task

Prescribe appropriate treatment, with reference to Figure 8.1.

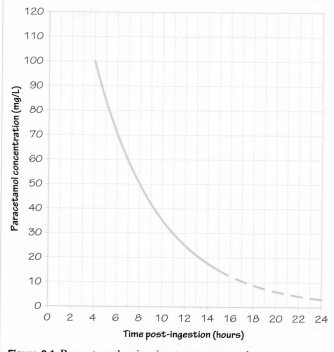

**Figure 8.1** Paracetamol poisoning treatment graph.

**Table 8.1** Case 8 investigation results

| Test | Value | Normal range |
|---|---|---|
| Hb | 140 g/L | 120–160 |
| MCV | 6.4 fL | 78–97 |
| Plt | 328 × 10$^9$/L | 150–400 × 10$^9$ |
| INR | 1.0 | 0.8–1.1 |
| Ur | 4.7 mmol/L | 2.5–8.0 |
| Creat | 58 μmol/L | 60–110 |
| Alb | 38 g/L | 35–48 |
| Bil | 10 μmol/L | <17 |
| ALT | 17 U/L | <40 |
| ALP | 48 U/L | 35–120 |
| CRP | <4 mg/L | <10 |
| Paracetamol | 118 mg/L (taken 4 h after paracetamol ingestion) | |

## 9 A 59-year-old man with acute pulmonary oedema

| | |
|---|---|
| **Patient name:** | Joel Jones |
| **ID number:** | 100009 |
| **Date of birth:** | 07/05/1955 |
| **Age:** | 59 years |
| **Weight:** | 82 kg |
| **Admission date:** | 07/01/2015 |
| **Date/time seen:** | 07/01/2015 12:00 |

### History

**PC** Shortness of breath.

**HPC** Mr Jones complains of 3 days of worsening shortness of breath at rest, ankle swelling and fatigue. He is unable to sleep because of his shortness of breath, which is worse lying flat. He has had no chest pain. He has not been taking his 'water tablets' as he has been on holiday for the past week and forgot to take them with him.

**PMH** Chronic heart failure 3 years ago based on an echocardiogram, which showed that his left ventricular ejection fraction was 35%. Myocardial infarction 5 years ago, hypertension and high cholesterol.

**DH** Aspirin 75 mg daily, atorvastatin 40 mg daily, bisoprolol 2.5 mg daily, furosemide 80 mg daily (not taken for 7 days), ramipril 5 mg daily. Intolerances: none known.

**SH** He is an ex-smoker, with a 30 pack year history, and quit 5 years ago.

### Examination

**General** He appears restless, anxious and short of breath.

**Obs** T 36.8°C, HR 108 beats/min regular, BP 160/100 mmHg, RR 28 breaths/min, $SpO_2$ 90% breathing air.

**CVS** His JVP is raised at 6 cm above the level of the sternal notch. He has normal first and second heart sounds but an additional third heart sound. There are no murmurs. His liver is palpable 2 cm beneath the costal margin and there is swelling of his lower limbs to just below his knees.

**RS** Bilateral crackles to the midzones.

### Investigations

For results of investigations, see Table 9.1.

### Task

A diagnosis of acute pulmonary oedema is made. Prescribe appropriate treatment.

**Table 9.1** Case 9 investigation results

| Test | Value | Normal range |
|---|---|---|
| ECG | Rate 90 beats/min, sinus rhythm, no acute ischaemic changes | |
| CXR | Upper lobe diversion and Kerley B lines | |
| $Na^+$ | 138 mmol/L | 135–145 |
| $K^+$ | 4.0 mmol/L | 3.5–4.7 |
| Ur | 7.8 mmol/L | 2.5–8.0 |
| Creat | 90 μmol/L | 60–110 |
| eGFR | >60 mL/min/1.73 m² | >60 |
| BNP | 1060 ng/L | <250 |

## 10 A 24-year-old woman with acute asthma

| | |
|---|---|
| **Patient name:** | Linda Powell |
| **ID number:** | 100010 |
| **Date of birth:** | 15/08/1990 |
| **Age:** | 24 years |
| **Weight:** | 70 kg |
| **Admission date:** | 07/01/2015 |
| **Date/time seen:** | 07/01/2015 10:00 |

### History

**PC** Shortness of breath.

**HPC** Miss Powell has had a non-productive cough for 1 week. Over the past 2 days she has also found it difficult to breathe. She ran out of her 'preventer' inhaler 1 month ago and has not had time to get to the GP to replace it. Her previous best peak expiratory flow rate (PEFR) is 450 L/min. She reports no fevers or muscle aches and pains. You are the first doctor to see her.

**PMH** She has had asthma since the age of 8 but has never taken oral steroids or been admitted to hospital before. She also has hay fever.

**DH** Clenil Modulite® (beclometasone dipropionate) 100 micrograms/metered dose, two puffs inhaled twice daily; salbutamol aerosol inhaler 100 micrograms/metered dose, one or two puffs inhaled as required. Intolerances: none known.

**SH** Lives alone in a first floor flat, non-smoker.

### Examination

**General** She is alert but is having difficulty completing sentences.

**Obs** T 36.5°C, HR 115 beats/min (regular), BP 125/90 mmHg, RR 28 breaths/min, $SpO_2$ 93% breathing air.

**RS** Good respiratory effort, no cyanosis. Normal percussion note. Good air entry throughout chest with diffuse expiratory wheeze. PEFR 200 L/min.

### Investigations

For results of investigations, see Table 10.1.

Miss Powell is diagnosed with an acute severe asthma attack and requires hospital admission.

### Task

Write an appropriate admission drug chart to address her acute condition.

**Table 10.1** Case 10 investigation results

| Test | Value | Normal range |
|---|---|---|
| Hb | 134 g/L | 120–160 g/L |
| WCC | $7.2 \times 10^9$/L | $4.0–11.0 \times 10^9$/L |
| Eos | $1.4 \times 10^9$/L | $0.1–0.8 \times 10^9$/L |
| Plt | $220 \times 10^9$/L | $150–400 \times 10^9$/L |
| Ur | 4.4 mmol/L | 2.5–8.0 mmol/L |
| Creat | 62 μmol/L | 60–110 μmol/L |
| CRP | <4 mg/L | 0–10 mg/L |
| CXR | Hyperinflation, no airspace abnormalities | |

## 11   A 57-year-old man who has suddenly deteriorated

| | |
|---|---|
| **Patient name:** | Robert Allen |
| **ID number:** | 100011 |
| **Date of birth:** | 04/03/1957 |
| **Age:** | 57 years |
| **Weight:** | 73 kg |
| **Admission date:** | 07/01/2015 |
| **Date/time seen:** | 07/01/2015 14:10 |

### History

**PC**    Acutely distressed.

**HPC**    Mr Allen presented to hospital about 3 hours ago with abdominal pain. He is suspected to have acute appendicitis. Treatment with intravenous fluid and antibiotics was started approximately 10 minutes ago, and arrangements are being made for his admission to a surgical ward. He has now become distressed. He says he feels light-headed, sick and, generally, 'like I'm going to die!'

**PMH**    Hay fever.

**DH**    Presently receiving intravenous (IV) infusions of a gelatin-based colloid (Gelofusine® 500 mL over 30 min) and co-amoxiclav (1.2 g in 20 mL water over 30 min).
Intolerances: none known.

**SH**    Non-smoker, drinks alcohol socially (about 8 units per week).

### Examination

**General**    He is alert but appears anxious and distressed. The skin over the whole of his upper body appears flushed.

**Obs**    T 38.2°C, HR 138 beats/min, BP 68/42 mmHg, RR 32 breaths/min, SpO$_2$ 94% breathing high-flow oxygen via non-rebreathe mask.

**Systems**    There is no stridor. Breath sounds can be heard bilaterally and there are no added sounds. His abdomen is tender but there is no guarding or rebound tenderness.

### Investigations

Results from initial blood tests are not yet available.

### Task

Document your immediate management of the situation on the prescription chart.

## 12   An 84-year-old man taking warfarin who has a headache

| | |
|---|---|
| **Patient name:** | James Fenton |
| **ID number:** | 100012 |
| **Date of birth:** | 15/02/1930 |
| **Weight:** | 75 kg |
| **Admission date:** | 07/01/2015 |
| **Date/time seen:** | 07/01/2015 18:00 |

### History

**PC**    Mr Fenton is seen in the emergency department with a headache.

**HPC**    At around 2pm, Mr Fenton was walking his dog when a deer ran in front of him. The dog gave chase and pulled him over. Mr Fenton banged the front of his head and he has had a gradually worsening headache ever since. He was warned when he started taking warfarin that should this ever happen, he should attend the emergency department immediately.

**PMH**    Transient ischaemic attack (2007), type 2 diabetes mellitus (diet controlled) and atrial fibrillation.

**DH**    Warfarin 3 mg daily (target INR 2–3; dosage stable over the past 3 years).
Erythromycin 500 mg four times daily for cellulitis of his left leg. Currently on day 7 of a 10-day course.
Intolerances: penicillin (anaphylaxis).

**SH**    Mr Fenton lives alone with his dog.

### Examination

**Obs**    HR 96 beats/min, BP 135/65 mmHg, RR 14 breaths/min, SpO$_2$ 98% breathing air.

**Legs**    Left leg is cool with some desquamation over previous area of cellulitis, but no active inflammation.

**NS**    No abnormal findings.

### Investigations

For results of investigations, see Table 12.1.

The emergency medicine registrar has discussed the case with the neurosurgical team who feel that no operative intervention is currently required. The haematology registrar has advised reversal of warfarin to prevent further bleeding with prothrombin complex concentrate and vitamin K in accordance with BNF guidelines.

### Task

Mr Fenton is now being admitted under the medical team. Write an admission drug chart to manage his subdural haematoma.

**Table 12.1** Case 12 investigation results

| Test | Value | Normal range |
|---|---|---|
| Hb | 145 g/L | 130–180 |
| WCC | 6.1 × 10$^9$/L | 4.0–11.0 |
| CRP | 5 mg/L | <10 |
| INR | 6.9 | 0.8–1.1 |
| CT brain | 3 cm left-sided acute subdural haematoma overlying the parietal lobe. No mass effect. No subarachnoid or intraventricular blood | |

## 13 A 66-year-old man with acute coronary syndrome

| | |
|---|---|
| **Patient name:** | Madhu Lakhani |
| **ID number:** | 100013 |
| **Date of birth:** | 28/07/1948 |
| **Age:** | 66 years |
| **Weight:** | 88 kg |
| **Admission date:** | 07/01/2015 |
| **Date/time seen:** | 07/01/2015 18:00 |

### History

**PC** Chest pain.

**HPC** Three hours ago Mr Lakhani developed sudden onset, central, crushing chest pain that radiated to his left arm and lasted 30 minutes. This was associated with nausea and sweating.

**PMH** Type 2 diabetes mellitus 5 years, hypertension 10 years.

**DH** Ramipril 2.5 mg twice daily, metformin 500 mg twice daily.
Intolerances: none known.

**SH** He has smoked 10 cigarettes a day for the past 40 years.

### Examination

**General** Uncomfortable and in pain.

**Obs** T 36.5°C, HR 90 beats/min, regular, BP 154/90 mmHg, RR 18 breaths/min, $SpO_2$ 96% breathing air.

**CVS** Capillary refill time less than 2 seconds, JVP 2 cm above the sternal angle, normal heart sounds.

**RS** Normal breath sounds.

### Investigations

For results of investigations, see Table 13.1.

### Task

A diagnosis of acute coronary syndrome is made. Prescribe appropriate treatment.

**Table 13.1** Case 13 investigation results

| Test | Value | Normal range |
|---|---|---|
| Hb | 130 g/L | 130–180 |
| WCC | $8.2 \times 10^9$/L | 4.0–11.0 |
| Plt | $240 \times 10^9$/L | 150–400 |
| INR | 1.0 | 0.8–1.1 |
| $Na^+$ | 140 mmol/L | 135–145 |
| $K^+$ | 4.0 mmol/L | 3.5–4.7 |
| Ur | 7.5 mmol/L | 2.5–8.0 |
| Creat | 80 μmol/L | 60–110 |
| eGFR | >60 mL/min/1.73 m² | >60 |
| Trop I | 152 ng/L | 0–50 |
| Gluc (random) | 7.8 mmol/L | 3.9–7.8 |
| ECG | 90 beats/min, sinus rhythm, normal axis, normal QRS complexes, ST segment depression in leads V4 to V6 | |

## 14 A 67-year-old man with an exacerbation of COPD

| | |
|---|---|
| **Patient name:** | Roland Harrison |
| **ID number:** | 100014 |
| **Date of birth:** | 13/07/1947 |
| **Weight:** | 59 kg |
| **Admission date:** | 07/01/2015 |
| **Date/time seen:** | 07/01/2015 18:00 |

### History

**PC** Shortness of breath.

**HPC** Over the past 3 days he has had a bad cough. His sputum has changed colour from grey to dark green. He has gone from being able to walk 100 yards to being breathless at rest.

**PMH** Chronic obstructive pulmonary disease (COPD) diagnosed 2013, ischaemic heart disease.

**DH** Tiotropium 18 micrograms one puff daily, Seretide 500 Accuhaler® one puff twice daily, salbutamol 100 micrograms two puffs as needed, aspirin 75 mg daily, simvastatin 20 mg daily.
Intolerances: none known.

**SH** He smokes 20 cigarettes per day.

### Examination

**General** Short of breath at rest, pursed lip breathing.

**Obs** T 37.8°C, HR 110 beats/min, BP 136/88 mmHg, RR 28 breaths/min, $SpO_2$ 92% breathing 28% oxygen via Venturi mask.

**CVS** Normal heart sounds.

**RS** Symmetrically reduced lung expansion, poor air entry, bilateral expiratory wheeze.

### Investigations

For results of investigations, see Tables 14.1 and 14.2.

### Task

A diagnosis of acute exacerbation of COPD is made. Prescribe appropriate treatment. Write appropriate admission medication on the drug chart provided for the management of Mr Harrison's acute and chronic conditions.

**Table 14.1** Case 14 investigation results

| Test | Value | Normal range |
|---|---|---|
| Hb | 154 g/L | 130–180 |
| WCC | $17.2 \times 10^9$/L | 4.0–11.0 |
| Plt | $233 \times 10^9$/L | 150–400 |
| Ur | 3.4 mmol/L | 2.5–8.0 |
| Crea | 98 μmol/L | 60–110 |
| CRP | 28 mg/L | <10 |
| CXR | Hyperinflated lungs, no consolidation | |

**Table 14.2** Case 14 arterial blood gas results while breathing 28% oxygen via Venturi mask

| Test | Value | Normal range |
|---|---|---|
| pH | 7.39 | 7.35–7.45 |
| $PaO_2$ | 8.8 kPa | 10.6–14.5 |
| $PaCO_2$ | 6.3 kPa | 4.0–6.0 |

# Answers

## 1    An 82-year-old woman who requires venous thromboembolism prophylaxis

### What should I consider when deciding what to prescribe?

In 2005, a report from the House of Commons Health and Select Committee stated that up to 25 000 people in the UK were dying each year from venous thromboembolism (VTE) acquired while in hospital. VTE risk assessment and management therefore forms an essential part of the care of every patient admitted to hospital.

### How do I determine the need for VTE prophylaxis?

You should consider whether the patient is at increased risk of VTE and, if they do, whether they have any contraindications to VTE prophylaxis.

*Assess risk of developing VTE.* Virchow's triad describes three categories of factors that increase the risk of venous thrombosis: reduced venous blood flow, e.g. due to reduced mobility or venous compression; vascular endothelial damage, e.g. due to trauma or surgery; and increased coagulability, e.g. due to acute illness, oestrogen therapy or cancer. Most hospitals will have a VTE risk assessment form that allows you to reflect on factors that increase a patient's risk of developing VTE based on national guidelines. If a patient meets **any** of the criteria for increased thrombosis risk, they should be offered treatment to prevent VTE, referred to as thromboprophylaxis, unless contraindicated.

Mrs Henshaw is at significantly increased risk of developing VTE. She has had leg trauma and an operative procedure, both of which may have caused vascular endothelial damage and stimulated increased coagulability. She has had a total anaesthetic time of longer than 60 minutes, will have significantly reduced postoperative mobility and is obese. All of these factors reduce venous blood flow. VTE is more common in older people, so her age (over 60 years old) is also associated with an increased risk of VTE. Therefore, she should be offered thromboprophylaxis.

*Assess risk of bleeding.* Assessment of bleeding risk is an essential part of the decision-making process when prescribing thromboprophylaxis. Patients at increased risk of bleeding, or of serious consequences from bleeding, should not be prescribed pharmacological prophylaxis except under senior or specialist guidance. Patients at particular risk of bleeding include those with acute stroke, active bleeding or bleeding disorders, thrombocytopenia, or those already taking anticoagulants (such as warfarin). Anticoagulant drugs are usually contraindicated for patients undergoing neurosurgical, spinal or eye surgery or lumbar puncture and specialist guidelines should be consulted before prescribing VTE prophylaxis

for these patients. A longer list of situations where patients are at increased risk of bleeding can be found in national guidelines.

Mrs Henshaw has undergone surgery in the last few hours, and may be at some risk of bleeding postoperatively. To reflect this, VTE prophylaxis is usually not started until 6 hours after surgery.

### What are the options for VTE prophylaxis?

Both mechanical and pharmacological methods are used to prevent venous thromboembolism.

*Mechanical VTE prophylaxis.* Mechanical thromboprophylaxis reduces the risk of VTE by mechanisms including reduction of venous diameter and improvements in venous flow and valvular function. The most commonly used mechanical devices are antiembolism stockings (thigh or knee length), which are elastic and compress the lower limb. Foot impulse devices and pneumatic compression devices (thigh or knee length), are slightly more sophisticated and prevent venous stasis by continuous movement or squeezing of the lower limb. Mechanical prophylaxis should be offered to all patients at increased risk of VTE (including those

| Surname HENSHAW | Hospital number 100001 | Weight 85 kg | Drug intolerances None known |
|---|---|---|---|
| First name MADELEINE | Date of birth 24/09/1932 | | |

**REGULAR PRESCRIPTIONS**

Circle / enter times below — Enter dates below — Month: January   Year: 2015 — 7 8 9

| DRUG PARACETAMOL | | | | (06) |
| Dose 1 g | Route Oral | Freq 6-hrly | Start date 7/1/15 | 08 / (12) |
| Signature A Doctor | Bleep 1234 | Review | | 16 / (18) |
| Additional instructions | | | | (24) |

| DRUG DALTEPARIN | | | | 06 |
| Dose 5000 units | Route SC | Freq Daily | Start date 7/1/15 | 08 / 12 |
| Signature A Doctor | Bleep 1234 | Review | | 16 / (18) |
| Additional instructions | | | | 22 |

**ONCE ONLY PRESCRIPTIONS**

| Date | Time to be given | DRUG | Dose | Route | Prescriber Signature | Prescriber Bleep | Administration Date given | Administration Time given | Administration Given by |
|---|---|---|---|---|---|---|---|---|---|
| | | | | | | | | | |
| | | | | | | | | | |

**OXYGEN**

| Target SpO₂ | ○ 94–98% ○ 88–92% |
| Mode of delivery | ○ Continuous ○ As required |
| Starting device | |
| Initials | Bleep | Date |

**AS REQUIRED MEDICATION**

| DRUG DIHYDROCODEINE | | | | Date / Time |
| Dose 30 mg | Route Oral | Max freq 4-hrly | Start date 7/1/15 | Dose |
| Signature A Doctor | Bleep 1234 | Review Daily | | Route / Given |
| Additional instructions For pain relief | | | | Check |

*Prescribing Scenarios at a Glance*, First Edition. Emma Baker, Daniel Burrage, Dagan Lonsdale, and Andrew Hitchings.

with increased risk of bleeding), provided no contraindications exist. Choice of device will depend on local availability, planned surgical intervention and patient preference.

Contraindications to mechanical interventions include peripheral arterial disease, peripheral neuropathy, fragile skin, severe limb oedema from cardiac failure, and unusual leg size or shape. Mrs Henshaw should **not** have a mechanical thromboprophylaxis device applied to the operated limb, although she could on the non-operative side. Some hospitals advocate prescribing mechanical prophylaxis on the drug chart. We have chosen not to do this.

*Pharmacological VTE prophylaxis.* Pharmacological agents recommended for VTE prophylaxis include heparin (low molecular weight or unfractionated), fondaparinux and novel oral anticoagulants (NOACs) including dabigatran and rivaroxaban. Currently, the most commonly used agent is low molecular weight heparin (LMWH), with other agents being reserved for use where LMWH is contraindicated or for specific patient groups. This is a rapidly developing field so local guidelines should be consulted.

### Heparin

Heparin is a naturally occurring polysaccharide that inhibits coagulation by activating the enzyme anti-thrombin III that, in turn, inactivates thrombin and factor Xa. Natural (unfractionated) heparin (UFH) consists of chains of molecules of different molecular weights. LMWH (e.g. dalteparin, enoxaparin, tinzaparin) is prepared by removing the larger molecules (>8000 Da). Compared with UFH, LMWH has greater bioavailability when given subcutaneously, is less plasma protein bound and has a more specific effect on factor Xa (less effect on thrombin). These properties make its anticoagulant activity more predictable. LMWH is eliminated almost entirely through renal clearance of the unmetabolised drug, whereas UFH is predominantly metabolised by the reticuloendothelial system and liver. UFH may therefore be preferred to LMWH for VTE prophylaxis or treatment in patients with renal failure.

Side effects of heparin include haemorrhage, thrombocytopenia, osteoporosis, injection site reactions and skin necrosis. As heparins are made from animal products, a synthetic alternative may be considered for patients with concerns about using animal products.

### Fondaparinux

Fondaparinux is a synthetic factor Xa inhibitor, with a mechanism of action similar to that of LMWH. It is administered subcutaneously for VTE prophylaxis. It is excreted unchanged via the kidney, meaning that caution should be used in patients with renal disease. Side effects include bleeding, purpura and anaemia. Thrombocytopenia is reported but this is less common than with LMWH and by a different mechanism. It is licensed for use as VTE prophylaxis in medical and surgical patients but is prescribed less commonly for this indication than LMWH.

### Novel oral anticoagulants (NOACs)

Dabigatran is an oral direct thrombin inhibitor that has been licensed as a method of VTE prophylaxis for patients undergoing hip and knee replacement. Side effects include abdominal pain, nausea and vomiting as well as haemorrhage. Rivaroxaban is an oral direct factor Xa inhibitor. It has a similar licence and side effect profile to dabigatran.

Unlike the coumarins (e.g. warfarin) there is no easily available monitoring test for NOACs, although dose response is more reliable and laboratory monitoring is unnecessary. No reversal agent is available.

NICE guidelines now advise NOACs as first line for VTE prophylaxis in patients undergoing hip and knee replacement.

## How do I write the prescription?

We have chosen to prescribe a LMWH, dalteparin. This is prescribed as a once daily dose of 5000 units given subcutaneously. 'Units' should be written out in full. The first dose should be given 6 hours after surgery and then once every 24 hours thereafter. As the operation finished at 11:30, it is safe to prescribe the first dose for 18:00 provided there are no ongoing concerns about postoperative haemorrhage. Mrs Henshaw has normal renal function so you do not need to prescribe UFH.

## Further reading

Medical Pharmacology at a Glance. Chapter 19: Drugs used to affect blood coagulation.

Prescribing at a Glance. Chapters 38 & 39: An approach to common prescribing requests.

Department of Health. Risk assessment for venous thromboembolism (2010). Available at: http://webarchive.nationalarchives.gov.uk/20130107105354/http://www.dh.gov.uk/prod_consum_dh/groups/dh_digitalassets/@dh/@en/@ps/documents/digitalasset/dh_113355.pdf (accessed 15 January 2014).

National Institute for Health and Care Excellence. CG92 Venous thromboembolism: reducing the risk (2010). Available at: http://guidance.nice.org.uk/CG92/NICEGuidance/pdf/English (accessed 15 January 2014).

## What should I consider when deciding what to prescribe?

Ms Gomez is a 104-year-old woman with chronic obstructive pulmonary disease (COPD) who presents with respiratory failure due to a non-infective exacerbation of COPD. She requires oxygen treatment to address this. However her history of COPD and prior need for non-invasive ventilation indicate that she is at risk of carbon dioxide retention, so oxygen prescribing must be approached with caution.

### Acute relief of breathlessness and hypoxia

It is essential that Ms Gomez is offered oxygen to correct her hypoxia and relieve her symptoms of breathlessness. You should prescribe oxygen by setting target oxygen saturations which should be achieved by oxygen administration. For most patients, target oxygen saturations should be set at 94-98%. However, for patients at risk of carbon dioxide retention this target may be too high, as demonstrated by Ms Gomez's ABG results. Breathing air, Ms Gomez is hypoxic (saturations 84%) with a normal carbon dioxide level. When her oxygen saturations are 'normalised' to 95% by breathing 35% oxygen, she becomes hypercapnic and acidotic. This tendency to retain carbon dioxide is thought to be due multiple pathophysiological mechanisms (including ventilation–perfusion mismatching and reduced 'hypoxic drive'). It is dangerous, as high carbon dioxide levels can lead to a reduced conscious level and even death.

The target oxygen saturation for patients with chronic lung disease should be set at 88-92%. Ms Gomez achieves oxygen saturations in this range (89%) breathing 28% oxygen. The corresponding arterial oxygenation is satisfactory (>8kPa) without significant hypercapnia. You should therefore prescribe 28% oxygen, a concentration which can be achieved with precision by specifying a Venturi mask as the starting device for administration.

When blood gas results are unavailable, you should use information from a patient's medical history to guide your prescription. In this case, the history of COPD with previous non-invasive ventilation suggests she may be at risk of hypercapnia. You should therefore prescribe oxygen therapy to target the lower oxygen saturation range (88–92%).

It is important to remember that hypoxia is dangerous. You should not avoid giving oxygen to a hypoxic patient just because you are worried about the possibility of hypercapnia. If you are ever in doubt, seek advice from senior colleagues.

### Treatment of the underlying cause

The cause of Ms Gomez's acute hypoxia is a non-infective exacerbation of her COPD and she should

| Surname GOMEZ | Hospital number 100002 | Weight 68 kg | Drug intolerances None known |
|---|---|---|---|
| First name MARIA | Date of birth 16/08/1910 | | |

**REGULAR PRESCRIPTIONS**

Month: January  Year: 2015

| DRUG SERETIDE 250 ACCUHALER | Circle / enter times below ↓ | 7 | 8 |
|---|---|---|---|
| Dose 2 puffs / Route Inh / Freq twice daily / Start date 7/1/15 | 06 | | |
| | 08 ⊗ | | |
| | 12 | | |
| Signature A Doctor / Bleep 1234 / Review | 16 | | |
| | 18 ⊗ | | |
| Additional instructions Salmeterol/fluticasone | 22 | | |
| DRUG TIOTROPIUM | 06 | | |
| Dose 18 micrograms / Route Inh / Freq Daily / Start date 7/1/15 | 08 ⊗ | OMIT | OMIT |
| | 12 | | |
| Signature A Doctor / Bleep 1234 / Review | 16 | | |
| | 18 | | |
| Additional instructions Omit while receiving ipratropium | 22 | | |
| DRUG SALBUTAMOL | 06 ⊗ | | |
| | 08 | | |
| Dose 2.5 mg / Route Neb / Freq 6-hrly / Start date 7/1/15 | 12 ⊗ | | |
| Signature A Doctor / Bleep 1234 / Review | 16 | | |
| | 18 ⊗ | | |
| Additional instructions Driven on air | 24 ⊗ | | |
| DRUG IPRATROPIUM BROMIDE | 06 ⊗ | | |
| | 08 | | |
| Dose 250 micrograms / Route Neb / Freq 6-hrly / Start date 7/1/15 | 12 ⊗ | | |
| Signature A Doctor / Bleep 1234 / Review | 16 | | |
| | 18 ⊗ | | |
| Additional instructions Driven on air | 24 ⊗ | | |
| DRUG PREDNISOLONE | 06 | | |
| | 08 ⊗ | | |
| Dose 30 mg / Route Oral / Freq Daily / Start date 7/1/15 | 12 | | |
| Signature A Doctor / Bleep 1234 / Review 7 days | 16 | | |
| | 18 | | |
| Additional instructions COPD exacerbation | 22 | | |
| DRUG DALTEPARIN | 06 | | |
| | 08 | | |
| Dose 5000 units / Route SC / Freq Daily / Start date 7/1/15 | 12 | | |
| Signature A Doctor / Bleep 1234 / Review | 16 | | |
| | 18 ⊗ | | |
| Additional instructions | 22 | | |

**ONCE ONLY PRESCRIPTIONS**

| Date | Time to be given | DRUG | Dose | Route | Prescriber Signature | Prescriber Bleep | Administration Date given | Administration Time given | Administration Given by |
|---|---|---|---|---|---|---|---|---|---|
| | | | | | | | | | |
| | | | | | | | | | |
| | | | | | | | | | |

**OXYGEN**

| Target SpO₂ | ○ 94-98%  ✓ 88-92% |
|---|---|
| Mode of delivery | ✓ Continuous  ○ As required |
| Starting device | 28% Venturi |
| Initials AD | Bleep 1234 | Date 7/1/15 |

**AS REQUIRED MEDICATION**

| DRUG SALBUTAMOL 100 MICROGRAMS | Date | | |
|---|---|---|---|
| | Time | | |
| Dose 2 puffs / Route INH / Max freq Hourly / Start date 7/1/15 | Dose | | |
| | Route | | |
| Signature A Doctor / Bleep 1234 / Review | Given | | |
| | Check | | |
| Additional instructions | | | |
| DRUG | Date | | |

continue on the acute treatment prescribed on her chart (see Case 14). She is prescribed nebulised salbutamol and ipratropium. As she is at risk of carbon dioxide retention with high flow oxygen these should be driven with air.

## How do I write the prescription?

### Oxygen

As a medical gas, oxygen requires a prescription. In accordance with British Thoracic Society guidelines, most hospital drug charts now include a section to enable you to do this. For Ms Gomez, you should prescribe oxygen to target saturations between 88 to 92%. This should be given continuously, with the 'as required' instruction being reserved, for example, for people who desaturate with physiotherapy. In the first instance you should administer this via a Venturi mask designed to deliver a specific oxygen concentration of 28% with an oxygen flow rate of 4 L/min. The concentration of oxygen and the delivery device should be reviewed regularly.

### Regular medications

You should note under additional instructions that her nebulisers should be driven with air. Supplementary oxygen can still be delivered concurrently by nasal cannulae. No further changes to her medications are required.

### Further reading/useful references

Prescribing at a glance: Chapter 29: Using drugs for the respiratory system

British Thoracic Society 2008. Guideline for Emergency Oxygen Use in Adults. http://www.brit-thoracic.org.uk/guidelines-and-quality-standards/emergency-oxygen-use-in-adult-patients-guideline/ (accessed 16 January 2014)

---

## 3  A 64-year-old man with severe acute abdominal pain

| Surname O'CONNOR | Hospital number 100003 | Weight | Drug intolerances None known |
|---|---|---|---|
| First name EOGHAN | Date of birth 18/10/1950 | 73 kg | |

**REGULAR PRESCRIPTIONS**

| | Circle / enter times below ↓ | ↘ Enter dates below | Month: January | Year: 2015 |
|---|---|---|---|---|
| | | 7 | | |
| DRUG PARACETAMOL | ✎ ④ ✎ ⑩ | | | |
| Dose 1 g / Route IV / Freq 6-hrly / Start date 7/1/15 | 12 | | | |
| Signature A Doctor / Bleep 1234 / Review | ⑯ AM | | | |
| | 18 | | | |
| Additional instructions | ㉒ | | | |
| DRUG AMOXICILLIN | 06 | | | |
| | 08 | | | |
| Dose 1 g / Route IV / Freq 8-hrly / Start date 7/1/15 | 12 | | | |
| Signature A Doctor / Bleep 1234 / Review 48 hr | ⑯ AM | | | |
| | 18 | | | |
| Additional instructions Abdominal sepsis | ㉒ | | | |
| DRUG METRONIDAZOLE | 06 | | | |
| | 08 | | | |
| Dose 500 mg / Route IV / Freq 8-hrly / Start date 7/1/15 | 12 | | | |
| Signature A Doctor / Bleep 1234 / Review 48 hr | ⑯ AM | | | |
| | 18 | | | |
| Additional instructions Abdominal sepsis | ㉒ | | | |

| GENTAMICIN | Level (μg/mL) | N/A | | |
|---|---|---|---|---|
| Indication Abdominal sepsis / Start date 7/1/15 | Time taken | N/A | | |
| | Dose | 360mg | | |
| Signature A Doctor / Bleep 1234 / Review 48 hr | Dr initials | AD | | |
| Trough levels should be taken 18–24 hours post-dose. The next dose is administered if the level is <1 mg/L. | Time given | 1600 | | |
| | Nurse initials | AM | | |
| DRUG | 06 | | | |

**ONCE ONLY PRESCRIPTIONS**

| Date | Time to be given | DRUG | Dose | Route | Prescriber | | Administration | | |
|---|---|---|---|---|---|---|---|---|---|
| | | | | | Signature | Bleep | Date given | Time given | Given by |
| 7/1/15 | 18:10 | ONDANSETRON | 4 mg | IV | A Doctor | 1234 | | | |
| 7/1/15 | 18:10 | MORPHINE – initial dose 4 mg IV then give 2 mg IV at 5 min intervals titrated to effect (max 10 mg) | | | A Doctor | 1234 | | | |

**OXYGEN**

| Target SpO₂ | ✔ 94–98%  ○ 88–92% |
|---|---|
| Mode of delivery | ✔ Continuous  ○ As required |
| Starting device | Facemask 10 L/min |
| Initials AD | Bleep 1234 | Date 7/1/15 |

### What should I consider when deciding what to prescribe?

Mr O'Connor is in severe pain and requires urgent effective analgesia using an agent that can rapidly be titrated to effect. In this situation, you should use a strong opioid, such as morphine. Mr O'Connor is 'nil by mouth' due to peritonitis and the need for urgent surgery. The drug should therefore be prescribed for parenteral (non-oral) administration. Other indications for parenteral administration of strong opioids include acute coronary syndromes, painful sickle cell crises, and major trauma.

### Routes of administration for morphine

Morphine is the drug most commonly used in the management of severe pain, although other strong opioids are available (e.g. diamorphine, oxycodone, fentanyl). Morphine can be given intravenously (IV), intramuscularly (IM), subcutaneously (SC) or orally (the latter in immediate- and modified-release forms; see Case 29), depending on the clinical situation.

*Intravenous administration* yields the most rapid effect (about 5 minutes). This relates both to the desired effect (analgesia) and potential undesirable effects (e.g. hypotension, respiratory and neurological depression). It is therefore only appropriate for use in high-dependency areas (e.g. the emergency department, operating theatres, postoperative recovery unit, and critical care units), and should be given under the supervision of an individual experienced in its use. When used appropriately, intravenous morphine is probably the most effective means of controlling severe acute pain.

*Intramuscular or subcutaneous administration* brings about a smoother onset and offset of effect, and is safer for use on general wards. The same analgesic effect can be obtained as with IV administration, but the delay between administration and peak effect is longer. You therefore need to take care to avoid 'dose stacking', where a repeat dose is administered before the previous one has been fully absorbed. To do this you should allow an interval of at least 1 hour between IM doses and 2 hours between SC doses. A longer interval may be required in patients with circulatory compromise, as absorption from poorly perfused tissue is slower. In this context, be alert to the patient who becomes drowsy after fluid resuscitation: it may be that a 'pool' of morphine has suddenly been absorbed as the tissue was re-perfused.

*Oral administration* is by far the safest and most appropriate route of administration for morphine and other strong opioids in chronic pain. However, in severe acute pain such as that associated with an acute abdomen, the delay between administration and onset of effect (about 30 minutes in a 'well' patient – much longer in a patient with acute illness) is too long to make it useful.

### Practical use of intravenous morphine in severe pain
As IV morphine has a rapid onset of effect, the dose can be titrated (given in small incremental amounts) until the desired level of analgesia is achieved or signs of opioid toxicity emerge. The magnitude of the incremental doses must be decided for the individual patient based on the severity of their pain and their likely sensitivity to the adverse effects of the opioid (which may be increased in advanced age, renal or hepatic impairment, and patients with acute haemodynamic instability). There is no single 'ideal dose' and you should consult local guidelines and more experienced colleagues to help you decide.

Mr O'Connor is in severe pain and has no major risk factors for increased opioid sensitivity. We have selected an initial dose of morphine 4 mg. We would assess the effect of this at about 5 minutes: if he is still in significant pain and has no signs of opioid toxicity (i.e. is awake with respiratory rate >8 breaths/minute and no hypotension), it would be appropriate to administer an additional dose, usually half that of the initial dose (2 mg in this case). This may then be repeated at 5-minute intervals until the pain is adequately controlled or signs of opioid toxicity emerge. If he is still in pain after 10 mg has been administered you should seek further advice from a senior colleague.

In patients with less severe pain or those who are more sensitive to the effects of opioids, you would use lower doses (e.g. morphine 2 mg initially followed by incremental doses of 1 mg at 5-minute intervals).

### Other analgesic considerations
If Mr O'Connor had not already received paracetamol, it would be appropriate to administer this now. Although paracetamol is generally perceived to be a 'weak' analgesic, it is an effective drug which works quickly (especially when given intravenously) and by a different mechanism to that of morphine. It may therefore reduce his pain and/or his requirement for morphine. Mr O'Connor has already been given paracetamol (at 16:00) and his next dose is therefore not due until 22:00. It is being given intravenously because he is nil by mouth and has likely bowel perforation.

The morphine we administer now will last for at least the next couple of hours, by which time it is to be hoped that he will be under general anaesthesia. He is likely to be in significant pain postoperatively. However, given the complexity of his immediate surgical and anaesthetic management, decisions regarding postoperative analgesia in this case are best made by the anaesthetist.

### Antiemetics and laxatives
Whenever you prescribe a strong opioid by a parenteral route you should also prescribe an anti-emetic (see Case 28). This should be administered with the first dose of the opioid. A reasonable choice for Mr O'Connor would be ondansetron 4 mg IV or cyclizine 50 mg IM or by slow IV injection. Metoclopramide should be avoided in patients with suspected gastrointestinal obstruction or perforation as it increases gut motility.

Laxatives are an important consideration in patients who require repeated doses of an opioid. However, given that Mr O'Connor is about to undergo major abdominal surgery, it is not appropriate to start this now. This issue should be readdressed in the postoperative period.

### Prescription chart review
Other aspects of Mr O'Connor's care are being dealt with by colleagues. Nevertheless, it is always a good idea to review the whole prescription chart. Mr O'Connor is being treated with antibiotics appropriate for abdominal sepsis and has no relevant allergies to these (note that the gentamicin prescription in this case is written on a 'sticker', which accommodates documentation of serum concentration measurements; see Case 26). Prophylaxis against venous thromboembolism has not yet been prescribed. This should be addressed once results from initial investigations are available to confirm there is no coagulopathy associated with his acute illness.

### How do I write the prescription?
In the model prescription, we have prescribed morphine and ondansetron in the once-only section of the prescription chart, as we intend only to provide acute symptom relief at this stage. As described above, the prescription calls for an initial dose of morphine 4 mg followed by incremental 2-mg doses, titrated to effect. You should discuss this prescription directly with the nurse who will administer it, to ensure it adequately conveys your intentions. In addition, while you are unfamiliar with the use of IV morphine you should always confirm the appropriateness of your prescription with a senior colleague.

This prescription of morphine is best administered by drawing morphine sulfate 10 mg (1 mL of a 10 mg/mL solution) into a 10-mL syringe, then drawing 9 mL of 0.9% sodium chloride into the same syringe (resulting solution volume 10 mL, containing morphine at a concentration of 1 mg/mL). Immediately label the syringe with details of its contents. The initial dose (4 mg) is contained in 4 mL of this solution, and subsequent doses (2 mg) in 2 mL.

### Further reading
Medical Pharmacology at a Glance. Chapter 29: Opioid analgesics.

# 4 A 55-year-old woman with atrial fibrillation

**REGULAR PRESCRIPTIONS**

| Surname SULLIVAN | Hospital number 100004 | Weight | Drug intolerances |
|---|---|---|---|
| First name EDNA | Date of birth 26/12/1959 | 78 kg | None known |

| DRUG METOPROLOL | | | | Circle/enter times below ↓ | Enter dates below | Month: January | | Year: 2015 |
|---|---|---|---|---|---|---|---|---|
| | | | | | 7 | | | |

Details:

**METOPROLOL**
Dose 50 mg | Route Oral | Freq 3 times daily | Start date 7/1/15
Signature A Doctor | Bleep 1234 | Review
Additional instructions: Do not give if heart rate <50 beats/min
Times: 06, (08), 12, (16) OMIT, 18, (22)

**DALTEPARIN**
Dose 15000 units | Route SC | Freq Daily | Start date 7/1/15
Signature A Doctor | Bleep 1234 | Review
Additional instructions:
Times: 06, 08, 12, 16, (18) OMIT, 22

**AMLODIPINE**
Dose 5 mg | Route Oral | Freq Daily | Start date 7/1/15
Signature A Doctor | Bleep 1234 | Review
Additional instructions: Do not give if BP <90/60
Times: 06, (08), 12, 16, 18, 22

**SIMVASTATIN**
Dose 40 mg | Route Oral | Freq Daily | Start date 7/1/15
Signature A Doctor | Bleep 1234 | Review
Additional instructions:
Times: 06, 08, 12, 16, 18, (22)

**ONCE ONLY PRESCRIPTIONS**

| Date | Time to be given | DRUG | Dose | Route | Prescriber Signature | Prescriber Bleep | Administration Date given | Administration Time given | Administration Given by |
|---|---|---|---|---|---|---|---|---|---|
| 7/1/15 | 15:00 | METOPROLOL | 50 mg | Oral | AD | 1234 | | | |
| 7/1/15 | 15:00 | DALTEPARIN | 15000 units | SC | AD | 1234 | | | |
| | | | | | | | | | |

**OXYGEN**

| Target SpO₂ | ○ 94–98% ○ 88–92% |
|---|---|
| Mode of delivery | ○ Continuous ○ As required |
| Starting device | |
| Initials | Bleep | Date |

## What should I consider when deciding what to prescribe?

Mrs Sullivan is a 55-year-old woman with atrial fibrillation that appears to have been present for at least 72 hours. She has a fast (>100 beats/min) ventricular rate and is experiencing palpitations relating to her arrhythmia. However, there are no features of severely impaired tissue perfusion (e.g. shock, syncope, myocardial ischaemia or pulmonary oedema). Reversible causes of atrial fibrillation, such as infection, hypovolaemia, thyroid disease and electrolyte disturbances, have not been identified by her investigations. In her treatment you therefore need to focus on control of ventricular rate, prevention of thromboembolism and consider whether an attempt should be made to restore sinus rhythm.

## Control of ventricular rate

Control of ventricular rate will relieve symptoms and reduce cardiac work and the risk of complications. Drug therapies available to control ventricular rate include:

- beta adrenoceptor blockers (e.g. metoprolol and bisoprolol)
- non-dihydropyridine calcium channel antagonists (e.g. verapamil and diltiazem)
- cardiac glycosides (digoxin)
- amiodarone (can be used for both rate and rhythm control).

Beta adrenoceptor blockers are the first-line choice for control of ventricular rate in stable atrial fibrillation. Beta adrenoceptor blockers commonly used for atrial fibrillation include metoprolol, bisoprolol and carvedilol. Your choice of beta adrenoceptor blocker will be determined by your patient's comorbidities, local guidelines, availability of medicines and your own experience. A shorter-acting beta adrenoceptor blocker such as metoprolol may be preferable in the first instance, as it will allow more rapid titration of the dose. You should target a ventricular rate of less than 110 beats/min in the first instance.

Non-dihydropyridine calcium channel antagonists are an effective alternative to beta adrenoceptor blockers for acute and chronic rate control. They may be used where beta adrenoceptor blockers are contraindicated, e.g. in patients with asthma. You should not prescribe them with beta adrenoceptor blockers without specialist supervision as, in combination, there is a risk of complete heart block.

The cardiac glycoside digoxin can also be used to control the ventricular rate. This effect is often lost during exertion, so digoxin monotherapy should usually be avoided unless the patient is very sedentary. However, digoxin is a useful option for add-on treatment if monotherapy with a beta adrenoceptor blocker or calcium channel blocker is inadequate. In addition, due to its positive inotropic effect, it may be useful in patients with heart failure.

Amiodarone can be used for rate control in patients with atrial fibrillation in special circumstance such as severe left ventricular failure. However, it should be avoided if possible as it can cause severe phlebitis when given intravenously though peripheral veins and in the longer term causes adverse effects on organs such as the thyroid gland and liver. As it can restore sinus rhythm it should be used with caution in patients with atrial fibrillation for >48 hours who are not treated with anticoagulation.

Mrs Sullivan has atrial fibrillation uncomplicated by comorbidities. She should therefore be prescribed a beta adrenoceptor blocker.

### Prevention of thromboembolism

Atrial fibrillation carries a significant risk of thromboembolic events, principally stroke. In the short term, we have elected to commence anticoagulation with 'treatment dose' low molecular weight heparin (LMWH). In the longer term, oral anticoagulation is likely to be recommended.

Drugs indicated for longer term anticoagulation in patients with atrial fibrillation include vitamin K antagonists (e.g. warfarin), novel oral anticoagulants (e.g. dabigatran) and antiplatelet agents (e.g. aspirin). Warfarin, with a target INR of 2–3, is superior (65% risk reduction) to aspirin (20% risk reduction) in reducing the risk of stroke.

## Restoration of sinus rhythm

Restoration of sinus rhythm has the benefits of controlling ventricular rate and reducing the risk of thromboembolic disease. In patients with signs of severely impaired tissue perfusion (e.g. shock, syncope, myocardial ischaemia or pulmonary oedema) immediate electrical cardioversion should be considered. Cardioversion is also an option for patients where onset of atrial fibrillation can clearly be identified as being <48 hours previously. In these patients, pharmacological cardioversion, e.g. using amiodarone, is also an option.

Cardioversion should not be attempted at this stage for Mrs Sullivan. As her atrial fibrillation appears to have commenced 3 days ago, there is a risk that cardiac thrombus may have developed and that cardioversion could trigger an embolus and stroke. The decision as to whether sinus rhythm should be restored should therefore be delayed until full anticoagulation is achieved and she can be seen by a specialist in an outpatient clinic.

## Continuing usual treatment

You should continue Mrs Sullivan's regular medications, with careful monitoring of her blood pressure.

## How do I write the prescription?
### Control of ventricular rate

You should prescribe a beta adrenoceptor blocker. We have prescribed metoprolol at the recommended dose for management of arrhythmias in the regular section of the drug chart: 50 mg three times daily. As you are seeing Mrs Sullivan at 15:00 and the next routine dose of metoprolol is due at 16:00, you should prescribe the initial dose in the once only section. Ensure it is clear that this is intended to replace the next scheduled dose, for example by writing 'OMIT' against this, as indicated. You should review her response in 2–3 hours as by this time the metoprolol dose should have been fully absorbed. If her rate is not adequately controlled, a further dose may be required. It is good practice to indicate any circumstances under which you would not want a medication given. In this scenario, we have indicated that metoprolol should not be given if the heart rate is less than 50 beats/min in the 'additional instructions' box.

## Prevention of thromboembolism

We have prescribed dalteparin (an LMWH) to prevent thromboembolism caused by atrial fibrillation. You will notice that the BNF does not give this as a specific prescribing indication for LMWHs. We have elected to use the dose recommended for the treatment of venous thromboembolic disease. Mrs Sullivan is 78 kg. The dalteparin dose for adults with body weight 69–82 kg is 15,000 units daily (make sure you write 'units' out in full). Again we have used the once only section to ensure timely administration before regular dalteparin is commenced. As the next dose of dalteparin is due 3 hours after the initial dose, the regular dose has been omitted as shown.

## Existing medications

Amlodipine should be prescribed at her usual dose of 5 mg daily in the regular medications section of the chart. As a new beta adrenoceptor blocker has been started it will be important to monitor Mrs Sullivan's blood pressure to ensure she does not become hypotensive. This has been indicated in the additional instructions box. Her simvastatin should also be prescribed.

## Further reading

Medical Pharmacology at a Glance. Chapter 17: Antiarrhythmic drugs.

Prescribing at a Glance. Chapters 26–28: Using drugs for the cardiovascular system.

NICE clinical guideline 36. Atrial Fibrillation. 2006. Available at: http://www.nice.org.uk/nicemedia/live/10982/30054/30054.pdf (accessed 16 January 2014).

# 5 A 32-year-old man with community-acquired pneumonia

| Surname HASDEU | Hospital number 100005 | Weight 85kg | Drug intolerances None known |
|---|---|---|---|
| First name DRAGOS | Date of birth 17/09/1982 | | |

**REGULAR PRESCRIPTIONS**

| | Circle / enter times below ↓ | Enter dates below | | | | | | | | Month: January | | Year: 2015 | |
|---|---|---|---|---|---|---|---|---|---|---|---|---|---|

| DRUG AMOXICILLIN | 06 |
|---|---|
| Dose 1 g / Route IV / Freq 8-hrly / Start date 7/1/15 | 08 |
| Signature A Doctor / Bleep 1234 / Review 48 hr | ✗⑭ 12 / 18 |
| Additional instructions For community-acquired pneumonia | 22 |

| DRUG CLARITHROMYCIN | 06 |
|---|---|
| Dose 500 mg / Route ORAL / Freq 12-hrly / Start date 7/1/15 | 08 / 12 |
| Signature A Doctor / Bleep 1234 / Review 7 days | 16 / ⑱ |
| Additional instructions For community-acquired pneumonia | 22 |

| DRUG DALTEPARIN | 06 |
|---|---|
| Dose 5000 units / Route SC / Freq Daily / Start date 7/1/15 | 08 / 12 |
| Signature A Doctor / Bleep 1234 / Review | 16 / ⑱ |
| Additional instructions | 22 |

| DRUG PARACETAMOL | 06 |
|---|---|
| Dose 1 g / Route ORAL / Freq 6-hrly / Start date 7/1/15 | 08 / ⑫ |
| Signature A Doctor / Bleep 1234 / Review | 16 / ⑱ |
| Additional instructions | ✗㉔ |

| DRUG IBUPROFEN | 06 |
|---|---|
| Dose 400 mg / Route ORAL / Freq 8-hrly / Start date 7/1/15 | ⑧ / 12 |
| Signature A Doctor / Bleep 1234 / Review 48 hr | ⑯ / 18 |
| Additional instructions With food | ✗㉔ |

## What should I consider when deciding what to prescribe?

Dragos Hasdeu has community-acquired pneumonia. This is a serious infection with an associated risk of death, which can be reduced by prompt and effective antibiotic prescribing and good supportive care.

## Which organism?

The most commonly identified pathogen in people with community-acquired pneumonia is *Streptococcus pneumoniae* (Gram-positive). Other common causative organisms are *Haemophilus influenzae* (Gram-negative) and atypical organisms including *Legionella* and *Mycoplasma* species. Pneumonia can also be caused by *Staphylococcus aureus*, other Gram-negative organisms and viruses such as influenza A. As a pathogen may not be immediately identifiable and the aetiology is diverse, selecting an appropriate antibiotic is difficult.

## Are there any clinical clues?

As *Legionella* tends to cause more severe forms of pneumonia, illness severity may point to aetiology. The CURB-65 score can be used as a simple severity assessment, with 1 point being allocated for each of new-onset **C**onfusion, **U**rea >7 mmol/l, **R**espiratory Rate ≥30 breaths/min, **B**lood Pressure <90 mmHg systolic or ≤60 mmHg diastolic and age ≥**65** years. Pneumonia is considered mild (CURB-65 0–1), moderate (CURB-65 2) or severe (CURB-65 3–5) and risk of death increases with severity.

Dragos Hasdeu has moderately severe pneumonia with a CURB-65 score of 2 (raised urea and respiratory rate).

## Which antibiotics?

Mild pneumonia is usually treated with a broad-spectrum antibiotic effective against relevant Gram-positive and Gram-negative organisms. A broad-spectrum penicillin (e.g. amoxicillin), a macrolide (e.g. clarithromycin) or a tetracycline (e.g. doxycycline) are all reasonable choices and antibiotics can be given orally if the patient is otherwise well.

Moderate and severe pneumonia are treated with a combination of antibiotics effective against Gram-positive, Gram-negative and atypical organisms. A common combination would be a broad-spectrum penicillin (e.g. amoxicillin) **with** a macrolide (e.g. clarithromycin). Where there are signs of sepsis (e.g. fever, tachycardia and signs of reduced tissue perfusion), antibiotics are usually given initially at high doses via the intravenous route, with a switch to oral antibiotics once the patient is apyrexial, has improved clinically and is able to take treatment orally. In severe pneumonia, co-amoxiclav (amoxicillin and clavulanic acid) may be prescribed instead of amoxicillin as co-amoxiclav is also effective against *S. aureus*, anaerobes and some organisms resistant to penicillin.

As Dragos Hasdeu has moderately severe pneumonia and no antibiotic allergies, you should prescribe amoxicillin and clarithromycin for him.

## Local antibiotic guidelines

Most hospitals and primary care practices have local antibiotic guidelines (see Appendix 1 for an example), which you should always follow when choosing antibiotic treatment. These guidelines aim to balance the benefits of antibiotics with minimising harm (antibiotic resistance, 'superbug' infections). For example, severe pneumonia could be treated with benzylpenicillin (highly active against *S. pneumoniae*) and clarithromycin (active against atypical organisms and some Gram-negative organisms) to reduce the risk of amoxicillin-associated *Clostridium difficile* infection (see Case 34).

## Any other treatment?

Dragos has hypoxia breathing room air and a raised urea with increased insensible fluid loss due to tachypnoea and pyrexia. He is in pain and has infection and reduced mobility. Supportive care should include oxygen prescription, fluid management, analgesia and prophylaxis against venous thromboembolism (see Case 1).

## How do I write the prescription?
### Antibiotics

Dragos has moderate severity pneumonia with systemic symptoms and a marked inflammatory response. You should therefore choose antibiotic doses at the upper end of the recommended ranges in the BNF. Intravenous administration would also be reasonable. On the model prescription, amoxicillin has been prescribed intravenously but clarithromycin has been prescribed orally. As intravenous (IV) infusion of macrolides can cause local tenderness and phlebitis and requires a large proximal vein, and their oral bio-availability is high, the IV route tends to be reserved for macrolide use in the most severe infections.

Dragos is seen at 10:00, which does not correspond to an administration time for regular prescriptions. You should therefore write the first dose of antibiotics on the once only section of the drug chart and hand this over to a nurse for immediate administration. Subsequent regular doses of antibiotics should be evenly spaced to ensure consistent plasma concentrations for effective eradication of infection.

When prescribing antibiotics, you should always indicate the reason for prescription and timing of review. In the model prescription, amoxicillin review has been set for 48 hours, when a switch to oral administration should be considered. Once intravenous administration is no longer required, oral administration is preferred as it is safer, cheaper and allows the patient to leave hospital.

### Oxygen

Dragos has hypoxia and hypocapnia with respiratory alkalosis. As adequate oxygenation is essential and he is not at risk of carbon dioxide retention (see Case 2), you should prescribe oxygen with target saturations of 94–98%. A simple face mask would be a reasonable first device for administering oxygen, as controlled oxygen delivery is not required.

### Fluids

Dragos has increased insensible fluid loss, tachycardia and a raised urea. He is able to eat and drink so you should encourage oral fluid intake. In the model prescription, 1 L of 0.9% sodium chloride with 20 mmol potassium chloride has prescribed to support oral fluid replacement over the first 8 hours. This should be reviewed. Further fluid therapy should not be prescribed without a review of the patient.

### Analgesia

Dragos has pleuritic chest pain, caused by inflammation of the pleura overlying the infected lung. You should consider short-term use of a non-steroidal anti-inflammatory drug (NSAID), which can be very effective for this type of pain. As Dragos is young and has no significant past medical history it is reasonable to prescribe the NSAID with food, but without other prophylaxis against peptic ulceration. In the model prescription, background analgesia with paracetamol (also anti-pyretic) and as required analgesia with codeine phosphate for breakthrough pain have also been prescribed.

### Venous thromboembolism prophylaxis

Dragos has acute infection, dehydration and reduced mobility, all of which are risk factors for venous thromboembolism. You should therefore prescribe low molecular weight heparin (LMWH) as standard thromboprophylaxis. Dalteparin is the LMWH selected for the model prescription.

### Further reading

Medical Pharmacology at a Glance. Chapters 38 and 39: Antibacterial drugs.
Prescribing at a Glance. Chapter 32: Using drugs for infection.
Community-acquired pneumonia guidelines from the British Thoracic Society. Available at: http://www.brit-thoracic.org.uk/guidelines-and-quality-standards/community-acquired-pneumonia-in-adults-guideline/ (accessed 21 January 2014).

**ONCE ONLY PRESCRIPTIONS**

| Date | Time to be given | DRUG | Dose | Route | Prescriber Signature | Prescriber Bleep | Administration Date given | Administration Time given | Administration Given by |
|---|---|---|---|---|---|---|---|---|---|
| 7/1/15 | 10:00 | AMOXICILLIN | 1 g | IV | AD | 1234 | | | |
| 7/1/15 | 10:00 | CLARITHROMYCIN | 500 mg | Oral | AD | 1234 | | | |

**OXYGEN**

| Target SpO₂ | ✓ 94–98% |
| | ○ 88–92% |
| Mode of delivery | ✓ Continuous |
| | ○ As required |
| Starting device | Face mask |

| Initials | Bleep | Date |
|---|---|---|
| AD | 1234 | 7/1/15 |

**AS REQUIRED MEDICATION**

| DRUG CODEINE PHOSPHATE | | | | Date | |
|---|---|---|---|---|---|
| | | | | Time | |
| Dose 30-60mg | Route Oral | Max freq 4-hrly | Start date 7/1/15 | Dose | |
| | | | | Route | |
| Signature A Doctor | Bleep 1234 | Review | | Given | |
| | | | | Check | |
| Additional instructions Maximum 240 mg per day | | | | | |

| DRUG | | | | Date | |
|---|---|---|---|---|---|
| | | | | Time | |
| Dose | Route | Max freq | Start date | Dose | |
| | | | | Route | |
| Signature | Bleep | Review | | Given | |
| | | | | Check | |
| Additional instructions | | | | | |

**INFUSION PRESCRIPTIONS**

| Date | Time | Fluid | Vol | Drug | Dose | Rate | Doctor initials | Nurse initials | Batch no | Start time | Stop time |
|---|---|---|---|---|---|---|---|---|---|---|---|
| 7/1/15 | 10:00 | SODIUM CHLORIDE 0.9% | 1 litre | POTASSIUM CHLORIDE | 20 mmol | 8 hr | AD | | | | |

| Surname YARWOOD | Hospital number 100006 | Weight | Drug intolerances |
|---|---|---|---|
| First name HELEN | Date of birth 03/12/1969 | 69 kg | None known |

**REGULAR PRESCRIPTIONS**

| | | | | | Circle / enter times below ↓ | ↘ Enter dates below | | | Month: January | | Year: 2015 |
|---|---|---|---|---|---|---|---|---|---|---|---|
| | | | | | | 7 | | | | | |
| DRUG CARBAMAZEPINE | | | | | 06 | | | | | | |
| | | | | | (08) | | | | | | |
| Dose 600 mg | Route Oral | Freq 12-hrly | Start date 7/1/15 | | 12 | | | | | | |
| Signature A Doctor | | Bleep 1234 | Review | | 16 | | | | | | |
| Additional instructions | | | | | ✗ (20) | | | | | | |
| DRUG | | | | | 22 | | | | | | |

**ONCE ONLY PRESCRIPTIONS**

| Date | Time to be given | DRUG | Dose | Route | Prescriber Signature | Prescriber Bleep | Administration Date given | Administration Time given | Administration Given by |
|---|---|---|---|---|---|---|---|---|---|
| 7/1/15 | 02:00 | LORAZEPAM | 4mg | IV | AD | 1234 | | | |
| 7/1/15 | | LORAZEPAM FOR CONVULSIONS >5 MIN | 4mg | IV | AD | 1234 | | | |

**OXYGEN**

| Target SpO₂ | ✓ 94–98% |
|---|---|
| | ○ 88–92% |
| Mode of delivery | ✓ Continuous |
| | ○ As required |
| Starting device | Non-rebreathe mask |

| Initials | Bleep | Date |
|---|---|---|
| AD | 1234 | 7/1/15 |

## What should I consider when deciding what to prescribe?

Status epilepticus is defined as one seizure lasting more than 5 minutes or two or more seizures without a return of consciousness in between. As Mrs Yarwood has had repeated seizures without full recovery of consciousness and her current seizure has lasted 9 minutes, she meets these diagnostic criteria. Status epilepticus is a life-threatening emergency associated with neurological damage and an increased risk of death. Mrs Yarwood therefore needs urgent supportive care and prompt and effective treatment to terminate the seizure.

## Urgent supportive care

Using the ABCDE approach for the critically ill patient, you can see that Mrs Yarwood has a nasal airway in place, is being nursed on her side and is oxygenating adequately despite her ongoing seizure. She is maintaining an adequate blood pressure and has a cannula in place for intravenous access. Trolley rails and padding have already been implemented to reduce the risk that Mrs Yarwood will injure herself during her seizure.

## Emergency seizure management

The first choice of anti-convulsant for treatment of status epilepticus is a benzodiazepine. Benzodiazepines potentiate the actions of the inhibitory neurotransmitter gamma-aminobutyric acid (GABA), which may account for their anti-epileptic activity.

You should only prescribe benzodiazepines for seizures lasting longer than 5 minutes, as seizures usually self-terminate within 3 minutes. Mrs Yarwood's current seizure has now lasted 9 minutes and she has not regained full consciousness between seizures, so

benzodiazepine treatment is appropriate. She already has an indwelling intravenous (IV) cannula, so you should prescribe IV lorazepam. Lorazepam is the IV benzodiazepine of choice in status epilepticus, as it has a longer anti-seizure effect and causes less thrombophlebitis than IV diazepam. Where IV access is not possible, you can prescribe buccal midazolam, administered into the oral cavity, or rectal diazepam.

After benzodiazepine administration, you should monitor Mrs Yarwood for efficacy (seizure termination, recovery of consciousness) and adverse effects (respiratory depression, hypoxia) of treatment.

If seizures persist, you can prescribe a second dose of lorazepam. However, lorazepam should not be given more than twice in a 24-hour period. If seizures continue despite benzodiazepines, IV phenytoin should be given. IV phenobarbitone is an alternative if phenytoin is already being taken or is contraindicated. Patients who continue in status epilepticus despite these measures require sedation and ventilation.

### Other emergency measures

*Metabolic abnormalities.* If status epilepticus is caused by a metabolic abnormality, such as hypoglycaemia or pyridoxine (vitamin B6) deficiency (malnutrition, isoniazid treatment), you should correct these immediately with IV glucose (20% or 50%) or Pabrinex® (high dose B and C vitamins including pyridoxine and thiamine). In patients at risk of thiamine deficiency (alcohol excess, malnutrition), Pabrinex® should be given before or with intravenous glucose to reduce the risk of glucose precipitating Wernicke's encephalopathy. Mrs Yarwood does not require intravenous glucose or Pabrinex® as she has normal capillary glucose and no risk factors for pyridoxine or thiamine deficiency.

### Further management

Mrs Yarwood has longstanding epilepsy, usually reasonably well controlled with carbamazepine. However, her blood test currently shows very low plasma carbamazepine concentrations. When she recovers, discussions should include adherence to treatment, any recent changes in prescription or dose and any other new medicines that could potentially interact with carbamazepine. Review by an epilepsy specialist may also be useful.

You should also check that Mrs Yarwood does not drive. People with epilepsy must be free of daytime seizures for 1 year or have had asleep-only attacks for 3 years before they can drive a motor vehicle. They cannot drive large goods or passenger vehicles.

### How do I write the prescription?
#### Lorazepam

Your most urgent task is to terminate her seizure. You should prescribe lorazepam on the once only section of the drug chart for immediate administration. The usual dose is 4mg given as a slow IV injection over 2 minutes.

A maximum of two doses of lorazepam can be given in 24 hours. As long as no other benzodiazepines have been given, e.g. in the ambulance, you should write a second lorazepam dose on the once only section of the drug chart. Note that in the model prescription we have stated that this second dose of lorazepam is for administration only if the seizure lasts >5 minutes (most self-terminate after 3 minutes). This second advance prescription allows rapid treatment of further seizures if the prescriber is not immediately available. An acceptable alternative would be to prescribe lorazepam in the as required section of the drug chart. However, it must be made clear that Mrs Yarwood should receive a maximum of one further dose today and subsequently should receive no more than two doses in any 24-hour period.

## Carbamazepine

You should prescribe her regular anti-convulsant treatment to start as soon as possible. On the model chart, carbamazepine has been prescribed at the dose that appeared to control her seizures in the past. When she has recovered from status epilepticus, further discussions may result in changes to her treatment. However, prescribing regular anti-convulsant therapy at this stage ensures that it is not forgotten and will help prevent further seizures.

## Other measures

You should prescribe oxygen to maintain saturations at 94–98%. You should carry out a venous thromboembolism assessment and consider whether prophylaxis is needed. Mrs Yarwood has reduced consciousness and is currently trolley-bound so her mobility is reduced. However, she has fallen out of bed, had several tonic–clonic convulsions and is experiencing unusual seizure activity. At this stage it would be reasonable to withhold low molecular weight heparin and impossible to apply anti-embolism stockings. The need for VTE prophylaxis should be reviewed once the seizures have been terminated and further clinical assessment has been performed.

## Further reading

Medical Pharmacology at a Glance. Chapters 25: Antiepileptic drugs.
Prescribing at a Glance. Chapter 30: Using drugs for the neurological system.
NICE epilepsy pathway. Available at: http://pathways.nice.org.uk/pathways/epilepsy (accessed 21 January 2014).

---

## 7   A 27-year-old woman with suspected bacterial meningitis

## What should I consider when deciding what to prescribe?

### Treatment of bacterial meningitis

Florence Menzes has bacterial meningitis, which is a life-threatening illness. You need to prescribe intravenous antibiotics and make sure they are administered as soon as the diagnosis is suspected, as urgent treatment saves life and reduces disability.

### Which organism?

The most common organisms that cause bacterial meningitis are *Neisseria meningitides* and *Streptococcus pneumoniae*. *Haemophilus influenzae* (*b*) meningitis has become less common in the UK since the introduction of an effective vaccine. *Listeria monocytogenes*, *Staphylococcus aureus* and Gram-negative bacilli are rarer causes of meningitis, which usually affect people who have underlying illness, are immunocompromised or have a cerebrospinal fluid leak.

### Which antibiotics?

Florence is 27 years old and has bacterial meningitis caused by an organism which is as yet unidentified. You should therefore prescribe intravenous cefotaxime, which is a broad-spectrum antibiotic that is active against both Gram-negative (*N. meningitides*, *H. influenzae*) and Gram-positive (*S. pneumoniae*) organisms.

There is nothing in Florence's clinical assessment that points to a specific causative organism to help

| Surname MENZES | Hospital number 100007 | Weight | Drug Intolerances |
|---|---|---|---|
| First name FLORENCE | Date of birth 01/02/1987 | 65 kg | None known |

**REGULAR PRESCRIPTIONS**

| | Circle / enter times below ↓ | ↘ Enter dates below | Month: **January** | | | Year: **2015** | |
|---|---|---|---|---|---|---|---|
| | | 7 | | | | | |
| DRUG **CEFOTAXIME** | 06 | | | | | | |
| | 08 | | | | | | |
| Dose 2 g / Route IV / Freq 6-hrly / Start date 7/1/15 | 12 | | | | | | |
| Signature A Doctor / Bleep 1234 / Review 10 days | 16 | | | | | | |
| | 18 | | | | | | |
| Additional instructions For bacterial meningitis | ✗ 24 | | | | | | |
| DRUG **DEXAMETHASONE** | 06 | | | | | | |
| | 08 | | | | | | |
| Dose 8 mg / Route IV / Freq 6-hrly / Start date 7/1/15 | 12 | | | | | | |
| Signature A Doctor / Bleep 1234 / Review 4 days | 16 | | | | | | |
| | 18 | | | | | | |
| Additional instructions Review with LP results | ✗ 24 | | | | | | |
| DRUG **PARACETAMOL** | 06 | | | | | | |
| | 08 | | | | | | |
| Dose 1 g / Route IV / Freq 6-hrly / Start date 7/1/15 | 12 | | | | | | |
| Signature A Doctor / Bleep 1234 / Review 48 hours | 16 | | | | | | |
| | 18 | | | | | | |
| Additional instructions Maximum 4 g in 24 hours | ✗ 24 | | | | | | |
| DRUG **DALTEPARIN** | 06 | | | | | | |
| | 08 | | | | | | |
| Dose 5000 units / Route S/C / Freq Daily / Start date 8/1/15 | 12 | | | | | | |
| Signature A Doctor / Bleep 1234 / Review | 16 | | | | | | |
| | 18 | | | | | | |
| Additional instructions | 22 | | | | | | |

**ONCE ONLY PRESCRIPTIONS**

| Date | Time to be given | DRUG | Dose | Route | Prescriber Signature | Prescriber Bleep | Administration Date given | Administration Time given | Administration Given by |
|------|------------------|------|------|-------|-----------|-------|------------|------------|----------|
| 7/1/15 | 23:00 | CEFOTAXIME | 2 g | IV | A Doctor | 1234 | | | |
| 7/1/15 | 23:00 | DEXAMETHASONE | 8 mg | IV | A Doctor | 1234 | | | |
| 7/1/15 | 23:00 | PARACETAMOL | 1 g | IV | A Doctor | 1234 | | | |

**OXYGEN**

| Target SpO₂ | ○ 94–98% |
|-------------|----------|
| | ○ 88–92% |
| Mode of delivery | ○ Continuous |
| | ○ As required |
| Starting device | |

| Initials | Bleep | Date |
|----------|-------|------|

**AS REQUIRED MEDICATION**

| DRUG CODEINE PHOSPHATE | | | | Date | | | | | | | |
|------|------|------|------|------|---|---|---|---|---|---|---|
| | | | | Time | | | | | | | |
| Dose 30–60 mg | Route Oral | Max freq 4-hrly | Start date 7/1/15 | Dose | | | | | | | |
| | | | | Route | | | | | | | |
| Signature A Doctor | | Bleep 1234 | Review | Given | | | | | | | |
| | | | | Check | | | | | | | |

Additional instructions
For pain relief. Maximum 240 mg daily.

| DRUG MORPHINE | | | | Date | | | | | | | |
|------|------|------|------|------|---|---|---|---|---|---|---|
| | | | | Time | | | | | | | |
| Dose 5–10 mg | Route SC | Max freq 2–4 hrly | Start date 7/1/15 | Dose | | | | | | | |
| | | | | Route | | | | | | | |
| Signature A Doctor | | Bleep 1234 | Review | Given | | | | | | | |
| | | | | Check | | | | | | | |

Additional instructions
For pain relief.

| DRUG CYCLIZINE | | | | Date | | | | | | | |
|------|------|------|------|------|---|---|---|---|---|---|---|
| | | | | Time | | | | | | | |
| Dose 50 mg | Route Oral/IV | Max freq 8-hrly | Start date 7/1/15 | Dose | | | | | | | |
| | | | | Route | | | | | | | |
| Signature A Doctor | | Bleep 1234 | Review | Given | | | | | | | |
| | | | | Check | | | | | | | |

Additional instructions

direct therapy. She does not have a non-blanching petechial rash (meningococcus), cerebrospinal fluid leak or ear disease (pneumococcus), travel or prior antibiotic exposure (antibiotic resistance) and is not immunocompromised or over 50 years (listeria). She has no antibiotic allergies. Treatment modifications for different organisms or clinical situations include:

- Proven meningococcus – cefotaxime might be changed to benzyl penicillin if sensitivities were known
- Prior antibiotic exposure/travel – consider adding vancomycin to treatment to cover penicillin- and cephalosporin-resistant pneumococci
- Listeria – add amoxicillin to cefotaxime treatment
- Antibiotic allergies – chloramphenicol can be used in penicillin and cephalosporin-allergic patients
- Seizure or other features to suggest viral encephalitis – add aciclovir.

All such treatment modifications should have input from a specialist in microbiology or infectious diseases.

### Any other treatment?

Even with optimal antibiotic treatment, ~20% of patients with bacterial meningitis die and ~20% of survivors have neurological complications such as hearing loss or epilepsy. This neurological damage is attributed to the inflammatory host response to infection, which can potentially be suppressed by corticosteroids. A large multicentre clinical trial found that administration of the corticosteroid dexamethasone to patients with suspected bacterial meningitis (starting with or just before the first dose of antibiotics) reduced death and disability. The benefit appeared most marked in patients with meningitis caused by *S. pneumoniae*. Most specialists would therefore now recommend giving dexamethasone with the first dose of an appropriate antibiotic for suspected bacterial meningitis. Dexamethasone should be continued for confirmed pneumococcal meningitis and stopped if bacterial infection is ruled out.

It is less clear whether dexamethasone is beneficial in non-pneumococcal bacterial meningitis, so you should ask for advice from your local specialist (infection or neurology).

### Relief of symptoms

You need to prescribe analgesia to relieve Florence's headache. One option would be regular paracetamol for background analgesia with a moderate (codeine) and/or strong (morphine) opioid analgesic. You should be aware of the side effects of opioid analgesia such as sedation and vomiting which could be confused with clinical deterioration due to worsening bacterial meningitis.

Florence has been vomiting. You should prescribe an anti-emetic, such as metoclopramide, cyclizine or prochlorperazine. This may enable her to take oral fluids and analgesia, which will make her condition easier to manage.

### Fluids

Her blood pressure, electrolytes and renal function are all normal, indicating that she is not significantly fluid depleted. Her fluid maintenance requirements are likely to be increased by pyrexia, which increases insensible losses. If possible she should be encouraged to take fluids orally. If this is prevented by vomiting, intravenous fluids should be prescribed.

### Prophylaxis against venous thromboembolism

Florence is at risk of venous thromboembolism (VTE) due to reduced mobility, sepsis and oral contraceptive use. However, she has just had a lumbar puncture, with some associated risk of bleeding. You should therefore prescribe low molecular weight heparin, but delay dosing for at least 4 hours after the lumbar puncture was performed. It is important to be sure that coagulation is normal before prescribing VTE prophylaxis as sepsis can lead to coagulopathy.

### How do I write the prescription?
### Cefotaxime

You must make sure that Florence receives her antibiotics immediately. One way of doing this is to write the first dose as a once only prescription to be given now (and hand this over to the responsible nurse to ensure immediate administration), with subsequent doses in the regular prescription section. In the model chart this has also been done for dexamethasone and paracetamol.

As bacterial meningitis is a severe infection, you should prescribe high-dose cefotaxime (2 g 6-hourly, as opposed to the usual dose of 1 g 6-hourly). It is important that the plasma concentrations of cefotaxime are consistently high to eradicate the infection. To achieve this, you should space cefotaxime doses evenly over 24 hours. This is shown on the model prescription, with doses at 6am, midday, 6pm and midnight.

When writing up antibiotic treatment you should specify the indication and duration of treatment as shown. Cefotaxime should usually be given intravenously for at least 10 days for bacterial meningitis, although treatment may be modified once the diagnosis is clarified.

### Dexamethasone

On the model prescription dexamethasone has been prescribed as recommended for bacterial meningitis in the British National Formulary. The dose and duration of treatment are those that were beneficial when tested in a multicentre clinical trial.

### Analgesia and anti-emetics

When writing up analgesia and anti-emetics for Florence, you should consider route of administration. Oral administration is convenient and acceptable to patients and generally safer than intravenous (risk of infection, toxicity from drug bolus) or intramuscular (risk of haematoma, unpredictable absorption) administration. However, oral administration may not be appropriate for Florence who has been vomiting. On the model drug chart this has been addressed by an intravenous prescription of regular paracetamol with a review date, when a change to oral and/or less frequent administration should be considered. The as required prescription of the anti-emetic cyclizine has been prescribed for either oral or intravenous administration at the discretion of the administering nursing staff. This is possible as cyclizine dose and frequency of administration is the same by either route.

### Low molecular weight heparin

You should prescribe this to start at least 4 hours after the lumbar puncture. On the model prescription an interval of 12 hours has been ensured.

### Oral contraception

While Florence is unwell with bacterial meningitis, maintenance of oral contraception is not a priority and may add to the risk of VTE. On recovery you should discuss issues around restarting oral contraception including timing and initial alternative precautions.

### Further reading

Medical Pharmacology at a Glance. Chapters 38: Antibacterial drugs.
Prescribing at a Glance. Chapter 32: Using drugs for infection.
Meningitis research foundation guidelines for management of meningitis and septicaemia. Available at: http://www.meningitis.org/health-professionals (accessed 21 January 2014).

---

## 8  A 31-year-old woman with paracetamol overdose

### What should I consider when deciding what to prescribe?

Eleanor Briggs is a 31-year-old woman who has presented 6 hours after a deliberate overdose of paracetamol. When planning management for a patient at risk of paracetamol poisoning, you need to obtain three key pieces of information:
- The time the first dose of paracetamol was ingested
- The time the last dose of paracetamol was ingested
- The total amount of paracetamol ingested.

If the interval between the first and last doses of paracetamol is less than 1 hour, and you know the time at which it was taken, your next step is to measure the serum paracetamol concentration. At least 4 hours must have elapsed since the time of ingestion before taking the blood sample. To interpret the result, you refer to a paracetamol poisoning treatment graph, such as that illustrated in Figure 8.1 (one can also be found in the BNF). If the concentration is above the treatment line, there is a significant risk of toxicity, and you should therefore offer treatment with the antidote, acetylcysteine.

Acetylcysteine works by supplementing the body's stores of glutathione. The body uses glutathione to detoxify *N*-acetyl-*p*-benzoquinone imine (NAPQI), a metabolite produced when paracetamol is taken in excess. Acetylcysteine is almost universally effective if started within 8 hours of paracetamol ingestion. Consequently, if you are working within this time frame, it is safe to wait until you know the result of the paracetamol concentration before starting treatment. By contrast, after 8 hours, you should start treatment

| Surname | Hospital number | Weight | Drug intolerances |
|---|---|---|---|
| BRIGGS | 100008 | | None known |
| First name | Date of birth | 65 kg | |
| ELEANOR | 04/04/1983 | | |

**INFUSION PRESCRIPTIONS**

| Date | Time | Fluid | Vol | Drug | Dose | Rate | Doctor initials | Nurse initials | Batch no | Start time | Stop time |
|---|---|---|---|---|---|---|---|---|---|---|---|
| 7/1/15 | 14:00 | 5% GLUCOSE | 200 mL | ACETYLCYSTEINE | 9750 mg | 249 mL/h | AD | | | | |
| 7/1/15 | To follow | 5% GLUCOSE | 500 mL | ACETYLCYSTEINE | 3250 mg | 129 ml/h | AD | | | | |
| 7/1/15 | To follow | 5% GLUCOSE | 1 L | ACETYLCYSTEINE | 6500 mg | 65 mL/h | AD | | | | |
| | | | | | | | | | | | |

with acetylcysteine immediately, then stop it if the concentration is later found to be below the treatment line.

If the interval between the first and last doses is greater than 1 hour (termed a staggered overdose), or if the time of ingestion is not known, you cannot use the paracetamol concentration to guide your management. In this case, you must base your decision on the amount of paracetamol taken. If it is more than 75 mg/kg of body weight, you should offer treatment with acetylcysteine.

In Eleanor Briggs's case, as she took all the tablets within 1 hour, and we know the time at which she took them, we will refer to the treatment graph. The sample was taken 4 hours after she ingested the tablets. At this time point, the treatment line is at 100 mg/L

(Figure 8.1). Her paracetamol concentration (118 mg/L) exceeds this, so we should offer treatment with acetylcysteine.

Acetylcysteine can cause an anaphylactoid reaction. This presents with similar features to an anaphylactic reaction (e.g. urticarial rash, nausea, tachycardia, wheeze), but it does not have an allergic basis. If this reaction occurs, you should stop the infusion temporarily and offer symptomatic treatment with an antihistamine (e.g. chlorphenamine 10 mg IV in adults). Once the patient's symptoms are improving, you should restart acetylcysteine treatment using the next infusion in the sequence.

### How do I write the prescription?

Acetylcysteine is administered by intravenous infusion. The drug is provided as a 200 mg/mL solution, which is diluted for administration, usually with 5% glucose. The infusion has three components, which should be given sequentially: 150 mg/kg (over 1 hour), 50 mg/kg (over 4 hours) then 100 mg/kg (over 20 hours). You should prescribe acetylcysteine in the infusion section of the drug chart.

Guidelines recommend the use of dosing tables (rather than calculation) to determine the correct acetylcysteine prescription. These are provided in the acetylcysteine package inserts, and reproduced in the BNF. Table 8.2 summarises the important data needed for the prescription of acetylcysteine for a patient in the weight band 60–69 kg, as applied in Ms Briggs's case.

The three infusions should be administered sequentially, with no breaks in between them. Once the third component has been infused, you should take blood to check the international normalised ratio (INR), alanine transaminase (ALT) and creatinine. You should refer to local guidelines determine how to act on these. However, in general, if they are normal, no further treatment is

**Table 8.2** Acetylcysteine dosing and administration for body weight 60–69 kg (dose calculation is based on the midpoint in the weight range)

|  | First infusion | Second infusion | Third infusion |
|---|---|---|---|
| Infusion duration | 1 hour | 4 hours | 20 hours |
| Diluent fluid | 5% glucose | 5% glucose | 5% glucose |
| Diluent volume | 200 mL | 500 mL | 1000 mL |
| Acetylcysteine dose | 9750 mg | 3250 mg | 6500 mg |
| Acetylcysteine solution volume | 49 mL | 17 mL | 33 mL |
| Infusion rate | 249 mL/h | 129 mL/h | 65 mL/h |

necessary. If they are abnormal (particularly the INR), acetylcysteine treatment should be continued by re-prescribing the third component of the infusion. The blood tests should then be repeated regularly (e.g. 12-hourly) until the results are seen to improve. Once the treatment is complete, Miss Briggs should be assessed by a liaison psychiatrist, so that the issues that lead to her overdose can be considered and addressed.

We do not anticipate that Miss Briggs's mobility is likely to be significantly restricted, and she has no other risk factors for venous thromboembolism. Consequently, we have elected not to prescribe low molecular weight heparin in this case.

### Further reading
Medical Pharmacology at a Glance. Chapter 46: Poisoning.

## What should I consider when deciding what to prescribe?

Mr Jones is a 59-year-old man who had a myocardial infarction 5 years ago. This left him with left ventricular impairment and requiring chronic diuretic therapy to control breathlessness and ankle swelling. He now presents with a severe exacerbation of his heart failure, which appears to have been precipitated by stopping his diuretics. He has pulmonary oedema. This is a life-threatening medical emergency. You should therefore use the ABCDE approach for initial assessment and support of Mr Jones, before starting more specific treatment for management of his heart failure.

Mr Jones is conscious, has a patent airway and is talking. He is breathing spontaneously but is hypoxic and therefore you should prescribe high-flow oxygen via a non-rebreathe mask. If this is not effective in improving his oxygenation, continuous positive airway pressure (CPAP) may be considered as the next step. You should ensure he has good intravenous access. His high blood pressure is likely due to the stress of this acute event and should improve as you begin to treat his acute heart failure.

## Management of acute heart failure

The goals of treatment are to relieve symptoms, including shortness of breath and associated anxiety, restore oxygenation and improve organ perfusion and haemodynamics. Cardiac function can be improved by:

1 Reducing venous return (preload), which optimises cardiac filling to allow efficient cardiac contraction
2 Reducing arterial pressure (afterload), which reduces the amount of work required in systole or
3 Increasing contractility of the cardiac muscle.

During treatment, Mr Jones should be monitored carefully using pulse, blood pressure, respiratory rate, oxygen saturations and urine output. Inadequate response should prompt senior medical review and intensification of treatment.

| Surname JONES | Hospital number 100009 | Weight | Drug intolerances |
| First name JOEL | Date of birth 07/05/1955 | 82 kg | None known |

**REGULAR PRESCRIPTIONS**

Month: January   Year: 2015

| DRUG | Circle/enter times below | 7 |
|---|---|---|
| **ASPIRIN** — Dose 75 mg, Route Oral, Freq Daily, Start date 7/1/15, Signature A Doctor, Bleep 1234 | 06, (08), 12, 16, 18, 22 | 08 |
| **ATORVASTATIN** — Dose 40 mg, Route Oral, Freq Daily, Start date 7/1/15, Signature A Doctor, Bleep 1234 | 06, 08, 12, 16, 18, (22) | 22 |
| **BISOPROLOL** — Dose 2.5 mg, Route Oral, Freq Daily, Start date 7/1/15, Signature A Doctor, Bleep 1234, Restart when acute heart failure is controlled | 06, (08), 12, 16, 18, 22 | OMIT |
| **RAMIPRIL** — Dose 5 mg, Route Oral, Freq Daily, Start date 7/1/15, Signature A Doctor, Bleep 1234 | 06, (08), 12, 16, 18, 22 | |
| **DALTEPARIN** — Dose 5000 units, Route SC, Freq Daily, Start date 7/1/15, Signature A Doctor, Bleep 1234 | 06, 08, 12, 16, (18), 22 | 18 |
| **FUROSEMIDE** — Dose 80 mg, Route Oral, Freq Daily, Start date 7/1/15, Signature A Doctor, Bleep 1234 | 06, (08), 12, 16, 18, 22 | 08 |

*Morphine.* There is no clinical trial evidence to support the use of morphine in acute heart failure. However, theoretical considerations and clinical experience suggest it may be helpful. It acts primarily by reducing the the sense of breathlessness and anxiety. This, in turn, reduces sympathetic outflow, promoting vasodilation and therefore reducing preload and afterload. Intravenous (IV) administration yields the most rapid onset of symptom relief (about 5 minutes) and will have a more predictable effect than intramuscular morphine as acute heart failure causes poor skeletal muscle perfusion. However, IV morphine can also cause a rapid onset of adverse effects including hypotension, respiratory and neurological depression. Morphine should therefore only be administered intravenously by experienced staff in a situation where there are intensive monitoring and resuscitation facilities

(such as the emergency department or high dependency area). The dose of morphine should be titrated carefully against symptoms and side effects. A method of doing this is described in Case 3. It is good practice to administer an anti-emetic, e.g. metoclopramide with morphine, to counteract side effects of nausea and vomiting.

*Nitrates.* You should prescribe a continuous intravenous infusion of glyceryl trinitrate (GTN) for Mr Jones. This acts as a vasodilator, predominantly reducing preload, but also has some beneficial effect on afterload. The main side effects of nitrates are hypotension and headache. You should start the GTN at a low infusion rate and slowly increase the rate, monitoring Mr Jones' blood pressure. The optimal dose is the highest infusion rate that can

## ONCE ONLY PRESCRIPTIONS

| Date | Time to be given | DRUG | Dose | Route | Prescriber | | Administration | | |
|------|------|------|------|------|------|------|------|------|------|
| | | | | | Signature | Bleep | Date given | Time given | Given by |
| 7/1/15 | 12:00 | FUROSEMIDE | 40 mg | IV | A Doctor | 1234 | | | |
| 7/1/15 | 12:00 | MORPHINE – initial dose 2.5 mg IV | | | A Doctor | 1234 | | | |
| | | then give 1.25 mg IV at 5 min intervals titrated to effect (max 10 mg) | | | | | | | |

## OXYGEN

| Target SpO₂ | ✓ 94–98% |
|------|------|
| | ○ 88–92% |
| Mode of delivery | ✓ Continuous |
| | ○ As required |
| Starting device | Non-rebreathe mask |

| Initials | Bleep | Date |
|------|------|------|
| AD | 1234 | 7/1/15 |

## AS REQUIRED MEDICATION

| DRUG METOCLOPRAMIDE | | | | Date | |
|------|------|------|------|------|------|
| | | | | Time | |
| Dose 10 mg | Route IV | Max freq 8-hrly | Start date 7/1/15 | Dose | |
| | | | | Route | |
| Signature A Doctor | | Bleep 1234 | Review | Given | |
| | | | | Check | |

Additional instructions
Give with morphine

| DRUG | | | | Date | |
|------|------|------|------|------|------|
| | | | | Time | |
| Dose | Route | Max freq | Start date | Dose | |
| | | | | Route | |
| Signature | | Bleep | Review | Given | |
| | | | | Check | |

Additional instructions

| DRUG | | | | Date | |
|------|------|------|------|------|------|
| | | | | Time | |
| Dose | Route | Max freq | Start date | Dose | |
| | | | | Route | |
| Signature | | Bleep | Review | Given | |
| | | | | Check | |

Additional instructions

| DRUG | | | | Date | |
|------|------|------|------|------|------|
| | | | | Time | |
| Dose | Route | Max freq | Start date | Dose | |
| | | | | Route | |
| Signature | | Bleep | Review | Given | |
| | | | | Check | |

Additional instructions

## INFUSION PRESCRIPTIONS

| Date | Time | Fluid | Vol | Drug | Dose | Rate | Doctor initials | Nurse initials | Batch no | Start time | Stop time |
|------|------|------|------|------|------|------|------|------|------|------|------|
| 7/1/15 | 12:00 | GLYCERYL TRINITRATE 1mg/mL | 50 mL | | | 1-10 mL/hr | AD | | | | |
| Start at 1 mL/hr and titrate to symptoms and systolic blood pressure (keep SBP >100 mmHg) | | | | | | | | | | | |

---

be achieved while maintaining the systolic blood pressure >90–100 mmHg. Nitrates should be used with caution in patients with hypotension, and particularly in patients with severe aortic stenosis; nitrates reduce the afterload, which can accentuate pressure gradients across a stenosed aortic valve, compromising cardiac output and coronary artery circulation.

*Loop diuretics.* You should prescribe a loop diuretic such as furosemide for Mr Jones, which will reduce preload by causing diuresis and venodilatation. As he has acute pulmonary oedema, he should be given the initial dose of furosemide intravenously, since absorption from the gut may be slow and erratic. You should monitor his response. Evidence for a good response will include reduction in his pulse rate and oxygen requirements, improvement in symptoms and increased urine output (e.g. 1–2 L of urine in 1–2 hours after furosemide dose). If the response is poor, a further single dose or a furosemide infusion may be required. Side effects to watch out for include hypotension, hypokalaemia and hyponatraemia. After initial treatment, Mr Jones will need to restart oral diuretic therapy to prevent future worsening of his cardiac failure. He may need a higher dose than usual for a week or two while fluid retention is cleared. Longer term diuretic therapy is monitored by weighing the

patient (1 L of water weighs 1 kg), looking for signs of heart failure (peripheral oedema, elevated JVP, pulmonary crepitations) and measuring renal function and electrolytes to detect side effects.

### Other acute measures

You should determine whether Mr Jones should receive prophylaxis against venous thromboembolism. He is a medical patient who is likely to have a significant reduction in his mobility while he is treated for acute heart failure and has significant cardiovascular comorbidities. He has no risk factors for bleeding and normal renal function. You should therefore prescribe a low molecular weight heparin.

### Continuing usual treatment

Ramipril, an angiotensin converting enzyme (ACE) inhibitor, reduces morbidity and mortality in patients with ischaemic heart disease and chronic heart failure. As Mr Jones is already established on ramipril and has no signs of hypotension or renal dysfunction, it is reasonable to continue this. However, this should be reviewed on a daily basis and, if signs of hypotension or renal failure develop, you should reduce the dose or omit it temporarily.

Bisoprolol, a competitive cardioselective beta adrenoreceptor antagonist, also reduces morbidity and mortality following myocardial infarction and in chronic heart failure. However, as beta adrenoreceptor antagonists reduce cardiac contractility, they can worsen cardiac failure in the acute situation. For Mr Jones it would be reasonable to omit the next dose of his bisoprolol, which can be restarted as soon as his acute cardiac failure is under control.

### How do I write the prescriptions?
### Oxygen

As Mr Jones has type 1 respiratory failure, you should prescribe continuous oxygen with target saturations of 94–98%. In the first instance, you should administer oxygen at a high flow rate (10–15 L/minute) via a non-rebreathe mask, and then titrate according to oxygen saturations.

### Morphine sulfate

Morphine is prescribed for titration against symptomatic improvement and side effects as described in Case 3.

### Metoclopramide

The usual dose of metoclopramide is 10 mg 8-hourly. It can be administered orally, intramuscularly or intravenously. As it is being prescribed here to prevent nausea and vomiting caused by intravenous morphine, intravenous administration will be the most appropriate route.

### Furosemide

You should prescribe the initial dose of intravenous furosemide as a once only prescription. The usual treatment dose in severe acute pulmonary oedema is 40–100 mg. Depending on Mr Jones' response to this initial dose you may need to prescribe an additional once only dose, or if significant fluid offloading is required he may need a furosemide infusion. At this stage you do not know how much 'maintenance' furosemide will be required. However, it would be sensible to restart his usual oral dose of furosemide (80 mg) so that this is not forgotten, and hand over that this should be reviewed depending on treatment response.

### Glyceryl trinitrate infusion

Mr Jones has heart failure, so it is important to minimise the volume of any solutions infused intravenously. GTN comes pre-prepared at a concentration of 1 mg/mL in 50-mL vials. The contents of one vial can be drawn up directly into a 50-mL syringe and administered via a syringe driver.

The recommended GTN dose for treatment of acute heart failure is 10–200 micrograms/min. You should start treatment at a low dose, e.g. 10 micrograms/min. You need to convert this dose into an infusion rate for administration; 10 micrograms/min is equivalent to 600 micrograms/hour. As there are 1000 micrograms in 1 mL, there are 600 micrograms in 0.6 mL. A pragmatic starting infusion rate is 1 mL/hr. This has been written up in the infusion section of the model prescription. It has also been indicated how the infusion rate should be increased and monitored. Good communication and handover between the prescriber and the nursing staff who will administer the drug is important.

### Other medications

Dalteparin and usual medications have been prescribed on the model prescription. The next dose of bisoprolol has been omitted, but there are clear indications for restarting it.

### Further reading

Medical Pharmacology at a Glance. Chapter 18: Drugs used in heart failure.

Prescribing at a Glance. Chapters 26–28: Using drugs for the cardiovascular system.

European Society of Cardiology. Guidelines for the diagnosis and treatment of acute and chronic heart failure 2008. European Heart Journal 2008;29,2388–2442. Available at: http://www.escardio.org/guidelines-surveys/esc-guidelines/Documents/CHF/guidelines-HF-FT.pdf (accessed 16 January 2014).

---

## 10  A 24-year-old woman with acute asthma

### What should I consider when deciding what to prescribe?

Miss Powell is a 24-year-old woman who is known to have asthma. She has presented with features of acute severe asthma. This is a serious condition for which she requires urgent treatment.

The key issues in managing her acute asthma are as follow.

### The ABCDE approach

As with most emergency situations, an ABCDE approach should be adopted when managing acute severe asthma. In this case, Miss Powell is alert and able to speak, indicating a secure airway. She is hypoxic, but does not have any circulatory compromise. The focus of this case therefore is in managing her respiratory problems, i.e. 'B'.

### Pathophysiology

In an acute exacerbation of asthma, the underlying pathology is inflammation of the airways, often triggered by allergen exposure or viral infection. Oedema of the airway walls, increased secretions and hyperreactivity, leading to bronchospasm and gas trapping, all contribute to airflow obstruction, which in turn can cause respiratory failure. Urgent treatment should therefore include supplementary oxygen to relieve hypoxia, bronchodilatation for rapid relief of bronchospasm and corticosteroids to address the underlying airway inflammation.

### Acute relief of hypoxia and breathlessness

*Oxygen.* Hypoxia in acute asthma exacerbations is potentially life-threatening. You should therefore

| Surname | Hospital number | Weight | Drug intolerances |
|---|---|---|---|
| POWELL | 100010 | | None known |
| First name | Date of birth | 70 kg | |
| LINDA | 15/08/1990 | | |

**REGULAR PRESCRIPTIONS**

Month: January   Year: 2015

Circle / enter times below: 7

| DRUG SALBUTAMOL | | | | Times | | | | | | |
|---|---|---|---|---|---|---|---|---|---|---|
| Dose 5 mg | Route NEB | Freq 4-hrly | Start date 7/1/15 | ✗ 02 | | | | | | |
| | | | | ✗ 06 | | | | | | |
| Signature A Doctor | Bleep 1234 | Review Daily | | ✗ 10 | | | | | | |
| | | | | ✗ 14 | | | | | | |
| | | | | ✗ 18 | | | | | | |
| Additional instructions Drive with oxygen | | | | ✗ 22 | | | | | | |

| DRUG IPRATROPIUM BROMIDE | | | | 06 | | | | | | |
|---|---|---|---|---|---|---|---|---|---|---|
| Dose 500 micrograms | Route NEB | Freq 6-hrly | Start date 7/1/15 | ✗ 02 | | | | | | |
| | | | | ✗ 08 | | | | | | |
| Signature A Doctor | Bleep 1234 | Review Daily | | ✗ 14 | | | | | | |
| | | | | ✗ 20 | | | | | | |
| Additional instructions Drive with oxygen | | | | 22 | | | | | | |

| DRUG CLENIL MODULATE (beclometasone) | | | | 06 | | | | | | |
|---|---|---|---|---|---|---|---|---|---|---|
| Dose 2 puffs | Route INH | Freq 12-hrly | Start date 7/1/15 | 08 | | | | | | |
| | | | | 12 | | | | | | |
| Signature A Doctor | Bleep 1234 | Review | | 16 | | | | | | |
| Additional instructions 100 micrograms/puff. Use spacer. | | | | ✗ 20 | | | | | | |
| | | | | 22 | | | | | | |

| DRUG PREDNISOLONE | | | | 06 | | | | | | |
|---|---|---|---|---|---|---|---|---|---|---|
| Dose 40 mg | Route Oral | Freq Daily | Start date 8/1/15 | 08 | | | | | | |
| | | | | 12 | | | | | | |
| Signature A Doctor | Bleep 1234 | Review 5 days | | 16 | | | | | | |
| | | | | 18 | | | | | | |
| Additional instructions For acute asthma | | | | 22 | | | | | | |

| DRUG DALTEPARIN | | | | 06 | | | | | | |
|---|---|---|---|---|---|---|---|---|---|---|
| Dose 5000 units | Route SC | Freq Daily | Start date 7/1/15 | 08 | | | | | | |
| | | | | 12 | | | | | | |
| Signature A Doctor | Bleep 1234 | Review | | 16 | | | | | | |
| Additional instructions | | | | 18 | | | | | | |
| | | | | 22 | | | | | | |

## ONCE ONLY PRESCRIPTIONS

| Date | Time to be given | DRUG | Dose | Route | Prescriber Signature | Prescriber Bleep | Administration Date given | Administration Time given | Administration Given by |
|------|------------------|------|------|-------|-----------|-------|------------|------------|----------|
| 7/1/15 | 10:00 | PREDNISOLONE | 40 mg | ORAL | AD | 1234 | | | |
| | | | | | | | | | |
| | | | | | | | | | |

**OXYGEN**

| | |
|--|--|
| Target SpO₂ | ✓ 94–98%  ◯ 88–92% |
| Mode of delivery | ✓ Continuous  ◯ As required |
| Starting device | Face mask 10 L/min |

| Initials | Bleep | Date |
|----------|-------|------|
| AD | 1234 | 7/1/15 |

## AS REQUIRED MEDICATION

| DRUG  SALBUTAMOL | | | | Date | | | | | | | | | | |
|---|---|---|---|---|---|---|---|---|---|---|---|---|---|---|
| | | | | Time | | | | | | | | | | |
| Dose 5 mg | Route NEB | Max freq 2-hrly | Start date 7/1/15 | Dose | | | | | | | | | | |
| | | | | Route | | | | | | | | | | |
| Signature A Doctor | | Bleep 1234 | Review daily | Given | | | | | | | | | | |
| | | | | Check | | | | | | | | | | |
| Additional instructions  Driven with oxygen. If requirement increases request urgent medical review. | | | | | | | | | | | | | | |

prescribe high flow oxygen aiming for SpO₂ 94–98%. If oxygen therapy does not correct hypoxia, you should call for urgent senior review as your patient may need intensive care admission and ventilatory support. You can monitor oxygen therapy using oxygen saturations, unless these are <92% or the patient is deteriorating clinically, when arterial blood gas measurement may be required to determine carbon dioxide concentrations.

*Bronchodilators.* You should prescribe high-dose bronchodilators by nebuliser driven by oxygen:

- *Beta 2 adrenoceptor agonists*, e.g. salbutamol, terbutaline. Beta 2 adrenoceptor agonists are standard therapy for acute asthma and reduce bronchospasm by relaxing smooth muscle in the airways. Their most common side effects are tachycardia and a fine tremor. Peripheral vasodilatation, myocardial ischaemia, nervousness and sleep disturbance can occur too. At higher doses, there is a risk of hypokalaemia and lactic acidaemia.
- *Muscarinic antagonists*, e.g. ipratropium. Addition of a nebulised anti-muscarinic to beta 2 adrenoceptor agonist treatment can enhance bronchodilatation, aid recovery and reduce length of hospital stay. You should therefore prescribe anti-muscarinics as part of initial treatment for acute severe or life-threatening asthma. Anti-muscarinic therapy is not considered beneficial in mild exacerbations of asthma, or once the acute exacerbation has stabilised. Ipratropium bromide relaxes smooth muscle by blocking muscarinic receptors at the neuromuscular junction. Side effects include dry mouth, blurred vision, urinary retention and constipation.

### Reducing the inflammatory response

*Corticosteroids.* Corticosteroid treatment is essential to address the airway inflammation underlying the acute attack. Early use of oral corticosteroids in acute asthma can prevent admission to hospital and subsequent relapse. Corticosteroids also decrease mortality and the requirement for beta 2 adrenoceptor agonist therapy.

In acute asthma, corticosteroids should be given orally, with intravenous administration reserved for patients who cannot swallow or are at risk of aspiration or who have malabsorption. Prednisolone is the oral corticosteroid of choice. Inhaled steroids should also be started or continued as soon as possible to commence the long-term management of the patient's asthma, although there is no clear evidence to suggest that inhaled steroids accelerate recovery in acute severe asthma.

Acute side effects of systemic corticosteroids include gastritis, hyperglycaemia and blurred vision. Patients may experience mood changes, including increased energy and well-being during treatment, which can change to low energy and mood on stopping treatment.

### Other measures to consider

*Magnesium sulfate.* A single dose of intravenous magnesium sulfate should be considered in patients with acute severe asthma who fail to respond to initial bronchodilator therapy. In Miss Powell's case, you should wait and assess her response to bronchodilator and corticosteroid therapy before prescribing magnesium.

*Antibiotics.* The majority of asthma exacerbations are caused by allergen exposure or viral infection. Antibiotics should not be commenced routinely in asthma exacerbations unless there is clear evidence of bacterial infection. Miss Powell has a non-productive cough, normal white cell count and CRP and no evidence of consolidation on chest X-ray, so you should not prescribe antibiotics for her.

*Escalation of care.* Crucially, you must review Miss Powell within 30 minutes of your initial management and therapies. If there is any deterioration or development of life-threatening signs then prompt senior review should be sought, potentially including referral to a critical care specialist. Clinical assessment alongside regular observations and frequent monitoring of PEFR will help track the course of a patient's exacerbation.

Once Miss Powell starts to improve, reduction in nebuliser therapy and return to her usual inhaled bronchodilators should occur gradually. Inhaler technique should be checked prior to discharge.

*Prophylaxis against venous thromboembolic (VTE) disease.* Miss Powell is breathless at rest with reduced mobility and airways inflammation and is therefore at increased risk of VTE. Do not forget to prescribe VTE prophylaxis (see Case 1).

### How do I write the prescription?

*Oxygen.* You should prescribe oxygen to target saturations of 94–98%. We would suggest starting with a simple face mask with review and modification of oxygen flow and/or delivery device if hypoxia is not corrected. Requirement of high flow oxygen via a non-rebreathe mask should prompt senior review.

*Salbutamol.* We have prescribed salbutamol at a dose of 5 mg via a nebuliser driven by oxygen. The frequency required is dependent on the response to the initial therapy. We have suggested you prescribe a dose every 4 hours with additional doses prescribed in the as required section for on-going breathlessness. Clear instructions should be given to indicate when medical review is needed, e.g. if a patient is increasingly breathless or has decreasing response to nebulisers. Dose and frequency required should be reviewed regularly.

It is worth noting that in patients without features of life-threatening asthma, high dose salbutamol may be administered using either a nebuliser *or* a metered dose inhaler via a spacer device. You should adhere to local guidelines.

*Ipratropium bromide.* This should be administered via a nebuliser driven by oxygen and you should prescribe it at a dose of 500 micrograms (these units must be written out in full) to be given every 6 hours. Additional doses of ipratropium should not be prescribed in the as required section as this is the maximum daily dose. The need for on-going therapy should be reviewed regularly, particularly as ipratropium is less efficacious once the acute exacerbation begins to settle.

*Prednisolone.* You should prescribe prednisolone at a dose of 40–50 mg once daily in the morning. Miss Powell has presented at 10:00 so the first dose is prescribed in the once only section, with subsequent doses prescribed regularly at 08:00 to coincide with the natural circadian steroid peak. You should specify the duration of therapy to be at least 5 days, although some patients may require a longer course, e.g. if symptoms are slow to settle. Provided inhaled corticosteroids are prescribed, treatment can be stopped abruptly. However, if oral prednisolone therapy has extended beyond 3 weeks or multiple courses have been taken recently, a tapered reduction should occur.

*Inhaled corticosteroids.* You should commence an inhaled corticosteroid as soon as possible and continue this for several weeks or months until the asthma is well controlled and treatment can be stepped down. Options include restarting the inhaled corticosteroid treatment that has previously maintained good control or changing to a combination high-dose inhaled corticosteroid/long-acting beta 2 adrenoceptor agonist (step 4 of the asthma guidelines), stepping treatment down when control improves. For Miss Powell, we have elected to restart her usual inhaled corticosteroids. We have advised that it be taken using a spacer to optimise drug delivery.

When prescribing CFC-free beclometasone dipropionate inhalers, you should use the proprietary names. This is because the different inhalers that are available do not all give equivalent doses and so are not interchangeable.

*Dalteparin.* We have prescribed dalteparin for Miss Powell. Local guidelines will differ in the choice of low molecular weight heparin for venous thromboembolism prophylaxis.

### Further reading

Medical Pharmacology at a Glance. Chapter 11: Asthma, hay fever and anaphylaxis.

Prescribing at a Glance. Chapter 29: Using drugs for the respiratory system.

British Thoracic Society asthma guidelines. Available at: http://www.brit-thoracic.org.uk/guidelines-and-quality-standards/asthma-guideline/ (accessed 15 January 2014).

| Surname | Hospital number | Weight | Drug intolerances |
|---|---|---|---|
| ALLEN | 100011 | | ~~None known~~ |
| First name | Date of birth | 73 kg | Anaphylactic reaction |
| ROBERT | 04/03/1957 | | to ?co-amoxiclav/gelatin |
| | | | A Doctor 7/1/15 |

**REGULAR PRESCRIPTIONS**

Month: January    Year: 2015

| | Circle / enter times below ↓ | 7 | | | | | | | |
|---|---|---|---|---|---|---|---|---|---|
| DRUG CO-AMOXICLAV | 06 | | | | | | | | |
| Dose 1.2 g / Route IV / Freq 8-hrly / Start date 7/1/15 | 08 | | Stopped due to anaphylactic reaction | | | | | | |
| | 12 | | A Doctor | | | | | | |
| Signature A Doctor / Bleep 1234 / 48 h | ✗ (14) AN | | 7/1/15 14:10 | | | | | | |
| | 18 | | 1234 | | | | | | |
| Additional instructions Abdominal sepsis | (22) | | | | | | | | |
| DRUG DALTEPARIN | 06 | | | | | | | | |
| Dose 5000 units / Route SC / Freq Daily / Start date 7/1/15 | 08 | | | | | | | | |
| | 12 | | | | | | | | |
| Signature A Doctor / Bleep 1234 / Review | 16 | | | | | | | | |
| | (18) | | | | | | | | |
| Additional instructions | 22 | | | | | | | | |
| DRUG PARACETAMOL | (06) | | | | | | | | |
| Dose 1 g / Route IV / Freq 6-hrly / Start date 7/1/15 | 08 | | | | | | | | |
| | (12) | | | | | | | | |
| Signature A Doctor / Bleep 1234 / Review | 16 | | | | | | | | |
| | (18) | | | | | | | | |
| Additional instructions | ✗ (24) | | | | | | | | |

## What should I consider when deciding what to prescribe?

Anaphylaxis is a life-threatening condition that requires emergency management. When you encounter a patient whom you suspect to be having an anaphylactic reaction, you should immediately call for help (e.g. call the resuscitation team). However, this is one of the few situations in which – whatever your specialty or level of seniority – you *must* know the details of immediate management by heart, and proceed to administer this before senior support arrives. The discussion below relates to adult patients; the principles of treatment for children are similar, but the drug doses differ.

### Immediate management

The following steps should ideally be performed in parallel, along with summoning help.

*ABCDE.* Rapidly assess his airway, breathing, circulation, level of consciousness and look for relevant exposures (see next paragraph). Administer high-flow oxygen if this is not already being done. To improve venous return, lay him on his back and elevate his legs (if he was in respiratory distress, you would put him in the most comfortable position to help his breathing; if he was vomiting or unconscious you would lay him on his side). Do not try to secure IV access at this stage as there are more pressing priorities.

*Stop the precipitant.* Quickly look for anything that might be precipitating the reaction (the allergen) and, if possible, remove this. Stop any infusion of a drug, colloid fluid or blood product (but do not remove the intravenous cannula if it is functional). In Mr

Allen's case, you should stop both the co-amoxiclav and Gelofusine® infusions, because both penicillins and gelatins are associated with a risk of anaphylaxis. By contrast, crystalloid fluid preparations (e.g. glucose, sodium chloride, compound sodium lactate) do not cause anaphylaxis, unless they or the infusion equipment are contaminated with another substance.

*Administer adrenaline.* Adrenaline must be given without delay, so you should know the dose, strength, route and injection volume without needing to look it up. In anaphylaxis, adrenaline is administered as a concentrated (1 : 1000 = 1 mg or 1000 micrograms per mL) solution by intramuscular injection. The initial dose in an adult is 500 micrograms (0.5 mL) IM. The preferred site of injection is the anterolateral aspect of the thigh. If there is inadequate response after 5 minutes, administer a second 500-microgram dose. You should *not* administer adrenaline intravenously unless cardiac arrest supervenes (although you may observe individuals who are skilled and experienced in the use of intravenous adrenaline – e.g. senior anaesthetists and intensive care specialists – using this route, with extreme care, in selected cases).

### Additional supportive care

Once the precipitant has been stopped and adrenaline administered, you may turn your attention to other aspects of urgent supportive care. Ensure good IV access is available. If you suspect that an IV infusion has precipitated the reaction, replace the giving set with a new one. If there is hypotension, administer a fluid challenge (e.g. 1 L 0.9% sodium chloride as quickly as possible – do not use a colloid, unless you are certain that it is not a potential allergen). If there is bronchospasm, administer salbutamol by nebuliser. At present, there is no reason to do this in Mr Allen's case. Monitor him closely throughout and beyond the reaction, as patients with anaphylaxis may rapidly progress to cardiac arrest.

### Subsequent management

The most important aspects of management of anaphylaxis are described above, and nothing should interfere with these. However, once the reaction is settling it is common to administer a histamine ($H_1$) receptor antagonist (e.g. chlorphenamine) and a corticosteroid (e.g. hydrocortisone). Anti-histamines help to relieve itch associated with the urticarial rash that is common with anaphylaxis. Corticosteroids may help to prevent a recurrence of anaphylaxis a few hours later (the biphasic reaction). However, neither offer any benefit in the immediate life-threatening phase of the reaction, so they are not considered further here. If the reaction is suspected to have been caused by a medicine, this should be indicated on the prescription chart. Any on-going prescription for the potential culprit medicine(s) must be stopped and, if necessary, alternative treatment prescribed. In Mr Allen's case, alternative antibiotic therapy will be needed. This must be with a non-beta-lactam antibiotic; it would be best to discuss this with the on-call microbiologist.

On hospital discharge, he should be given advice about anaphylaxis and, as appropriate, strategies for avoiding allergens. Unless it is absolutely clear that the allergen was a substance only encountered in the medical setting (e.g. a drug class that can only be given parenterally), he should be provided with an adrenaline auto-injector (e.g. Anapen®, EpiPen®) for self-administration, and advised on when and how to use this. Once he fully recovers, he should ideally be referred to an allergist for further assessment and advice on long-term management.

### How do I write the prescription?

Provision of life-saving treatment takes priority over prescription writing. Therefore it is appropriate to administer treatment first then write the prescriptions as soon as a suitable opportunity arises.

In real life, you should have already given adrenaline 500 micrograms by IM injection. You must now write a prescription and record its administration: do this in the once only section of the drug chart, as shown (if additional doses were given, these should be recorded separately in the once only section). Adrenaline is an exception to the usual rule that you should prescribing drugs by their international non-proprietary name (INN). As the INN for adrenaline ('epinephrine') is less familiar to many healthcare professionals, combined with the fact that the drug is generally used in emergency situations, the Medicines and Healthcare products Regulatory Agency (MHRA) currently recommends that 'adrenaline' is still used in prescription writing. On product labelling, the drug is identified as 'adrenaline (epinephrine)'.

The fluid challenge should be prescribed in the fluid section. It is better to prescribe the infusion duration specifically, rather than to use the imprecise term 'stat'. You should have stopped the drugs that may have precipitated the reaction, and recorded this on the drug chart. Exactly how you do this is not important, provided it is clear (an example is shown in the model prescription).

If you elected to give an anti-histamine and/or corticosteroid (noting that these should not interfere with the provision of more urgent treatment), typical choices would be chlorphenamine 10 mg IV or IM, and hydrocortisone 100 mg IV or IM. The initial doses should be prescribed in the once only section. However, as this is not part of the immediate management, these have not been prescribed on the model chart.

Finally, you should have added details of the reaction and the suspected triggers to the record of his drug intolerances, both on the prescription chart and in his medical notes. An alternative antibiotic is likely to be required. However, as the choice should be determined in consultation with a microbiologist and senior decision maker, this has not yet been prescribed on the model chart.

### Further reading

Resuscitation Council UK. Emergency treatment of anaphylactic reactions (2008). Available at: http://www.resus.org.uk/pages/reaction.pdf (accessed 21 January 2014).

National Institute for Health and Clinical Excellence. Anaphylaxis: NICE guideline (CG134; 2011). Available at: http://guidance.nice.org.uk/CG134 (accessed 21 January 2014).

Medical Pharmacology at a Glance. Chapter 11: Asthma, hay fever and anaphylaxis.

**ONCE ONLY PRESCRIPTIONS**

| Date | Time to be given | DRUG | Dose | Route | Prescriber Signature | Prescriber Bleep | Administration Date given | Administration Time given | Administration Given by |
|------|------|------|------|------|------|------|------|------|------|
| 7/1/15 | 14:10 | ADRENALINE | 500 micrograms | IM | A Doctor | 1234 | 7/1/15 | 14:10 | AD / AN |

**OXYGEN**

| Target SpO₂ | ✓ 94–98% ○ 88–92% |
|------|------|
| Mode of delivery | ✓ Continuous ○ As required |
| Starting device | Non-rebreather mask |

| Initials | Bleep | Date |
|------|------|------|
| AD | 1234 | 7/1/15 |

**AS REQUIRED MEDICATION**

| DRUG MORPHINE | | | | Date | |
| | | | | Time | |
| Dose 2.5–10mg | Route IV/IM | Max freq 4-hrly | Start date 7/1/15 | Dose | |
| | | | | Route | |
| Signature A Doctor | | Bleep 1234 | Review | Given | |
| | | | | Check | |
| Additional instructions | | | | | |

| DRUG CYCLIZINE | | | | Date | |
| | | | | Time | |
| Dose 50 mg | Route IV/IM | Max freq 8-hrly | Start date 7/1/15 | Dose | |
| | | | | Route | |
| Signature A Doctor | | Bleep 1234 | Review | Given | |
| | | | | Check | |
| Additional instructions | | | | | |

| DRUG | | | | Date | |
| | | | | Time | |
| Dose | Route | Max freq | Start date | Dose | |
| | | | | Route | |
| Signature | | Bleep | Review | Given | |
| | | | | Check | |
| Additional instructions | | | | | |

| DRUG | | | | Date | |
| | | | | Time | |
| Dose | Route | Max freq | Start date | Dose | |
| | | | | Route | |
| Signature | | Bleep | Review | Given | |
| | | | | Check | |
| Additional instructions | | | | | |

*Stopped due to anaphylactic reaction*
*A Doctor, 7/1/15 14:10 (1234)*

**INFUSION PRESCRIPTIONS**

| Date | Time | Fluid | Vol | Drug | Dose | Rate | Doctor initials | Nurse initials | Batch no | Start time | Stop time |
|------|------|------|------|------|------|------|------|------|------|------|------|
| 7/1/15 | 14:00 | GELOFUSINE | 500 mL | - | - | 30 min | AD | AN AN | 1234-567 | 14:00 | 14:10 |
| 7/1/15 | 14:10 | 0.9% SODIUM CHLORIDE | 1 L | - | - | 20 min | AD | | | | |

| Surname FENTON | Hospital number 100012 | Weight | Drug intolerances |
|---|---|---|---|
| First name JAMES | Date of birth 15/02/1930 | 75 kg | Penicillin - anaphylaxis |

**REGULAR PRESCRIPTIONS**

| | Circle / enter times below ↓ | ⊠ Enter dates below | | | Month: January | | | Year: 2015 |
|---|---|---|---|---|---|---|---|---|
| | | 7 | 8 | 9 | | | | |
| DRUG PARACETAMOL | 06 | | | | | | | |
| Dose 1 g / Route Oral / F 4 times daily / Start date 7/1/15 | 08 | | | | | | | |
| | 12 | | | | | | | |
| Signature A Doctor / Bleep 1234 / Review | 16 | | | | | | | |
| Additional instructions | 18 | | | | | | | |
| | 22 | | | | | | | |
| DRUG | 06 | | | | | | | |

**ONCE ONLY PRESCRIPTIONS**

| Date | Time to be given | DRUG | Dose | Route | Prescriber Signature | Prescriber Bleep | Administration Date given | Administration Time given | Administration Given by |
|---|---|---|---|---|---|---|---|---|---|
| 7/1/15 | 18:00 | PROTHROMBIN COMPLEX CONCENTRATE | 3750 Units | IV | AD | 1234 | | | |
| 7/1/15 | 18:00 | PHYTOMENADIONE | 5 mg | IV | AD | 1234 | | | |
| | | | | | | | | | |

**OXYGEN**

| Target SpO₂ | ○ 94–98% ○ 88–92% |
|---|---|
| Mode of delivery | ○ Continuous ○ As required |
| Starting device | |

| Initials | Bleep | Date |
|---|---|---|
| | | |

**AS REQUIRED MEDICATION**

| DRUG DIHYDROCODEINE | Date | | | | |
|---|---|---|---|---|---|
| | Time | | | | |
| Dose 30 mg / Route Oral / Max freq 4-hrly / Start date 7/1/15 | Dose | | | | |
| | Route | | | | |
| Signature A Doctor / Bleep 1234 / Review | Given | | | | |
| Additional instructions | Check | | | | |

## What should I consider when deciding what to prescribe?

Mr Fenton is an 84-year-old man taking warfarin to prevent thromboembolic complications of atrial fibrillation. The major complication of warfarin therapy is haemorrhage. He has now been admitted with a subdural haematoma, caused by a minor head injury and excessive anticoagulation (INR 6.9). His subdural haematoma is not large enough to require neurosurgery, but he requires urgent reversal of anti-coagulation to prevent ongoing bleeding.

## Management of subdural haematoma

### Anticoagulation with warfarin

Warfarin works by inhibiting the formation of functional coagulation factors (II, VII, IX, X, and the anticoagulants protein C and protein S – the vitamin K dependent factors). Warfarin prolongs the time taken for blood to clot, an effect that can be measured using the prothrombin time. The prothrombin time of a patient taking warfarin is divided by the prothrombin time in a normal control to calculate the international normalised ratio (INR).

Mr Fenton is taking warfarin to prevent thromboembolic complications of atrial fibrillation. He has a target INR of 2–3, which means that he should take enough warfarin to prolong his prothrombin time to 2–3 times normal. He has come into hos-

pital with an INR of 6.9, i.e. with a dangerous delay in his blood clotting. The effect of warfarin needs to be reversed to prevent worsening of his subdural bleed.

### Reversal of warfarin effect

In a patient who is bleeding as a result of warfarin therapy, you need both to provide an immediate supply of functional coagulation factors and to prescribe vitamin K to overcome the effects of warfarin and allow the patient to synthesise their own new coagulation factors. You should therefore prescribe prothrombin complex concentrate and phytomenadione (vitamin $K_1$) for Mr Fenton, as advised by the haematologist.

*Prothrombin complex concentrate* (PCC) contains concentrated clotting factors II, VII, IX and X, and proteins C and S. It is produced from pooled donor plasma. It provides rapid and effective reversal of warfarin-induced anti-coagulation, acting within about 1 hour. Possible side effects of PCC include anaphylaxis, myocardial infarction, venous thrombosis and disseminated intravascular coagulation. PCC undergoes rigorous measures to prevent transmission of infection from donors. An alternative to PCC is fresh frozen plasma (FFP). However, FFP has a number of disadvantages: a larger volume must be administered, it works less quickly, provides less effective reversal of anticoagulation and contains a number of factors that are not required.

*Phytomenadione (vitamin $K_1$).* This acts more slowly than PCC (it takes up to 24 hours to exert its effect), but it is required for optimal performance of PCC, and to sustain normal clotting once the effect of PCC has waned. Side effects relate mainly to allergic reactions, including anaphylaxis, although this is rare.

### Is it safe to reverse warfarin treatment?

Mr Fenton is on warfarin to prevent thromboembolic complications of atrial fibrillation, primarily cerebrovascular events such as stroke or transient ischaemic attack (TIA). As he has had a TIA previously, he is at high risk of a further cerebrovascular event and this risk is increased by his type 2 diabetes mellitus and age. However, this future risk is greatly outweighed by the current risk of further intracranial bleeding. Warfarin treatment should therefore be reversed immediately. Specialist advice, e.g. from cardiology or haematology colleagues, may be needed in weighing up the risks and benefits of restarting warfarin once the intracranial haemorrhage has resolved.

## Management of symptoms

Mr Fenton has a headache. As well as reversing anticoagulation, you should prescribe simple analgesics, such as paracetamol and dihydrocodeine. If possible you should avoid strong opioids. Mr

Fenton needs regular neurological assessment to detect any expansion of his haematoma, and the sedative effects of such drugs may cause confusion. Non-steroidal anti-inflammatory drugs should also be avoided as they inhibit platelet function and may further impair clotting. Additionally they may cause gastrointestinal ulceration, which may be dangerous in a patient receiving anticoagulation.

## Drug interactions

Mr Fenton usually has an INR of 2–3 and has been stable on a warfarin dose of 3 mg for the past 3 years. His INR has suddenly increased to 6.9. This is due to a drug interaction between erythromycin, prescribed for cellulitis, and warfarin.

### Cytochrome P450 system

The cytochrome P450 system is a group of enzymes found in the liver and other organs, which is responsible for the metabolism of many drugs to eliminate them from the body. The activity of these enzymes can be altered by some drugs, e.g. enzyme inhibitors: erythromycin, ciprofloxacin, sodium valproate, omeprazole; enzyme inducers: carbamazepine, rifampicin, alcohol (chronic consumption), phenytoin. If a patient takes a drug metabolised by the cytochrome P450 system (the 'substrate' drug) with a drug that inhibits or induces these enzymes, then the plasma concentration of the substrate drug will be altered. Some substrate drugs, such as warfarin, have a narrow therapeutic range, which means that their effective plasma concentration is close to their toxic plasma concentration. If a substrate drug with a narrow therapeutic range is taken with a drug that alters cytochrome P450 enzyme activity, then a clinically-significant drug interaction may occur.

Mr Fenton has taken erythromycin (a cytochrome P450 inhibitor), which has inhibited the metabolism of warfarin. The resulting increased plasma concentration of warfarin has further inhibited synthesis of clotting factors and prolonged the prothrombin time (now 6.9 times normal).

### Antibiotics and warfarin

Gut flora produce vitamin K, which to some extent counters the effect of warfarin. Broad-spectrum antibiotics of all classes kill gut flora, reducing vitamin K synthesis and this can potentiate the effects of warfarin.

## What should you do about his cellulitis?

Mr Fenton was prescribed erythromycin for cellulitis, which has led to a drug interaction with warfarin. You need to decide whether he needs a further prescription for a different antibiotic or whether he can stop this treatment. He has completed 7 days of treatment, his leg is no longer inflamed and his inflammatory markers are normal. It would therefore be reasonable to stop antibiotics and observe for recurrence.

## How do I write the prescription?
## Allergies

Do not forget to document his anaphylaxis to penicillin, even though it is not directly relevant to the current treatment.

## Reversal of warfarin effect

You have been asked to prescribe specialist drugs that you are likely to be unfamiliar with. In this situation it is important to pay close attention to up-to-date guidelines and re-consult the specialist if you are unsure about any aspect of the prescription.

The BNF currently (2014) provides clear advice on the treatment of haemorrhage for a patient on warfarin, based on the recommendations of the British Society for Haematology. You have been advised to consult these guidelines.

### Deciding which advice to follow

The first question to address is which situation is applicable to Mr Fenton's case. The BNF divides recommendations into guidance for: major bleeding; INR >8.0 with minor or no bleeding; INR 5.0–8.0 with minor or no bleeding; and unexpected bleeding at therapeutic levels. Although Mr Fenton has an INR of 6.9, any intracranial haemorrhage should be considered to be major bleeding and you should follow the major bleeding recommendations for him.

### Phytomenadione (vitamin $K_1$)

You should prescribe phytomenadione at a dose of 5 mg via slow intravenous injection in the once only section of the drug chart. It is good practice to use the correct pharmacological name (phytomenadione) rather than the less specific term, vitamin K. Mr Fenton should be monitored for signs of allergic or anaphylactic reaction during and after the injection.

### Prothrombin complex concentrate (e.g. Beriplex®/Octaplex®)

The BNF recommends prescribing prothrombin complex at a dose of 25–50 units/kg. This leaves you with the difficult task of picking a dose from this range. As Mr Fenton has had an intracranial bleed and worsening of this could have life-threatening consequences, it would be reasonable to choose a dose of 50 units/kg for him. Consult local guidelines or specialist advice if in doubt. Mr Fenton weighs 75 kg, so prescribe 3750 units (50 × 75) in the once only section of the drug chart. Beriplex® and Octaplex® also contain heparin, so caution must be used in patients with heparin allergy.

## Analgesia

On the model drug chart, we have chosen to prescribe regular paracetamol at a dose of 1 g, four times per day with dihydrocodeine at a dose of 30 mg up to 4-hourly as required for breakthrough pain. You should review Mr Fenton in a few hours to make sure his headache is settling with this treatment. If not you may need to prescribe the opioids regularly or increase the dose. If he is requiring regular opioids for a prolonged period, consider co-prescription of a laxative such as docusate sodium in the regular or as required section of the chart, as appropriate.

## Further reading

Medical Pharmacology at a Glance. Chapter 19: Drugs used to affect blood coagulation.

Prescribing at a Glance. Chapter 22: Dealing with adverse drug reactions.

## Drug Chart

| Surname | Hospital number | Weight | Drug intolerances |
|---|---|---|---|
| LAKHANI | 100013 | 88 kg | None known |
| **First name** MADHU | **Date of birth** 28/07/1948 | | |

**REGULAR PRESCRIPTIONS**

Chart 1 of 2

Circle / enter times below ↓ — Enter dates below — Month: **January** — Year: **2015**

Dates: 7, 8, 9

**DRUG ASPIRIN**
- Dose: 75 mg | Route: Oral | Freq: Daily | Start date: 8/1/15
- Signature: A Doctor | Bleep: 1234 | Review:
- Times: 06, (08), 12, 16, 18, 22
- Additional instructions: ACS, to continue lifelong

**DRUG CLOPIDOGREL**
- Dose: 75 mg | Route: Oral | Freq: Daily | Start date: 8/1/15
- Signature: A Doctor | Bleep: 1234 | Review:
- Times: 06, (08), 12, 16, 18, 22
- Additional instructions: ACS, to continue for 12 months

**DRUG FONDAPARINUX**
- Dose: 2.5 mg | Route: SC | Freq: Daily | Start date: 7/1/15
- Signature: A Doctor | Bleep: 1234 | Review:
- Times: 06, 08, 12, 16, (18) OMIT, 22
- Additional instructions: ACS, to continue until discharge

**DRUG RAMIPRIL**
- Dose: 2.5 mg | Route: Oral | Freq: 12-hrly | Start date: 7/1/15
- Signature: A Doctor | Bleep: 1234 | Review:
- Times: 06, (08), 12, 16, ✗ (20), 22
- Additional instructions:

**DRUG ATORVASTATIN**
- Dose: 40 mg | Route: Oral | Freq: Daily | Start date: 7/1/15
- Signature: A Doctor | Bleep: 1234 | Review:
- Times: 06, 08, 12, 16, 18, (22)
- Additional instructions: Check LFTs in 3 and 12 months

**DRUG LANSOPRAZOLE**
- Dose: 30 mg | Route: Oral | Freq: Daily | Start date: 7/1/15
- Signature: A Doctor | Bleep: 1234 | Review:
- Times: 06, (08), 12, 16, 18, 22
- Additional instructions: Gastric protection for dual antiplatelet therapy

## What should I consider when deciding what to prescribe?

Mr Lakhani is a 66-year-old man who has been admitted with central chest pain that radiated to his left arm, and was associated with nausea and sweating. He has significant risk factors for cardiovascular disease that include type 2 diabetes mellitus, hypertension and smoking. He has a significantly raised troponin level after 3 hours and an abnormal ECG showing regional ST segment depression, which together confirm the diagnosis of a non-ST elevation myocardial infarction (NSTEMI). The key issues in managing Mr Lakhani's NSTEMI are acute relief of his pain, treatment of acute cardiac ischaemia and measures to prevent future complications.

## Acute relief of chest pain

Measures should be taken as soon as possible to relieve Mr Lakhani's chest pain. You should initially prescribe a fast-acting nitrate, such as sublingual glyceryl trinitrate (GTN). GTN reduces preload, reducing myocardial oxygen demand and ischaemia. It provides symptomatic relief from angina lasting up to 30 minutes, and dosing can be repeated after 5 minutes if necessary. Common side effects include headache, reflex tachycardia and hypotension. You should be aware that tolerance to nitrates can occur, although this normally follows sustained or recurrent use. If chest pain persists despite two to three doses of a nitrate, the next step would be to administer intravenous morphine (see Case 3). In addition to its analgesic properties, morphine can help to reduce the oxygen demand of the myocardium by reducing the heart rate and blood pressure. It is good practice to offer an anti-emetic agent, such as metoclopramide, alongside strong opioids to reduce the side effects of nausea and vomiting.

## Treatment of the underlying cause

The principal aim of treatment for acute coronary syndrome is to optimise blood flow to the heart.

*Antiplatelet therapy.* NSTEMI occurs when platelet-rich thrombus forms in atheromatous coronary arteries. Antiplatelet drugs help to prevent further coronary artery occlusion by reducing platelet aggregation. Following acute myocardial infarction, antiplatelet treatment increases survival and can halve the risk of further myocardial infarction.

*Aspirin* irreversibly inhibits cyclo-oxygenase, reducing the production of the pro-aggregatory factor, thromboxane. It should be administered to all patients with acute coronary syndrome (ACS), including those with unstable angina, NSTEMI and ST elevation myocardial infarction (STEMI).

*Clopidogrel* blocks adenosine diphosphate (ADP) receptors on the surface of platelets and acts synergistically with aspirin to reduce platelet aggregation. Clopidogrel should be prescribed to all but the lowest risk patients with ACS; i.e. anyone with a predicted 6-month mortality of greater than 1.5%. The risk of mortality can be calculated using the Global Registry of Acute Cardiac Events (GRACE) score.

Low doses of aspirin and clopidogrel require up to a week to reach their full antiplatelet effect, so you should prescribe an immediate loading dose, in addition to regular treatment from day 2.

*Antithrombin therapy.* You should prescribe antithrombin therapy, such as fondaparinux or heparin, to all patients with ACS, unless they have a high bleeding risk. Risk factors for bleeding include increasing age, known bleeding complications, low body weight and renal impairment. Fondaparinux, a factor Xa inhibitor, is preferred to low molecular weight heparin as it has been shown to be as effective at reducing mortality in ACS, with a lower risk of bleeding. In patients with significant renal impairment (serum creatinine concentration $>265\,\mu mol/L$) you should prescribe unfractionated heparin instead of fondaparinux.

Aspirin, clopidogrel and fondaparinux are indicated in this case as Mr Lakhani's GRACE score predicts a high mortality risk; his score is 119, which is associated with an 8% risk of death over the next 6 months. In addition to medical therapy Mr Lakhani's high GRACE score suggests he will need prompt review by a cardiologist to arrange for coronary angiography within the next 96 hours.

## Other measures to prevent complications

Mr Lakhani has been started on dual antiplatelet therapy that could predispose him to gastrointestinal ulceration and bleeding. You should therefore prescribe gastric protection for the duration of the dual antiplatelet therapy. There is some evidence that proton pump inhibitors (PPIs), particularly omeprazole, reduce the antiplatelet effect of clopidogrel by decreasing its activation by cytochrome P450 enzymes. Understanding continues to evolve on this issue, but current evidence suggests that lansoprazole and pantoprazole have a lower propensity to interact with clopidogrel. As such, these are the preferred PPIs in this setting.

## Minimising future complications

Prior to discharge, all patients who have had an acute myocardial infarction should be offered long-term treatment with aspirin, a beta adrenoceptor blocker, a statin and an angiotensin converting enzyme (ACE) inhibitor (or angiotensin receptor blocker). These drugs have all been shown to improve prognosis for this patient group.

A *beta adrenoceptor blocker*, such as metoprolol or bisoprolol, should be introduced as soon as the patient is clinically stable. Usual practice is to commence a beta adrenoceptor blocker 24 hours after admission and then titrate up to the maximum tolerated dose. The beta adrenoceptor blocker should be continued indefinitely aiming for a heart rate between 50 and 60 beats/min.

*Statin therapy* should be offered as soon as possible to any patient with evidence of cardiovascular disease. You should choose a statin indicated for use in myocardial infarction (refer to the BNF), choosing generic low cost preparations where available.

*ACE inhibitors.* Unless there are signs of cardiogenic shock, ongoing treatment with ramipril will be important for secondary prophylaxis.

## Continuing usual treatment

*Metformin* should be withheld in the context of a recent myocardial infarction, as there is an increased risk of lactic acidosis if contrast nephropathy occurs following angiography. You should therefore withhold it until 48 hours after the angiogram. If his blood glucose concentration exceeds 11 mmol/L you should prescribe a variable rate insulin infusion (see Case 30).

## How do I write the prescription?
### Glyceryl trinitrate

Glyceryl trinitrate can be administered as a sublingual tablet or spray in the as required section of the drug chart. We have elected to prescribe the spray, which delivers 400 micrograms per metered dose; the patient should spray 1–2 doses under the tongue. It is good practice to avoid using abbreviated drug names and units when prescribing, so you should avoid abbreviating glyceryl trinitrate to 'GTN', and write the word 'micrograms' in full.

| Surname LAKHANI | Hospital number 100013 | Weight 88 kg | Drug intolerances None known |
| First name MADHU | Date of birth 28/07/1948 | | |

Circle / enter times below — Enter dates below — Month: January — Year: 2015

| DRUG METFORMIN | Dose 500 mg | Route Oral | Freq Twice daily | Start date 7/1/15 | Signature A Doctor | Bleep 1234 | Review | Additional instructions: Restart 48 hours after angiogram if renal function stable |
| --- |

Times: 06, 08 (circled), 12, 16, 18 (circled), 22 — 7, 8, 9
- 08: OMIT (8), OMIT (9)
- 18: OMIT (7), OMIT (8), OMIT (9)

| DRUG METOPROLOL | Dose 12.5 mg | Route Oral | Freq 8-hrly | Start date 7/1/15 | Signature A Doctor | Bleep 1234 | Review | Additional instructions: Target heart rate 50-60 beats/min |
| --- |

Times: 06, 08 (circled), 12, 16 (circled), 18, 22, 24 (circled) — OMIT

### ONCE ONLY PRESCRIPTIONS

| Date | Time to be given | DRUG | Dose | Route | Prescriber Signature | Prescriber Bleep | Administration Date given | Administration Time given | Administration Given by |
| --- | --- | --- | --- | --- | --- | --- | --- | --- | --- |
| 7/1/15 | 18:00 | ASPIRIN | 300mg | Oral | AD | 1234 | | | |
| 7/1/15 | 18:00 | CLOPIDOGREL | 300mg | Oral | AD | 1234 | | | |
| 7/1/15 | 18:00 | FONDAPARINUX | 2.5mg | SC | AD | 1234 | | | |

### OXYGEN

| Target SpO₂ | ○ 94–98% / ○ 88–92% |
| Mode of delivery | ○ Continuous / ○ As required |
| Starting device | |

| Initials | Bleep | Date |
| --- | --- | --- |

### AS REQUIRED MEDICATION

| DRUG GLYCERYL TRINITRATE SPRAY | Dose 1-2 sprays | Route SL | Max freq 5 min | Start date 7/1/15 | Signature A Doctor | Bleep 1234 | Review |
| --- |

Additional instructions: 400 micrograms/spray. For chest pain. Contact doctor if more than 2 consecutive doses required.

| DRUG MORPHINE | Dose 2.5-5 mg | Route IM/IV | Max freq 4-hrly | Start date 7/1/15 | Signature A Doctor | Bleep 1234 | Review |
| --- |

Additional instructions: If chest pain not relieved by glyceryl trinitrate

| DRUG METOCLOPRAMIDE | Dose 10 mg | Route IV | Max freq 8-hrly | Start date 7/1/15 | Signature A Doctor | Bleep 1234 | Review |
| --- |

Additional instructions: Give with morphine to relieve nausea and vomiting

## Morphine sulfate

Morphine sulfate should be prescribed as required for relief of ischaemic chest pain as repeated doses may be needed. An initial dose of 2.5–5 mg would be appropriate every 4 hours, and adjusted according to the patient's response. It is good practice to state when this should be considered, for example 'for pain not controlled with glyceryl trinitrate', and to monitor for respiratory depression, hypotension and bradycardia. We have written this up to be given by IM or IV routes, depending on the expertise of the staff administering treatment and where the patient is. For discussion of issues around safe prescribing of intravenous morphine (see Case 3).

## Metoclopramide

The usual dose of metoclopramide is 10 mg 8-hourly. It can be administered orally, IM or IV. As it is being prescribed here to prevent nausea and vomiting caused by morphine, IV administration will be the most appropriate route.

## Oxygen

Oxygen is not required for Mr Lakhani as he achieves the target oxygen saturations of 94–98% breathing air, but should be considered for patients with acute myocardial infarction with oxygen saturations <94%.

## Antiplatelet agents

Aspirin is prescribed as a once only loading dose of 300 mg orally and then continued indefinitely at a dose of 75 mg daily. Clopidogrel is also prescribed as a once only loading dose of 300 mg orally and should be continued for 12 months at a dose of 75 mg daily. It is good practice to write the indication and intended duration of antiplatelet therapy in the additional instructions and in the discharge summary. To avoid the risk of overdosage, make sure you check that aspirin and clopidogrel have not already been administered by the ambulance crew or emergency department staff.

## Fondaparinux

Fondaparinux is prescribed as a dose of 2.5 mg subcutaneously on admission, and daily thereafter until discharge or up to a maximum of 8 days, whichever is sooner. It is usual practice in most hospitals to administer anticoagulants in the early evening.

## Atorvastatin

Atorvastatin is prescribed regularly at a nightly dose of 40 mg orally.

## Lansoprazole

Lansoprazole is prescribed in the regular section at a dosage of 30 mg daily for oral administration, and its indication stated in the additional instructions.

## Metoprolol

Metoprolol should be started at a low dose of 12.5 mg three times daily when the patient is clinically stable. If tolerated, this can later be switched to a longer acting beta adrenoceptor blocker such as bisoprolol 2.5 mg once daily. In the additional instructions it is good practice to note the target heart rate of 50–60 beats/min.

## Other medications

Ramipril should be continued by prescription in the regular section of the chart. It is reasonable to continue Mr Lakhani's current dose initially, although this should be titrated to achieve optimal blood pressure control prior to discharge. If the dose is increased, you should ask his GP to monitor serum electrolytes and blood pressure in 1–2 weeks.

Metformin has been withheld, but there are clear instructions that it should be reintroduced 48 hours after Mr Lakhani's angiogram provided his renal function remains stable.

### Further reading

Medical Pharmacology at a Glance. Chapter 16: Drugs used in angina.
Prescribing at a Glance. Chapters 26–28: Using drugs for the cardiovascular system.
GRACE. Available at: http://www.outcomes-umassmed.org/grace/ (accessed 16 January 2014).
NICE clinical guideline 94. Unstable angina and NSTEMI (2010). Available at: http://www.nice.org.uk/nicemedia/live/12949/47924/47924.pdf (accessed 16 January 2014).

## What should I consider when deciding what to prescribe?

Mr Harrison is a 67-year-old man with chronic obstructive pulmonary disease (COPD). He has been admitted with increasing shortness of breath, cough and green sputum, which are the key symptoms of an acute exacerbation of COPD. This diagnosis is backed up by the clinical findings of increased respiratory rate, hypoxia and expiratory wheeze.

### Urgent supportive measures

Using the ABCDE approach, you can see that Mr Harrison has a patent airway and is adequately oxygenated on current treatment. As Mr Harrison has COPD and $PaCO_2$ above the normal range, he is at risk of worsening $CO_2$ retention with high flow oxygen treatment, so you should prescribe oxygen with target $SpO_2$ 88–92% (see Case 2). Breathlessness during COPD exacerbations is caused by increased bronchospasm and air trapping with hyperinflation. You can manage this with bronchodilator nebulisers including salbutamol (beta 2 adrenoceptor agonist) and ipratropium (anti-muscarinic). He has no evidence of circulatory compromise.

### Antibiotics

Mr Harrison has green sputum (indicating the presence of neutrophils) and is pyrexial with raised C-reactive protein and white cell count (inflammatory markers). Taken together these findings indicate that his exacerbation may have been triggered by a bacterial infection, which may respond to antibiotics.

*Which organism?* The absence of consolidation on Mr Harrison's chest X-ray indicates that this is a COPD exacerbation (infection of the airways) rather than pneumonia (infection of the lung parenchyma). As these different diseases are caused by different infecting organisms, correct interpretation of the chest X-ray helps you to choose an appropriate antibiotic regimen. Bacteria most likely to cause COPD exacerbations are *Haemophilus influenzae* and *Moraxella catarrhalis* (Gram-negative) and *Streptococcus pneumonia* (Gram-positive).

*Which antibiotic?* First-line antibiotics for COPD exacerbation therefore include tetracyclines, amoxicillin and macrolides, which have a broad spectrum of action. Most hospitals have antibiotic guidelines and it is important to get to know and to follow these (see Appendix 1 for an example).

### Other measures to speed recovery and prevent complications

*Oral corticosteroid treatment* (prednisolone) for acute exacerbations speeds up improvement in lung function, breathlessness and hypoxia, probably by reducing pulmonary inflammation. In hospi-

talised patients, corticosteroids reduce length of stay by ~1 day. They also reduce the likelihood of treatment failure.

*Prophylaxis against venous thromboembolic disease (VTE).* Mr Harrison is breathless at rest and his mobility is reduced. He has infection and inflammation and is at increased risk of VTE. You should therefore prescribe prophylaxis.

### Continuing usual treatment

Mr Harrison takes aspirin and simvastatin for ischaemic heart disease and you should continue these during admission. There is some evidence that COPD exacerbations trigger cardiac events and so this is a particularly important time for him to be taking cardiac prophylaxis.

Gastrointestinal ulceration and bleeding are important side effects of aspirin and the risk of these side effects will be increased

| Surname HARRISON | Hospital number 100014 | Weight | Drug intolerances |
|---|---|---|---|
| First name ROLAND | Date of birth 13/07/1947 | 59 kg | None known |

**REGULAR PRESCRIPTIONS** Chart 1 of 2

| | Circle / enter times below ↓ | Enter dates below | Month: January | Year: 2015 |
|---|---|---|---|---|
| | | 7 | 8 | 9 | | | |
| DRUG **SALBUTAMOL** — Dose 2.5 mg, Route Neb, 6 times daily, Start date 7/1/15 — Signature A Doctor, Bleep 1234, Review Daily — Additional instructions: Driven by air | 06, 08, 12, 16, 18, 22 | | | | | | |
| DRUG **IPRATROPIUM** — Dose 250 micrograms, Route Neb, 4 times daily, Start date 7/1/15 — Signature A Doctor, Bleep 1234, Review Daily — Additional: Driven by air. Restart tiotropium when stopping ipratropium nebs | 06, 08, 12, 16, 19, 22 | | | | | | |
| DRUG **PREDNISOLONE** — Dose 30 mg, Route Oral, Freq Daily, Start date 7/1/15 — Signature A Doctor, Bleep 1234, Review 10 days — Additional instructions | 06, 08, 12, 16, 18, 22 | | | | | | |
| DRUG **DOXYCYCLINE** — Dose 100 mg, Route Oral, Freq Daily, Start date 7/1/15 — Signature A Doctor, Bleep 1234, Review 5 days — Additional instructions: For COPD exacerbation | 06, 08, 12, 16, 18, 22 | OMIT | | | | | |
| DRUG **SERETIDE 500 ACCUHALER** — Dose 1 puff, Route Inh, Freq 12-hrly, Start date 7/1/15 — Signature A Doctor, Bleep 1234, Review — Additional instructions | 06, 08, 12, 16, 18, 22 | | | | | | |
| DRUG **TIOTROPIUM** — Dose 18 micrograms, Route Inh, Freq Daily, Start date 7/1/15 — Signature A Doctor, Bleep 1234, Review — Additional instructions: Withhold while on ipratropium | 06, 08, 12, 16, 18, 22 | OMIT | OMIT | OMIT | | | |

Chart 2 of 2

| Surname HARRISON | Hospital number 100014 | Weight | Drug intolerances |
|---|---|---|---|
| First name ROLAND | Date of birth 13/07/1947 | 59 kg | None known |

**REGULAR PRESCRIPTIONS**

| | Circle / enter times below ↓ | Enter dates below | 7 | 8 | 9 | Month: January | | Year: 2015 |
|---|---|---|---|---|---|---|---|---|

| DRUG ASPIRIN | 06 |
|---|---|
| Dose 75 mg / Route Oral / Freq Daily / Start date 7/1/15 | (08) |
| Signature A Doctor / Bleep 1234 / Review | 12 / 16 / 18 |
| Additional instructions With food | 22 |

| DRUG OMEPRAZOLE | 06 |
|---|---|
| Dose 20 mg / Route Oral / Freq Daily / Start date 7/1/15 | (08) |
| Signature A Doctor / Bleep 1234 / Review 10 days | 12 / 16 / 18 |
| Additional instructions While on prednisolone | 22 |

| DRUG SIMVASTATIN | 06 / 08 |
|---|---|
| Dose 20 mg / Route Oral / Freq Daily / Start date 7/1/15 | 12 / 16 / 18 |
| Signature A Doctor / Bleep 1234 / Review | (22) |
| Additional instructions | |

| DRUG DALTEPARIN | 06 / 08 |
|---|---|
| Dose 5000 units / Route SC / Freq Daily / Start date 7/1/15 | 12 / 16 |
| Signature A Doctor / Bleep 1234 / Review | (18) |
| Additional instructions | 22 |

**ONCE ONLY PRESCRIPTIONS**

| Date | Time to be given | DRUG | Dose | Route | Prescriber Signature | Prescriber Bleep | Administration Date given | Administration Time given | Administration Given by |
|---|---|---|---|---|---|---|---|---|---|
| 7/1/15 | 18:00 | DOXYCYCLINE | 200 mg | Oral | AD | 1234 | | | |

**OXYGEN**

| Target SpO₂ | ○ 94–98% / ☑ 88–92% |
|---|---|
| Mode of delivery | ☑ Continuous / ○ As required |
| Starting device | 28% Venturi |
| Initials AD | Bleep 1234 | Date 7/1/15 |

**AS REQUIRED MEDICATION**

| DRUG SALBUTAMOL | Date / Time |
|---|---|
| Dose 2.5 mg / Route Neb / Max freq 2-hrly / Start date 7/1/15 | Dose / Route |
| Signature A Doctor / Bleep 1234 / Review | Given / Check |
| Additional instructions | |

---

while Mr Harrison is also taking prednisolone. You should therefore consider prescribing a proton pump inhibitor (PPI) for gastric protection while he is on prednisolone, making sure to review and consider stopping the PPI at the end of the course of corticosteroids.

## How do I write the prescription?
### Bronchodilators
#### Nebulisers
During an acute COPD exacerbation, you should prescribe bronchodilators by the nebulised route. As Mr Harrison has COPD and $PaCO_2$ above the normal range, he is at risk of worsening $CO_2$ retention with high-flow oxygen treatment. You should therefore state on the prescription that his nebulisers should be driven by air, not oxygen.

Salbutamol, a beta 2 adrenoreceptor agonist, is prescribed at a dose of 2.5 mg to relieve bronchospasm, hyperinflation and breathlessness. A higher dose is unlikely to have further benefit and will cause more side effects, including tremor and tachycardia. Note that salbutamol has been written up both regularly 4-hourly and on the as required side of the drug chart to allow administration as often as needed for breathlessness.

Ipratropium, an anti-muscarinic, is a bronchodilator with a different mechanism of action to salbutamol, so has additional benefit for COPD patients during exacerbations. Side effects include a dry mouth, blurred vision and urinary retention, so a reasonable dose to balance benefits and side effects is 250 micrograms 6-hourly. There is no additional benefit from extra doses of ipratropium so this is not written on the as required side.

### Inhalers
It is good practice to write up the patient's usual inhalers. Seretide® is a combination of long-acting beta 2 adrenoreceptor agonist (salmeterol) and inhaled corticosteroid (fluticasone). Seretide® comes as a dry powder inhaler (Accuhaler) or a metered dose inhaler (Evohaler). Accuhaler prescribing is currently encouraged for COPD as it is cheaper than the Evohaler. Seretide® accuhalers come in three strengths: 100, 250 and 500. The numbers refer to the amount of fluticasone in micrograms per inhaled dose. In a Seretide® Accuhaler, there is 50 micrograms salmeterol per puff irrespective of the amount of fluticasone. Seretide® can be continued during exacerbation and may have on-going benefit. As there is no recognised compound name, it should be prescribed by brand name. Tiotropium, a long-acting anti-muscarinic drug, should be withheld during ipratropium treatment. This can be indicated in the administration boxes with a note in the additional instructions area as shown.

### Antibiotics
Doxycycline, a tetracycline antibiotic, has been chosen for Mr Harrison. An initial dose of 200 mg is prescribed in the once only section for the day of admission, with a dose of 100 mg daily prescribed in the regular section for subsequent days (can be increased to 200 mg daily for severe infections). You should always write the indication for antibiotics in the additional instructions box, along with a date when the prescription should be reviewed or stopped. In the model prescription, doxycycline has deliberately been prescribed at lunchtime. Doxycycline is best taken with food, as on an empty stomach it can cause nausea, vomiting and oesophageal irritation. However, the food should not include dairy products (e.g. breakfast cereals with milk), because calcium binds to doxycycline and prevents its absorption and anti-microbial effects.

### Prednisolone
Side effects of systemic corticosteroids include hyperglycaemia, blurred vision and mood changes, including increased energy and

well-being during treatment, which can change to low energy and mood on stopping treatment. As prednisolone has limited efficacy and multiple side effects in COPD exacerbations, it is usually prescribed at a dose of 30 mg/day for 7–14 days.

### Low molecular weight heparin
As Mr Harrison has normal renal function, he can receive low molecular weight heparin, which is renally excreted, for prophylaxis against venous thromboembolism.

### Further reading
Medical Pharmacology at a Glance. Chapters 38 and 39. Antibacterial drugs.
Prescribing at a Glance. Chapter 29: Using drugs for the respiratory system.

# Section 2: On call in the hospital

# Cases

## 15 A 91-year-old man with hypoglycaemia

| | |
|---|---|
| **Patient name:** | Alec Robinson |
| **ID number:** | 100015 |
| **Date of birth:** | 26/02/1923 |
| **Age:** | 91 years |
| **Weight:** | 82 kg |
| **Admission date:** | 06/01/2015 03:00 |
| **Date/time seen:** | 07/01/2015 20:00 |

### History
**Problem**   Found unresponsive.

**History**   Mr Robinson, who was admitted yesterday with suspected osteomyelitis of his right foot, has been found unresponsive by the nursing staff. They report that his blood glucose concentration is low.

**PMH**   Type 2 diabetes mellitus, hypercholesterolaemia, peripheral vascular disease.

**DH**   Aspirin 75 mg daily, gliclazide 80 mg twice daily, metformin 850 mg three times daily, simvastatin 40 mg nightly.

Intolerances: none known.

**SH**   Non-smoker; drinks 35–40 units of alcohol per week.

### Examination
**General**   Airway patent; breathing spontaneously; pulse palpable. Unresponsive to voice; localises and groans in response to a noxious stimulus. Pupils 4 mm and reactive.

**Obs**   T 38.1°C, HR 100 beats/min, BP 136/81 mmHg, RR 20 breaths/min, SpO$_2$ 93% breathing 10 L/min oxygen via facemask.

**Systems**   A brief focused examination is unremarkable. He has one peripheral intravenous cannula, which is functional.

### Investigations
CBG    2.1 mmol/L    3.9–7.8 mmol/L

### Task
Prescribe appropriate treatment for hypoglycaemia.

## 16 A 60-year-old woman requesting night sedation

| | |
|---|---|
| **Patient name:** | Katherine Horton |
| **ID number:** | 100016 |
| **Date of birth:** | 14/03/1954 |
| **Age:** | 60 years |
| **Weight:** | 63 kg |
| **Admission date:** | 07/01/2015 15:45 |
| **Date/time seen:** | 07/01/2015 21:15 |

### History
**Problem**   Mrs Horton is requesting 'a tablet to help her sleep'.

**History**   Mrs Horton was admitted electively this afternoon for a right mastectomy and sentinel node biopsy tomorrow morning. She was found to have adenocarcinoma of the right breast 2 weeks ago. She is very anxious about the operation. Despite appropriate explanation and reassurance, she is concerned that she is going to be 'up all night with worry'.

**PMH**   Hypothyroidism.

**DH**   Levothyroxine 50 micrograms daily.

Intolerances: none known.

**SH**   Non-smoker, drinks approximately 10 units of alcohol per week.

### Examination
**General**   She looks well.

**Obs**   T 37.0°C, HR 80 beats/min, BP 132/86 mmHg, RR 17 breaths/min, SpO$_2$ 98% breathing air.

**Systems**   Normal cardiorespiratory examination earlier today. Clinically euthyroid.

### Investigations
Normal full blood count and renal profile from pre-admission clinic 1 week ago.

### Task
Address her request for night sedation.

*Prescribing Scenarios at a Glance*, First Edition. Emma Baker, Daniel Burrage, Dagan Lonsdale, and Andrew Hitchings.

## 17 A 62-year-old man with suspected opioid toxicity

**Patient name:** Samuel Johnson
**ID number:** 100017
**Date of birth:** 04/04/1952
**Age:** 62 years
**Weight:** 67 kg
**Admission date:** 06/01/2015
**Date/time seen:** 07/01/2015 14:30

### History

Problem | Reduced level of consciousness.
History | Mr Johnson was admitted yesterday with severe back pain due to myeloma. His analgesic treatment regimen was escalated from co-codamol to morphine sulfate. He has reportedly been 'intermittently drowsy' since yesterday afternoon.
PMH | Myeloma, chronic kidney disease.
DH | At admission: co-codamol 30/500 two tablets orally 6-hourly.
Since admission: paracetamol 1 g 6-hourly, Oramorph® (morphine sulfate solution, 10 mg/5 mL) 2.5 mg orally 4-hourly, metoclopramide 10 mg orally 8-hourly, senna 15 mg nightly, dalteparin 5000 units SC daily.
Intolerances: none known.
SH | He is a non-smoker and drinks approximately 12 units of alcohol per week.

### Examination

General | He is unresponsive, but his airway is patent.
Obs | T 36.5°C, HR 55 beats/min, BP 112/65 mmHg, RR 6 breaths/min, SpO$_2$ 94% breathing air.
Systems | Glasgow coma score 9 (E2 M5 V2), pupils 2 mm and minimally reactive; the rest of the examination is normal.

### Investigations

For results of investigations, see Table 17.1.

### Task

Opioid toxicity is suspected. Prescribe appropriate immediate treatment.

**Table 17.1** Case 17 investigation results

| Test | Value | Normal range |
|------|-------|--------------|
| Creat | 144 μmol/L | 60–110 |
| CBG | 6.2 mmol/L | 3.9–7.8 |

## 18 A 58-year-old man who has low blood pressure

**Patient name:** Thomas Stone
**ID number:** 100018
**Date of birth:** 11/04/1956
**Weight:** 79 kg
**Admission date:** 02/01/2015
**Date/time seen:** 07/01/2015 15:00

### History

Problem | Low blood pressure.
History | Mr Stone was admitted 5 days ago for an elective left hemicolectomy and defunctioning stoma for colorectal cancer. He has been recovering well with good urine and stoma output for the past 24 hours.
Today he felt light-headed when standing up after lunch. The nursing staff helped him back to bed and laid him flat, with resolution of his symptoms. His blood pressure is usually between 118/68 and 122/74 mmHg. It was 86/52 mmHg when he felt light-headed, improving to 102/84 mmHg on returning to bed. His postoperative pain is well controlled.
PMH | Hypertension, angina, colorectal cancer.
DH | Amlodipine 5 mg daily, aspirin 75 mg daily, bisoprolol 5 mg daily, glyceryl trinitrate 400 micrograms sublingually as required.
Intolerances: none known.
SH | He has smoked 5 cigarettes a day for 30 years, and drinks 6 pints of bitter each week.

### Examination

General | He is now back in bed. He is not pale or cyanosed.
Obs | T 36.8°C, HR 88 beats/min, BP 102/84 mmHg lying flat, RR 16 breaths/min, SpO$_2$ 96% breathing air, urine output 50 mL/h.
Systems | Capillary refill <2 seconds.
Abdomen soft, with mild tenderness around a healthy-looking stoma site. Bowel sounds present.

### Investigations

For results of investigations, see Table 18.1.

### Task

Review Mr Stone's drug chart and make any changes to his medications to prevent further hypotension.

**Table 18.1** Case 18 investigation results

| Test | Value | Normal range |
|------|-------|--------------|
| Hb | 132 g/L | 130–180 |
| Neut | 7.8 × 10$^9$/L | 1.7–8.0 |
| Plt | 365 × 10$^9$/L | 150–400 |
| Na$^+$ | 138 mmol/L | 135–145 |
| K$^+$ | 3.8 mmol/L | 3.5–4.7 |
| Ur | 7.2 mmol/L | 2.5–8.0 |
| Creat | 87 μmol/L | 60–110 |

## 19 A 44-year-old woman who is 'nil by mouth'

| | |
|---|---|
| **Patient name:** | Virginia de la Cruz |
| **ID number:** | 100019 |
| **Date of birth:** | 19/03/1970 |
| **Age:** | 44 years |
| **Weight:** | 80 kg |
| **Admission date:** | 07/01/2015 18:45 |
| **Date/time seen:** | 07/01/2015 20:00 |

### History

Problem   Asked to prescribe fluids.

History   She was admitted earlier this evening after a fall from a ladder. She fell from a height of about 2 m while painting her staircase. On arrival in the emergency department she was found to have significant facial injuries and a fracture of her right radius. She will require surgery, but it is uncertain when this will be done. She is currently unable to take any food or water by mouth, as she finds this too painful, and a nasogastric tube cannot be inserted due to her injuries. It is anticipated that she will be able to resume oral intake in about 2–3 days.

PMH   None of relevance.

DH   No regular medication.
Intolerances: none known.

SH   She has never smoked; she consumes 7–10 units of alcohol per week.

### Examination

General   There are significant facial injuries.

Obs   T 36.4°C, HR 88 beats/min, BP 138/82 mmHg, RR 18 breaths/min, SpO$_2$ 98% breathing air.

Systems   Capillary refill time <3 sec; jugular venous pressure normal; no significant postural drop in blood pressure.

### Investigations

For results of investigations, see Table 19.1.

### Task

The nurse has bleeped you to ask if you would prescribe intravenous fluids. Write a prescription to cover the next 24 hours.

**Table 19.1** Case 19 investigation results

| Test | Value | Normal range |
|---|---|---|
| Hb | 145 g/L | 120–160 |
| MCV | 82 fL | 78–97 fL |
| WCC | 9.8 × 10$^9$/L | 4.0–11.0 × 10$^9$ |
| Plt | 338 × 10$^9$/L | 150–400 × 10$^9$ |
| Na$^+$ | 139 mmol/L | 135–145 |
| K$^+$ | 4.6 mmol/L | 3.5–4.7 |
| Ur | 5.6 mmol/L | 2.5–8.0 |
| Creat | 81 μmol/L | 60–110 |

## 20 A 59-year-old man with circulatory compromise

| | |
|---|---|
| **Patient name:** | Emmanuel Hoyles |
| **ID number:** | 100020 |
| **Date of birth:** | 03/02/1955 |
| **Age:** | 59 years |
| **Weight:** | 71 kg |
| **Admission date:** | 06/01/2015 23:45 |
| **Date/time seen:** | 07/01/2015 14:00 |

### History

Problem   Generally unwell.

History   He presented yesterday with right flank pain. The clinical presentation was suggestive of pyelonephritis. Antibiotic treatment was started and he was admitted to the urology ward. He now says that although his pain and nausea have improved, he feels 'spaced-out' and generally unwell.

PMH   None.

DH   None.
Intolerances: none known.

SH   He is an ex-smoker of 20 pack-years' duration. He drinks 20–30 units of alcohol per week.

### Examination

General   He looks unwell.

Obs   T 38.4°C, HR 115 beats/min, BP 86/60 mmHg, RR 23 breaths/min, SpO$_2$ 95% breathing air.

Systems   Capillary refill time 5 sec; jugular venous pressure level not visible. Right renal angle tenderness with no rebound tenderness or guarding. Urine output 15 mL in last hour.

### Task

Prescribe appropriate initial treatment pending urgent review by a senior colleague.

## 21 | A 15-month-old girl with gastroenteritis

| | |
|---|---|
| **Patient name:** | Rani Jaswal |
| **ID number:** | 100021 |
| **Date of birth:** | 16/10/2013 |
| **Weight:** | 12 kg |
| **Date/time seen:** | 07/01/2015 17:30 |

### History
Problem   Dehydration.

History   Rani was admitted earlier today with vomiting and diarrhoea due to viral gastroenteritis. The rate of gastrointestinal fluid loss is now negligible, but she cannot tolerate oral or nasogastric rehydration.

PMH   Born at term with no perinatal complications. Growing and developing well.

DH   No medication; up to date with immunisations. Intolerances: none known.

SH   Lives with her parents and 4-year-old brother (well).

### Examination
General   She is quiet. Her peripheries are warm but her capillary refill time is slightly prolonged at 3 sec.

Obs   T 36.9°C, HR 110 beats/min (normal for age).

### Investigations
For results of investigations, see Table 21.1.

### Task
Rani has been assessed by the paediatric registrar who estimates that she is 5% dehydrated. He asks you to prescribe IV fluid to cover her maintenance requirements and to correct her fluid deficit over the next 24 hours (see Box 21.1).

**Table 21.1** Case 21 investigation results

| Test | Value | Normal range |
|---|---|---|
| Na$^+$ | 142 mmol/L | 135–145 |
| K$^+$ | 3.6 mmol/L | 3.5–4.7 |
| Ur | 2.5 mmol/L | 2.5–8.0 |
| Creat | 56 μmol/L | 60–110 |
| CBG | 4.0 mmol/L | 3.9–7.8 |

---

### Box 21.1 Fluid prescribing in children

#### Calculating maintenance requirements
**A** 100 mL/day for each kg of body weight up to 10 kg
**B** 50 mL/day for each kg between 10 and 20 kg
**C** 20 mL/day for each kg above 20 kg

Maintenance requirement = **A** + **B** + **C** (cap at 80 mL/hr in girls and 100 mL/hr in boys)

#### Adjusting for additional ongoing losses
Measure accurately and add to maintenance requirements

#### Calculating existing deficits
Deficit (mL) = dehydration severity (%) × weight (kg) × 10

#### Fluid choice
Use 0.45% sodium chloride with 5% glucose with electrolyte additives as needed

---

## 22 | A 5-year-old boy with a painful right arm

| | |
|---|---|
| **Patient name:** | Charlie Hewett |
| **ID number:** | 100022 |
| **Date of birth:** | 11 June 2009 |
| **Age:** | 5 years |
| **Weight:** | 22 kg |
| **Admission date:** | 06/01/2015 |
| **Date/time seen:** | 07/01/2015 16:00 |

### History
Problem   Charlie has a painful right arm.

History   He fell from a swing yesterday afternoon. He was reviewed by the orthopaedic registrar and found to have fracture of his distal radius, which was operated on this morning. The surgery was uneventful and he has returned to the ward with his arm in a back-slab. He was given morphine in recovery at 14:00 but has vomited three times and is still complaining of 'bad' pain.

PMH   He has no past medical history of note and is up to date with his vaccinations.

DH   Nil.
Intolerances: none known.

SH   Charlie lives with his mother, stepdad and half-sister Julia.

### Examination
General   Alert and chatty.

Obs   T 36.9°C, HR 130 beats/min, BP 90/40 mmHg, RR 28 breaths/min, SpO$_2$ 98% breathing air. These are normal for a 5-year-old child.

Systems   His hand is slightly swollen but has normal colour, temperature and sensation. The remainder of examination is normal.

### Task
Review Charlie's drug chart and prescribe appropriate medication.

### Suggested resource
BNF for Children (BNFc). http://www.evidence.nhs.uk/formulary/bnfc/current

## 23  A 12-hour-old boy with signs of sepsis

| | |
|---|---|
| **Patient name:** | Amos Jones |
| **ID number:** | 100023 |
| **Date of birth:** | 06/01/2015 |
| **Age:** | 12 hours |
| **Weight:** | 4.22 kg |
| **Admission date:** | 06/01/2015 |
| **Date/time seen:** | 07/01/2015 10:00 |

### History

**Problem**  Amos has a temperature and is not feeding well.

**History**  Amos was born at term by spontaneous vaginal delivery 12 hours ago. He was in good condition and did not require any resuscitation. He was placed under observation as the maternal membranes ruptured 36 hours before delivery. His mother had no evidence of group B streptococci on high-vaginal swab, did not receive any intrapartum antibiotics and has remained well.

**PMH**  Normal pregnancy and normal routine prenatal scans.

**DH**  Nil.
Intolerances: none known.

**SH**  He is the first baby of non-consanguineous parents.

### Examination

**General**  He appears quiet.

**Obs**  T 38.5°C, HR 180 beats/min (age-specific reference range, 120–160 beats/min), RR 72 breaths/min (30–60 beats/min), SpO$_2$ 92% breathing air.

**Systems**  Amos has increased work of breathing (subcostal and intercostal recession with intermittent grunting). The remainder of his newborn examination is unremarkable.

Amos has been reviewed by the registrar and she is concerned he is showing signs of severe early neonatal sepsis. She has asked you to prescribe an urgent dose of antibiotics while she puts in a cannula and takes blood. She tells you that the trust guidelines recommend gentamicin and benzylpenicillin for early neonatal sepsis (within the first 48 hours of life).

The BNF for Children (BNFc) gives the following guidance regarding antibiotic dosing in neonatal sepsis:

*Gentamicin.* For neonates ≥32 weeks postmenstrual age, 4–5 mg/kg every 24 hours by slow intravenous injection or intravenous infusion.

*Benzylpenicillin.* For neonates aged <7 days, 25 mg/kg 12-hourly (dose doubled in severe infection).

### Task

Prescribe an urgent dose of gentamicin and benzylpenicillin for Amos.

---

## 24  A 60-year-old man who has developed a hot joint

| | |
|---|---|
| **Patient name:** | Mr Juan Gonzalez |
| **ID number:** | 100024 |
| **Date of birth:** | 19/10/1954 |
| **Age:** | 60 years |
| **Weight:** | 82 kg |
| **Admission date:** | 07/01/2015 |
| **Date/time seen:** | 07/01/2015 20:00 |

### History

**Problem**  Swollen right big toe.

**History**  Juan Gonzalez was admitted electively this evening for a left total hip replacement, which is scheduled for tomorrow morning. He was reviewed in the pre-admission clinic 2 weeks ago, where he was advised to take a new anti-hypertensive drug to achieve better blood pressure control. You have been called to see him as he is complaining of a swollen and painful right big toe. The toe has become increasingly swollen over the past 24 hours. It is now exquisitely tender, to the point that even contact with the bed sheets is intolerable. In himself, he feels well. There is no recent history of trauma.

**PMH**  Gout, hypertension, osteoarthritis.

**DH**  Allopurinol 100 mg daily, amlodipine 10 mg daily, bendroflumethiazide 2.5 mg daily, ramipril 10 mg daily, co-codamol 30/500 one or two tablets as required every 4 hours, maximum 8 tablets in 24 hours.
Intolerances: none known.

**SH**  He works in finance. He drinks half a bottle of Rioja Gran Reserva per day. He is a non-smoker.

### Examination

**General**  He appears generally well.

**Obs**  T 36.5°C, HR 88 beats/min, BP 138/65 mmHg, RR 16 breaths/min, SpO$_2$ 98% breathing air.

**MSS**  The right first metatarsophalangeal joint is hot, swollen, erythematous and tender. There are gouty tophi on the pinnae of his ears.

A presumptive diagnosis of acute gout is made.

### Task

Prescribe appropriate treatment for Mr Gonzalez to address his inflamed toe.

## 25 A 65-year-old man with hypokalaemia

| | |
|---|---|
| **Patient name:** | Derek MacGee |
| **ID number:** | 100025 |
| **Date of birth:** | 19/03/1959 |
| **Age:** | 65 years |
| **Weight:** | 82 kg |
| **Admission date:** | 07/01/2015 16:00 |
| **Date/time seen:** | 07/01/2015 20:00 |

### History

Problem  Found to have hypokalaemia on routine blood tests.

History  Mr MacGee was admitted earlier today with a 2-day history of diarrhoea and vomiting, suspected to have an infective aetiology. He is unable to keep food and drink down. On admission, IV fluid was administered to correct dehydration. You have just been called by the biochemistry lab technician, who informs you that his admission blood tests indicated hypokalaemia.

PMH  Hypertension, atrial fibrillation.

DH  Aspirin 75 mg daily, amlodipine 5 mg daily, bisoprolol 10 mg daily.

Intolerances: none known.

SH  Non-smoker, consumes about 28 units of alcohol per week, fully independent.

### Examination

General  Looks well.

Obs  T 37.5°C, HR 75 beats/min, rhythm irregular, BP 122/82 mmHg, RR 16 breaths/min, SpO$_2$ 96% breathing air.

Systems  Normal other than for the findings of atrial fibrillation and mild non-peritonitic abdominal tenderness.

### Investigations

For results of investigations, see Table 25.1.

### Task

Prescribe appropriate treatment.

**Table 25.1** Case 25 investigation results

| Test | Value | Normal range |
|---|---|---|
| Na$^+$ | 135 mmol/L | 135–145 |
| K$^+$ | 2.7 mmol/L | 3.5–4.7 |
| Ur | 8.4 mmol/L | 2.5–8.0 |
| Creat | 82 µmol/L | 60–110 |
| eGFR | >60 mL/min/1.73 m$^2$ | >60 |
| ECG | Rate 75 beats/min; rhythm atrial fibrillation; left ventricular hypertrophy by voltage criteria | |

## 26 A 69-year-old woman being treated with gentamicin

| | |
|---|---|
| **Patient name:** | Patricia Hull |
| **ID number:** | 100026 |
| **Date of birth:** | 25/11/1945 |
| **Age:** | 69 years |
| **Weight:** | 71 kg |
| **Admission date:** | 06/01/2015 19:00 |
| **Date/time seen:** | 07/01/2015 19:00 |

### History

Problem  You are asked to review Mrs Hull's gentamicin level.

History  Mrs Hull was admitted with neutropenic sepsis. Antibiotic therapy with Tazocin® and gentamicin was started. Clinically, she appears to be improving, but the microbiology consultant has advised that both antibiotics should be continued at present pending results of a blood culture.

PMH  Myelodysplastic syndrome.

DH  Tazocin® (a combined preparation of tazobactam and piperacillin) 4.5 g IV 8-hourly and gentamicin 300 mg (5 mg/kg) IV given yesterday at 19:00.

Intolerances: none known.

SH  Non-smoker, does not drink alcohol, usually independent at home.

### Examination

General  She looks well.

Obs  T 37.8°C, HR 90 beats/min, BP 122/69 mmHg, RR 17 breaths/min, SpO$_2$ 98% breathing air.

Systems  No relevant findings.

### Investigations

For results of investigations, see Table 26.1.

### Task

As appropriate, prescribe the next dose of gentamicin based upon this information.

**Table 26.1** Case 26 investigation results

| Test | Value | Normal range |
|---|---|---|
| Ur | 9.9 mmol/L | 2.5–8.0 |
| Creat | 125 µmol/L | 60–110 |
| Gentamicin (at 15:00) | 1.8 µg/mL | <1 (trough) |

## 27 A 69-year-old man anticoagulated with warfarin

**Patient name:** Funsani Mzimba
**ID number:** 100027
**Date of birth:** 19/08/1945
**Age:** 69 years
**Weight:** 85 kg
**Admission date:** 03/01/2015
**Date/time seen:** 07/01/2015 19:00

### History

Problem | You have been called by the ward staff to prescribe Mr Mzimba's warfarin.

History | Mr Mzimba was admitted 4 days ago with pneumonia.

PMH | Mitral valve replacement 2007 (mechanical), atrial fibrillation.

DH | Bisoprolol 5 mg daily, warfarin usual dose 5 mg daily. Target INR 2.5–3.5.
New on this admission: amoxicillin 500 mg 8-hourly, clarithromycin 500 mg 12-hourly.
Intolerances: none known.

### Examination

General | There are no signs of bleeding.

Obs | T 36.5°C, HR 68 beats/min (irregularly irregular), BP 126/82 mmHg, RR 14 breaths/min, SpO$_2$ 98% breathing air.

### Investigations

For results of investigations, see Table 27.1.

### Task

Prescribe appropriate anticoagulant treatment for Mr Mzimba.

**Table 27.1** Case 27 investigation results

| Date of test | INR | Target range |
| --- | --- | --- |
| 3/1/2015 | 2.2 | 2.5–3.5 |
| 4/1/2015 | 2.3 | |
| 7/1/2015 | 4.6 | |

## 28 A 28-year-old woman with nausea

**Patient name:** Aarya Bokhari
**ID number:** 100028
**Date of birth:** 14/05/1986
**Age:** 28 years
**Weight:** 69 kg
**Admission date:** 07/01/2015
**Date/time seen:** 07/01/2015 19:30

### History

Problem | Mrs Bokhari is complaining of nausea following an operation to repair a broken wrist.

History | She was admitted today having fallen and sustained a wrist fracture. Her operation was straightforward and she returned to the ward at 17:30. Her pain is adequately controlled by the analgesia provided. However, she has begun to feel increasingly sick.

PMH | Schizophrenia.

DH | Olanzapine 10 mg daily.
Intolerances: haloperidol – neuroleptic malignant syndrome.

### Examination

General | She looks uncomfortable, but not unwell.

Obs | T 36.5°C, HR 85 beats/min, BP 118/75 mmHg, RR 12 breaths/min, SpO$_2$ 97% breathing air.

Systems | Normal examination. No signs of operative complications.

### From the anaesthetic chart

Uncomplicated anaesthetic.
Cyclizine 50 mg, intravenous, given at 17:00.
Morphine 5 mg, intravenous, given at 17:00.

### Task

Prescribe appropriate therapy to control Mrs Bokhari's nausea.

## 29   A 29-year-old man who is in pain following an operation

| | |
|---|---|
| **Patient name:** | Rory Bulwer |
| **ID number:** | 100029 |
| **Date of birth:** | 12/04/1985 |
| **Age:** | 29 years |
| **Weight:** | 75 kg |
| **Admission date:** | 05/01/2015 |
| **Date/time seen:** | 07/01/2015 08:00 |

### History
Problem   Mr Bulwer is complaining of pain in his leg.

History   Two days ago he was knocked off his bicycle and sustained a fracture to his left femur. This was repaired on the same day with the insertion of a femoral nail. The procedure was uncomplicated. He has had pain since the operation. He reports that the pain is relieved slightly when he takes the medications that the nurses give him regularly, but that it never fully goes and comes back before the next tablet is due. He has had to ask for extra pain relief frequently but says that even this does not entirely relieve the pain. He describes the pain at worse as being 7 out of 10 in severity.

PMH   None.

DH   None prior to admission. Current analgesia: paracetamol 1 g four times daily, ibuprofen 400 mg three times daily, Oramorph® (oral morphine solution 10 mg/5 mL) 2.5 mg as required max 2-hourly.
Intolerances: none known.

### Examination
General   Uncomfortable from pain.

Obs   T 36.5°C, HR 95 beats/min, BP 118/85 mmHg, RR 16 breaths/min, SpO$_2$ 98% breathing room air.

Ankle   The wound is clean with a small amount of blood on the dressing. Swelling in the limb is as expected for the procedure. There are no signs of compartment syndrome.

### Task
Prescribe appropriate analgesia for Mr Bulwer.

## 30   A 49-year-old man due to undergo surgery

| | |
|---|---|
| **Patient name:** | Ranjit Patel |
| **ID number:** | 100030 |
| **Date of birth:** | 01/02/1965 |
| **Age:** | 49 years |
| **Weight:** | 81 kg |
| **Admission date:** | 07/01/2015 14:00 |
| **Date/time seen:** | 07/01/2015 22:00 |

### History
Problem   Asked to prescribe variable rate intravenous insulin infusion.

History   Mr Patel has been admitted for a laparoscopic radical prostatectomy to treat prostate cancer. This is scheduled to begin at 08:00 tomorrow and is anticipated to be a difficult procedure, likely to take at least 4 hours. In view of this, and because his pre-operative glycaemic control has been poor, the diabetes team have advised that a variable rate intravenous insulin infusion be started pre-operatively.

PMH   Type 2 diabetes mellitus, hypercholesterolaemia, hypertension, obesity.

DH   Amlodipine 10 mg daily, metformin 1 g twice daily, simvastatin 40 mg daily; his usual insulin treatment comprises glargine 18 units SC at bedtime, and NovoRapid® 10 units with breakfast, lunch and dinner.
Intolerances: none known.

SH   Ex-smoker of 30 pack-years' duration, does not drink alcohol.

### Examination
General   He looks well.

Obs   T 36.8°C, HR 80 beats/min, BP 132/89 mmHg, RR 14 breaths/min, SpO$_2$ 95% breathing air.

Systems   Normal.

### Investigations
For results of investigations, see Table 30.1.

### Task
Prescribe the variable rate intravenous insulin infusion on the chart provided.

**Table 30.1** Case 30 investigation results

| Test | Value | Normal range |
|---|---|---|
| K$^+$ | 4.3 mmol/L | 3.5–4.7 |
| Gluc (random) | 11.3 mmol/L | 3.9–7.8 |
| HbA$_{1C}$ | 73 mmol/mol | 22–44 |

## 31 A 79-year-old woman with acute kidney injury

**Patient name:** Dorothy Harmsworth
**ID number:** 100031
**Date of birth:** 14/04/1935
**Age:** 79 years
**Weight:** 74 kg
**Admission date:** 02/01/2015 17:30
**Date/time seen:** 07/01/2015 21:15

### History

Problem    Abnormal renal profile.
History    Due to problems with the phlebotomy service, Mrs Harmsworth has not had any blood tests for several days. Samples were taken late this afternoon and you were asked to review them during your evening on-call shift. You have identified some abnormalities (detailed below). Mrs Harmsworth was admitted 5 days ago with a fracture of her right femoral neck. A hemiarthroplasy was performed, and she is now awaiting a bed in a rehabilitation unit. She is asymptomatic. On direct questioning, she says she has passed very little urine today.
PMH    Transient ischaemic attack 3 years ago.
DH    Aspirin 75 mg daily, dalteparin 5000 units SC daily, naproxen 250 mg 8-hourly, ramipril 5 mg daily, atorvastatin 10 mg nightly, tramadol 100 mg 6-hourly as required.
Intolerances: none known.
SH    Non-smoker, rarely consumes alcohol, lives alone with once-daily carer support.

### Examination

General    Looks well.
Obs    T 37.5°C, HR 92 beats/min, BP 132/72 mmHg, RR 18 breaths/min, SpO$_2$ 94% breathing air.
CVS    JVP 4 cm, no postural blood pressure change, normal heart sounds, no oedema.
RS    Normal.
Abdo    Normal, with no palpable masses.

### Investigations

For results of investigations, see Table 31.1.

### Task

Review her prescription chart and modify her treatment appropriately pending senior review.

**Table 31.1** Case 31 investigation results

| Test | Today | On admission | Normal range |
|---|---|---|---|
| Na$^+$ | 133 mmol/L | 136 mmol/L | 135–145 |
| K$^+$ | 5.3 mmol/L | 4.8 mmol/L | 3.5–4.7 |
| Ur | 29.6 mmol/L | 11.5 mmol/L | 2.5–8.0 |
| Creat | 289 μmol/L | 98 μmol/L | 60–110 |
| eGFR | 15 mL/min/1.73m$^2$ | 50 mL/min/1.73 m$^2$ | >60 |
| pH | 7.36 | | 7.35–7.45 |
| PaO$_2$ (breathing air) | 11.5 kPa | | 10.6–14.5 |
| PaCO$_2$ | 4.1 kPa | | 4.0–6.0 |
| HCO$_3^-$ (arterial) | 22 mmol/L | | 22–29 |
| BE | –2 mmol/L | | –2 to +2 |

## 32 An 85-year-old woman with hospital-acquired pneumonia

**Patient name:** Doris Nuttall
**ID number:** 100032
**Date of birth:** 01/11/1929
**Age:** 85 years
**Weight:** 75 kg
**Admission date:** 04/01/2015
**Date/time seen:** 07/01/2015 23:00

### History
Problem   You are asked to see Doris Nuttall who has become increasingly short of breath over the past 4 hours.

History   Mrs Nuttall was admitted 4 days ago with a left hemiplegia, secondary to an ischaemic stroke affecting the right middle cerebral artery territory.

PMH   Hypertension.

DH   Amlodipine 5 mg daily, clopidogrel 75 mg daily, dalteparin 5000 units subcutaneously daily, ramipril 5 mg daily.
Intolerances: none known.

SH   Ex-smoker with a 50 pack-year smoking history. She does not drink alcohol. She lives alone and was fully independent before the stroke.

### Examination
General   In bed, slumped to the right.

Obs   T 38.2°C, HR 104 beats/min, BP 112/68 mmHg (was 136/86 mmHg at 18:00), RR 36 breaths/min, SpO$_2$ 84% breathing oxygen 2 L/min via nasal cannula.

RS   Right lung base dull to percussion with bronchial breathing and coarse inspiratory crackles on auscultation.

NS   Left hemiplegia and facial droop. Left-sided neglect. Glasgow coma score E4, V4, M6.

### Investigations
For results of investigations, see Tables 32.1 and 32.2.

A diagnosis of hospital-acquired pneumonia is made, possibly secondary to aspiration.

### Task
Review her inpatient chart and make any changes to treatment you consider necessary.

**Table 32.1** Case 32 investigation results

| Test | Value | Normal range |
| --- | --- | --- |
| Hb | 118 g/L | 120–160 |
| WCC | 23.5 × 10$^9$/L | 4.0–11.0 |
| Plt | 346 × 10$^9$/L | 150–400 |
| Na$^+$ | 136 mmol/L | 135–145 |
| K$^+$ | 4.1 mmol/L | 3.5–4.7 |
| Ur | 10.8 mmol/L | 2.5–8.0 |
| Creat | 62 μmol/L | 60–110 |
| eGFR | >60 mL/min/1.73 m$^2$ | >60 |
| Gluc (random) | 4.4 mmol/L | 3.9–7.8 |
| CRP | 236 mg/L | <10 |
| CXR | Normal on admission, now right lower lobe consolidation | |

**Table 32.2** Case 32 arterial blood gas results (breathing oxygen 2 L/min via nasal cannula)

| Test | Value | Normal range |
| --- | --- | --- |
| pH | 7.52 | 7.35–7.45 |
| PaO$_2$ | 6.8 kPa | 10.6–14.5 kPa |
| PaCO$_2$ | 3.6 kPa | 4.0–6.0 kPa |
| HCO$_3^-$ (arterial) | 23 mmol/L | 22–29 mmol/L |
| BE | −1 mmol/L | −2 to +2 mmol/L |

## A 47-year-old man who has developed an abnormal liver profile

**Patient name:** Kazim Qureshi
**ID number:** 100033
**Date of birth:** 01/12/1967
**Age:** 47 years
**Weight:** 98 kg
**Admission date:** 31/12/2014
**Date/time seen:** 07/01/2015 12:00

### History

Problem   You are called to see Mr Qureshi to review his abnormal blood results.

History   Kazim Qureshi is an inpatient on a surgical ward. He was admitted as an emergency 7 days ago with an acute abdomen. An urgent laparotomy showed small bowel infarction secondary to a strangulated hernia. He underwent small bowel resection and hernia repair on 01/01/2015. He has had a stormy postoperative course with sepsis and delirium. He is now feeling better, is eating and mobilising to the bathroom and has no pain.

PMH   Psoriasis, hypercholesterolaemia.

DH   Prior to admission: methotrexate 15 mg once weekly, folic acid 5 mg daily, simvastatin 40 mg daily.
Added since admission: co-amoxiclav 1.2 g IV 8-hourly, paracetamol 1 g four times daily, dalteparin 5000 units SC daily.
As needed: morphine 10 mg 4-hourly, codeine phosphate 30–60 mg 4-hourly, haloperidol 2 mg 8-hourly.
Intolerances: none known.

SH   Non-smoker who does not drink alcohol.

### Examination

General   Orientated in time and place, looks well. No jaundice.

Obs   T 36.4°C, HR 64 beats/min, BP 134/78 mmHg, RR 12 breaths/min, SpO$_2$ 99% breathing air.

Abdo   Soft, non-tender. Wound healing well. No hepatomegaly or stigmata of chronic liver disease.

Skin   He has a small patch of psoriasis on each elbow.

### Investigations

For results of investigations, see Tables 33.1 and 33.2.

### Task

Review Mr Qureshi's inpatient chart and make any changes you consider necessary.

**Table 33.1** Case 33 investigation results

| Test | 13 October 2014 | 31 December 2014 | 4 January 2015 | 7 January 2015 | Normal range |
|---|---|---|---|---|---|
| Hb | 165 g/L | 186 g/L | 125 g/L | 129 g/L | 130–180 |
| WCC | 5.2 × 10$^9$/L | 24.1 × 10$^9$/L | 12.2 × 10$^9$/L | 4.6 × 10$^9$/L | 4.0–11.0 |
| Plt | 256 × 10$^9$/L | 599 × 10$^9$/L | 643 × 10$^9$/L | 366 × 10$^9$/L | 150–400 |
| INR | Not measured | 1.1 | 1.2 | 1.2 | 0.8–1.1 |
| Bil | 14 μmol/L | 16 μmol/L | 18 μmol/L | 22 μmol/L | <17 |
| Alb | 46 g/L | 35 g/L | 32 g/L | 34 g/L | 35–48 |
| ALT | 98 U/L | 102 U/L | 144 U/L | 188 U/L | <52 |
| ALP | 74 U/L | 68 U/L | 269 U/L | 480 U/L | 35–120 |
| GGT | 102 U/L | 112 U/L | 278 U/L | 466 U/L | <64 |
| CRP | 3 mg/L | 289 mg/L | 72 mg/L | 12 mg/L | <10 |

**Table 33.2** Case 33 investigation results

| Test | Result |
|---|---|
| Abdominal ultrasound (06/1/2015) | Diffuse changes consistent with hepatic inflammation. No gallstones, biliary dilatation, hepatic or subphrenic collections. The appearance has a wide differential, but given the clinical picture, drug-induced liver injury would seem the most likely diagnosis |
| Serology | Hepatitis A, B, C, EBV, CMV and HIV negative |
| Autoimmune screen | Anti-mitochondrial and anti-smooth muscle antibodies negative |

| | |
|---|---|
| **Patient name:** | Frederick George |
| **ID number:** | 100034 |
| **Date of birth:** | 21/10/1931 |
| **Age:** | 83 years |
| **Weight:** | 55 kg |
| **Admission date:** | 01/01/2015 |
| **Date/time seen:** | 07/01/2015 20:00 |

### History

| | |
|---|---|
| Problem | You are called to see Mr George who has developed diarrhoea. |
| History | He was admitted to hospital 6 days ago with a cough and shortness of breath and was found to have community-acquired pneumonia. His cough is now better and his breathing is back to normal. He was constipated for the first 5 days in hospital but opened his bowels yesterday, and today has had liquid (type 7) stools on six occasions. He has some associated abdominal pain but no nausea or vomiting and is able to drink freely. |
| PMH | Ischaemic heart disease, myocardial infarction, congestive cardiac failure, gastritis. |
| DH | Amoxicillin 1 g 8-hourly, aspirin 75 mg daily, bisacodyl 10 mg at night, bisoprolol 2.5 mg daily, dalteparin 5000 units daily, furosemide 80 mg daily, ispaghula husk one sachet daily, lansoprazole 30 mg daily, sertraline 50 mg daily, simvastatin 40 mg daily. |
| | Intolerances: none known. |
| SH | He lives with his wife and was previously independent. He is a non-smoker. He drinks 10 units of alcohol per week. |

### Examination

| | |
|---|---|
| General | Anxious and uncomfortable. |
| Obs | T 37.2°C, HR 80 beats/min, BP 136/78 mmHg, RR 14 breaths/min, SpO$_2$ 96% breathing air. |
| CVS | JVP 2 cm above the sternal angle, normal heart sounds, no pitting ankle or sacral oedema. |
| RS | Normal expansion, percussion and auscultation. |
| Abdo | Mildly tender, active bowel sounds, liquid stool on rectal examination, with no faecal impaction. |

### Investigations

For results of investigations, see Table 34.1.

The nursing staff are planning to move Mr George to a side room as they suspect he has *Clostridium difficile* infection.

### Task

Review his inpatient chart and make any changes to his treatment that are required.

**Table 34.1** Case 34 investigation results

| Test | Admission | 05/01/2015 | 07/01/2015 | Normal range |
|---|---|---|---|---|
| Hb | 14.2 g/L | 13.4 g/L | 15.1 g/L | 130–180 |
| WCC | 19.3 × 10$^9$/L | 6.6 × 10$^9$/L | 13.2 × 10$^9$/L | 4.0–11.0 |
| Plt | 396 × 10$^9$/L | 280 × 10$^9$/L | 344 × 10$^9$/L | 150–400 |
| Na$^+$ | 143 mmol/L | 140 mmol/L | 136 mmol/L | 135–145 |
| K$^+$ | 3.6 mmol/L | 3.4 mmol/L | 3.3 mmol/L | 3.5–4.7 |
| Ur | 6.2 mmol/L | 5.9 mmol/L | 9.4 mmol/L | 2.5–8.0 |
| Creat | 98 μmol/L | 94 μmol/L | 99 μmol/L | 60–110 |
| CRP | 238 mg/L | 25 mg/L | 78 mg/L | <10 |

**Patient name:**   Marco Alberici
**ID number:**      100035
**Date of birth:**  12/01/1926
**Age:**            88 years
**Weight:**         79 kg
**Admission date:** 02/01/2015
**Date/time seen:** 07/01/2015 13:15

## History

Problem   You received a handover to review Mr Alberici's blood tests. You have identified hyperkalaemia. This is a new finding.

History   Mr Alberici was admitted 5 days ago following a fall. This was thought to have been precipitated by a urinary tract infection, for which trimethoprim was started. He is now well and plans are being made for discharge in the next few days.

PMH       Paroxysmal atrial fibrillation, heart failure, hypertension, ischaemic heart disease.

DH        Bisoprolol 5 mg daily, furosemide 20 mg daily, ramipril 10 mg daily, simvastatin 40 mg daily, trimethoprim 200 mg 12-hourly, warfarin dosed according to INR (prescribed separately on an anti-coagulation chart).
          Intolerances: none known.

SH        Ex-smoker of 40 pack-years' duration, consumes 24 units of alcohol per week. He is supported by three times daily carers at home due to general debility.

## Examination

General   He does not look acutely unwell.
Obs       T 36.8°C, HR 60 beats/min, rhythm regular, BP 124/70 mmHg, RR 18 breaths/min, SpO$_2$ 94% breathing air.
Systems   Moderate pedal pitting oedema.

## Investigations

For results of investigations, see Table 35.1.

## Task

Review his prescription chart and modify his treatment appropriately pending senior review.

**Table 35.1** Case 35 investigation results

| Test | Value | Normal range |
|---|---|---|
| Na$^+$ | 133 mmol/L | 135–145 |
| K$^+$ | 6.6 mmol/L | 3.5–4.7 |
| Ur | 9.0 mmol/L | 2.5–8.0 |
| Creat | 144 µmol/L | 60–110 |
| Venous blood gas results | | |
| pH | 7.38 | 7.35–7.45 |
| HCO$_3^-$ | 23 mmol/L | 22–29 |
| BE | +1 mmol/L | −2 to +2 |
| ECG | Rate 60 beats/min. Sinus rhythm with first-degree heart block (PR interval 240 msec). Axis normal. QRS duration prolonged at 140 msec. Tall T-waves. At admission, the ECG was normal | |
| Urine MC&S | Moderate growth of *Escherichia coli* (sensitive to nitrofurantoin and trimethoprim, resistant to amoxicillin) | |

# 36 A 69-year-old woman with acute alcohol withdrawal

**Patient name:** Maureen Beatty
**ID number:** 100036
**Date of birth:** 12/09/1945
**Age:** 69 years
**Weight:** 54 kg
**Admission date:** 05/01/2015
**Date/time seen:** 07/01/2015 03:40

## History

Problem    You are called to the ward to see Maureen Beatty who has become acutely confused. She is anxious, shouting and trying to leave. She complains that staff are trying to poison her.

History    She was admitted just over 24 hours ago with abdominal pain, thought to be secondary to chronic pancreatitis. She has not previously been confused, although she was shaky and sweaty yesterday evening and has not been sleeping well.

PMH    Pancreatitis.

DH    Dalteparin 5000 units daily, co-codamol 30/500 two tablets 6-hourly, lactulose 10 mL 12-hourly. Intolerances: none known.

SH    She drinks one 700 mL bottle of vodka and smokes 30 cigarettes per day. Her consumption has been at this level over the past 5 years since her husband died.

## Examination

General    She is agitated, tremulous and sweaty. She looks thin.

Obs    T 36.7°C, HR 116 beats/min, regular, BP 146/94 mmHg, RR 18 breaths/min, SpO$_2$ 96% breathing air, Glasgow Coma Score E4 V4 M6.

Systems    Systems examination is unremarkable. There are no focal neurological deficits.

## Investigations

For results of investigations, see Table 36.1.

After appropriate assessment and consideration of other causes, her confusion is attributed to acute alcohol withdrawal.

## Task

Review her inpatient chart and prescribe appropriate treatment.

**Table 36.1** Case 36 investigation results

| Test | Value | Normal range |
| --- | --- | --- |
| Hb | 154 g/L | 120–160 |
| MCV | 104 fL | 78–97 |
| WCC | 10.6 × 10$^9$/L | 4.0–11.0 |
| Plt | 126 × 10$^9$/L | 150–400 |
| INR | 1.1 | 0.8–1.1 |
| Na$^+$ | 137 mmol/L | 135–145 |
| K$^+$ | 3.7 mmol/L | 3.5–4.7 |
| Ur | 2.1 mmol/L | 2.5–8.0 |
| Creat | 54 μmol/L | 60–110 |
| Alb | 36 g/L | 35–48 |
| Bil | 14 μmol/L | <17 |
| ALP | 98 U/L | 35–120 |
| GGT | 124 U/L | <38 |
| CRP | 8 mg/L | <10 |
| CBG | 6.9 mmol/L | 3.9–7.8 |
| Urine MC&S | Negative for blood, protein, leukocytes and nitrates | |
| CXR | Normal | |
| ECG | Shows sinus tachycardia | |

## 15 · A 91-year-old man with hypoglycaemia

### What should I consider when deciding what to prescribe?

The most common cause of hypoglycaemia (defined as a blood glucose concentration <4 mmol/L) in patients with diabetes mellitus is the administration of insulin or a sulphonylurea. This may be compounded by impairment of the counter-regulatory responses to hypoglycaemia (e.g. glucagon and adrenaline secretion), either as a direct effect of diabetes mellitus or due to concurrent treatment with a beta blocker. Alcohol consumption is also a risk factor for hypoglycaemia. Metformin generally does not cause hypoglycaemia. Non-drug causes of hypoglycaemia include critical illness and insulin secreting tumours, which are rare. In Mr Robinson's case, much the most likely explanation for hypoglycaemia is his gliclazide treatment, in conjunction with a change in his diet associated with hospital admission.

The management of hypoglycaemia may be divided into three main scenarios:

1 *Conscious patient able to swallow:* treat with glucose by mouth (e.g. Lucozade®)

2 *Conscious patient able to swallow but uncooperative:* treat with a glucose gel squeezed into the space between the teeth and the buccal mucosa, or if this is not possible, with glucagon IM

3 *Unconscious, aggressive or seizing:* address airway, breathing and circulation. If an intravenous cannula is available or can be sited quickly, administer 10% or 20% glucose by rapid IV infusion. If no IV access is available, administer glucagon by IM injection.

When administering IV glucose, take care to ensure the cannula is correctly sited, as glucose solutions are irritant if allowed to leak out of the vein into the tissues (extravasate). Glucagon, which works by stimulating gluconeogenesis and glycogenolysis, has the advantages of being quicker and easier to administer than IV glucose. However, it may be less effective in patients who are malnourished and those taking a sulphonylurea.

You should stay with the patient until he has regained consciousness.

Once the acute attack has been averted, you must ensure that the patient eats food containing a starchy carbohydrate to prevent relapse (e.g. at least one slice of bread or a sandwich; twice this amount is required in patients treated with glucagon, so as to replenish their glycogen stores). You should then review the patient's treatment to determine whether any changes are necessary. Detailed discussion is beyond the scope of this case study, but some general guidance points are offered:

| Surname ROBINSON | Hospital number 100015 | Weight 82 kg | Drug intolerances None known |
|---|---|---|---|
| First name ALEC | Date of birth 26/02/1923 | | |

**REGULAR PRESCRIPTIONS**

Month: January   Year: 2015

| DRUG | times | 6 | 7 |
|---|---|---|---|
| **METFORMIN** 850 mg ORAL 3-times daily Start date 7/1/15 Signature A Doctor Bleep 1234 Additional instructions With meals | 06 08 12 16 18 22 | AH AH AH | AH AH AH |
| **GLICLAZIDE** 80 mg ORAL Twice daily Start date 7/1/15 Signature A Doctor Bleep 1234 Additional instructions With meals | 06 08 12 16 18 22 | AH AH | AH AH |
| **ASPIRIN** 75 mg ORAL Daily Start date 7/1/15 Signature A Doctor Bleep 1234 | 06 08 12 16 18 22 | AH | AH |
| **SIMVASTATIN** 40 mg ORAL Nightly Start date 7/1/15 Signature A Doctor Bleep 1234 Additional instructions Withhold while on sodium fusidate | 06 08 12 16 18 22 | | |
| **FLUCLOXACILLIN** 1.2 g IV 6-hrly Start date 7/1/15 Signature A Doctor Bleep 1234 Review 14 days Additional instructions Osteomyelitis | 06 08 12 16 18 22 (24) | AH AH AH AH | AH AH AH |
| **SODIUM FUSIDATE** 500 mg ORAL 8-hrly Start date 7/1/15 Signature A Doctor Bleep 1234 Review 14 days Additional instructions Osteomyelitis | 06 08 12 (14) 16 18 22 | AH AH AH | AH AH |

**ONCE ONLY PRESCRIPTIONS**

| Date | Time to be given | DRUG | Dose | Route | Prescriber Signature | Prescriber Bleep | Administration Date given | Administration Time given | Administration Given by |
|---|---|---|---|---|---|---|---|---|---|
| 7/1/15 | 20:00 | GLUCOSE 10% | 100 mL | IV | A Doctor | 1234 | | | |

**OXYGEN**

| Target SpO₂ | ○ 94–98% ○ 88–92% |
|---|---|
| Mode of delivery | ○ Continuous ○ As required |
| Starting device | |
| Initials | Bleep | Date |

**AS REQUIRED MEDICATION**

| DRUG GLUCOSE 10% 100 mL IV Max freq See below Start date 7/1/15 Signature A Doctor Bleep 1234 Review Additional instructions For use in accordance with hypoglycaemia management protocol. Alert doctor if administered. | Date Time Dose Route Given Check |
|---|---|

*Prescribing Scenarios at a Glance*, First Edition. Emma Baker, Daniel Burrage, Dagan Lonsdale, and Andrew Hitchings.

- Never start a variable rate intravenous insulin infusion ('sliding scale') in response to a hypoglycaemic episode
- Do not omit insulin following a hypoglycaemic episode (although it is appropriate to delay its administration until the attack has been fully treated)
- If there is a pattern of hypoglycaemic attacks at a particular time of day, reduce the dose of insulin (or sulphonylurea) scheduled for administration *before* the time of hypoglycaemia.

All patients who have had a hypoglycaemic attack should have their blood glucose concentration levels monitored closely for the next 24–48 hours. Ensure the episode is clearly documented in the clinical notes.

### How do I write the prescription?

A typical treatment for severe hypoglycaemia is to give 100 mL glucose 10% (or 50 mL glucose 20%), administered as fast as the cannula will allow (usually over about 1–3 minutes). As the intention is for rapid administration (the exact rate of which is not important) this may be prescribed in the once only or as required sections of the drug chart (this contrasts with the prescription of glucose for fluid replacement, which should be prescribed in the infusion section). Indeed, it is recommended by some that glucose should routinely be prescribed in the as required section of the drug chart for all inpatients with diabetes, for administration by nursing staff if required in accordance with a hospital protocol. Both approaches are illustrated on the model chart.

If you elected to treat with glucagon, you should have prescribed this in a dose of 1 mg IV (or IM if no functioning cannula was available) in the once only section. If your patient fails to respond within 10 minutes of receiving glucagon, further treatment should be with IV glucose.

### Further reading

Medical Pharmacology at a Glance. Chapter 36: Antidiabetic agents.
Stanisstreet D, Walden E, Jones C, Graveling A. The Hospital Management of Hypoglycaemia in Adults with Diabetes Mellitus. NHS Diabetes (2010). Available at: http://www.diabetes.org.uk/About_us/What-we-say/Improving-diabetes-healthcare/The-hospital-management-of-Hypoglycaemia-in-adults-with-Diabetes-Mellitus/ (accessed 24 January 2014).

## 16 A 60-year-old woman requesting night sedation

**Surname:** HORTON
**Hospital number:** 100016
**Weight:** 63 kg
**Drug intolerances:** None known
**First name:** KATHERINE
**Date of birth:** 14/03/1954

### REGULAR PRESCRIPTIONS

Circle / enter times below ↓ — Enter dates below — 7 | Month: January | Year: 2015

| DRUG DALTEPARIN | | | | |
|---|---|---|---|---|
| Dose 5000 units | Route SC | Freq Daily | Start date 8/1/15 | 06 / 08 / 12 / 16 / (18) / 22 |
| Signature A Doctor | Bleep 1234 | Review | | |
| Additional instructions | | | | |

| DRUG LEVOTHYROXINE | | | | |
|---|---|---|---|---|
| Dose 50 micrograms | Route ORAL | Freq Daily | Start date 7/1/15 | 06 / (08) / 12 / 16 / 18 / 22 |
| Signature A Doctor | Bleep 1234 | Review | | |
| Additional instructions | | | | |

DRUG

### ONCE ONLY PRESCRIPTIONS

| Date | Time to be given | DRUG | Dose | Route | Prescriber Signature | Prescriber Bleep | Administration Date given | Administration Time given | Administration Given by |
|---|---|---|---|---|---|---|---|---|---|
| 7/1/15 | 21:30 | TEMAZEPAM | 10 mg | ORAL | A Doctor | 1234 | | | |
| | | | | | | | | | |
| | | | | | | | | | |

### OXYGEN

| Target SpO₂ | ○ 94–98% ○ 88–92% |
|---|---|
| Mode of delivery | ○ Continuous ○ As required |
| Starting device | |
| Initials | Bleep | Date |

### What should I consider when deciding what to prescribe?

The use of sedative drugs, such as benzodiazepines, to induce sleep (hypnosis) and alleviate anxiety (anxiolysis) is generally best avoided. Potential problems can arise both from their short-term use in hospital (their respiratory-depressant and sedative effects can be problematic in the context of acute illness), and in longer-term use (due to the development of a dependence state if used regularly for more than a few weeks). There are usually better non-pharmacological means of dealing with insomnia and anxiety. However, in selected cases, short-term pharmacological treatment for disabling symptoms may be reasonable. A single dose of an appropriate drug the night before elective surgery, in an otherwise well patient, is one such example.

Having determined that a sedative drug is indicated, you should next check that it is safe. Ensure that the patient is not at risk of harm from the drug's respiratory-depressant effects (e.g. COPD with chronic respiratory failure) or its sedative effects (e.g. severe hepatic or renal impairment). Avoid administering benzodiazepines to women who are pregnant or breast feeding, as the drug may cross the placenta or be excreted in breast milk, respectively.

You then need to select an appropriate drug. Benzodiazepines are preferred over other sedating drug classes. The effects of midazolam are too short-lived for effective night sedation, while long-acting agents such as diazepam may have a 'hangover-effect' the following morning. Therefore, it is best to select a drug with an intermediate duration of action, such as temazepam (a benzodiazepine) or zopiclone (a closely related 'Z'-drug). Always administer the drug orally and at the dose listed in the BNF (where a range is specified, generally use the lowest dose in this range). Elderly patients may be more susceptible to the effects of sedative drugs, so the dose should usually be reduced.

## How do I write the prescription?

Except under senior or specialist advice, never prescribe sedative drugs regularly. It is usually best to prescribe a single dose in the once only section of the drug chart. The example given here is of a single dose of temazepam 10 mg orally. Zopiclone 7.5 mg or zolpidem 10 mg orally would be equally acceptable alternatives.

## Further reading

Medical Pharmacology at a Glance. Chapter 24: Anxiolytics and hypnotics.

Prescribing at a Glance. Chapters 30 & 31: Using drugs for the neurological system.

---

## 17 A 62-year-old man with suspected opioid toxicity

## What should I consider when deciding what to prescribe?

Opioids are strong analgesic agents. In overdose, their main effects are respiratory depression, reduced level of consciousness and constricted pupils. All these features are evident in Mr Johnson's case. Notably, he also has impaired renal function (a common consequence of myeloma). This is relevant because morphine and its metabolites depend on the kidneys for their elimination. This probably explains why he appears to have developed opioid toxicity while taking what would otherwise be a reasonable starting dosage of morphine.

The specific antidote for opioid toxicity is *naloxone*. This works by displacing opioids from their receptor sites. Naloxone may be administered by the IV, SC or IM route. In the context of opioid toxicity associated with respiratory and neurological depression, IV injection is usually preferred, as this has the fastest onset of action. It is important to note that the duration of effect of naloxone (about 30 min with IV administration) is shorter than that of most opioids (e.g. about 4 hours for orally administered immediate-release morphine sulfate). Consequently, after initial IV injection, it is essential that you monitor the patient closely for at least the next hour, in case opioid toxicity recurs when the effect of naloxone wears off. Further doses of naloxone may then be necessary. These might be administered by SC or IM injection (as these provide a more sustained effect) or, more commonly, by IV infusion. These decisions are complex and should always be taken in consultation with a senior colleague, so will not be discussed further here.

The dosage of naloxone depends on the context. In a patient who was not previously taking a strong opioid, and who has signs of respiratory depression (as is the case for Mr Johnson), a typical dose would be 400 micrograms, repeated every 2–3 min until the patient is conscious and has a normal respiratory rate. If this is not achieved with 5–10 mg naloxone, you should consider alternative diagnoses. In patients on long-term regular opioid treatment – particularly in a palliative care setting – you should usually use lower incremental doses of naloxone (40–200 micrograms), so as not to precipitate an acute withdrawal state ('cold turkey'). In these cases, aim just to restore and maintain a normal respiratory rate.

After the acute situation has been dealt with, his regular opioid treatment should be reviewed. A reasonable course of action may be to halve his current morphine dosage, subject to ongoing monitoring and review. For ease of administration, we have prescribed 1 mg (0.5 mL of morphine sulfate oral solution).

| Surname JOHNSON | Hospital number 100017 | Weight 67 kg | Drug intolerances None known |
| First name SAMUEL | Date of birth 04/04/1952 | | |

**REGULAR PRESCRIPTIONS**

Month: January  Year: 2015

| | Circle / enter times below ↓ | 6 | 7 | | | | | | |
|---|---|---|---|---|---|---|---|---|---|
| **DRUG** ORAMORPH (10 mg/5 mL) | 06 ②② | AM | | | | | | A Doctor Bleep 1234 7/1/15 | |
| | 08 ⑥⑥ | AM | | | | | | | |
| Dose 2.5 mg  Route Oral  Freq 4-hrly  Start date 6/1/15 | 11 ⑩ | AM | | | | | | | |
| Signature A Doctor  Bleep 1234  Review | 16 ⑭ | AM | AM | | | | | | |
| | 18 ⑱ | AM | | | | | | | |
| Additional instructions Morphine sulfate immediate release | 22 ㉒ | AM | | | | | | | |
| **DRUG** METOCLOPRAMIDE | 06 | | AM | | | | | | |
| | 08 | | | | | | | | |
| Dose 10 mg  Route Oral  Freq 8-hrly  Start date 6/1/15 | 12 | | | | | | | | |
| Signature A Doctor  Bleep 1234  Review | 16 ⑭ | AM | AM | | | | | | |
| | 18 | | | | | | | | |
| Additional instructions | ㉒ | AM | | | | | | | |
| **DRUG** DALTEPARIN | 06 | | | | | | | | |
| | 08 | | | | | | | | |
| Dose 5000 units  Route SC  Freq Daily  Start date 6/1/15 | 12 | | | | | | | | |
| Signature A Doctor  Bleep  Review | 16 | | | | | | | | |
| Additional instructions | ⑱ | AM | | | | | | | |
| | 22 | | | | | | | | |
| **DRUG** PARACETAMOL | 06 | AM | AM | | | | | | |
| | 08 | | | | | | | | |
| Dose 1 g  Route Oral  Freq 6-hrly  Start date 6/1/15 | 12 | AM | AM | | | | | | |
| Signature A Doctor  Bleep 1234  Review | 16 | | | | | | | | |
| | ⑱ | AM | | | | | | | |
| Additional instructions | 22 ㉔ | AM | | | | | | | |
| **DRUG** SENNA | 06 | | | | | | | | |
| | 08 | | | | | | | | |
| Dose 15 mg  Route Oral  Freq Nightly  Start date 6/1/15 | 12 | | | | | | | | |
| Signature A Doctor  Bleep 1234  Review | 16 | | | | | | | | |
| | 18 | | | | | | | | |
| Additional instructions | ㉒ | AM | | | | | | | |
| **DRUG** ORAMORPH (10mg/5mL) | 06 ②② | | | | | | | | |
| | 08 ⑥⑥ | | | | | | | | |
| Dose 1 mg  Route Oral  Freq 4-hrly  Start date 7/1/15 | 12 ⑩ | | | | | | | | |
| Signature A Doctor  Bleep 1234  Review | 16 ⑭ | | | | | | | | |
| | 18 ⑱ | | | | | | | | |
| Additional instructions Morphine sulfate immediate release | 22 ㉒ | | | | | | | | |

## ONCE ONLY PRESCRIPTIONS

| Date | Time to be given | DRUG | Dose | Route | Prescriber Signature | Prescriber Bleep | Administration Date given | Administration Time given | Administration Given by |
|------|------|------|------|-------|------|------|------|------|------|
| 7/1/15 | 14:35 | NALOXONE | 400 micrograms | IV | AD | 1234 | 7/1/15 | 14:35 | AD/AN |
| 7/1/15 | 14:38 | NALOXONE | 400 micrograms | IV | AD | 1234 | 7/1/15 | 14:38 | AD/AN |
| | | | | | | | | | |

## OXYGEN

| Target SpO₂ | ○ 94–98% |
|---|---|
| | ○ 88–92% |
| Mode of delivery | ○ Continuous |
| | ○ As required |
| Starting device | |

| Initials | Bleep | Date |
|---|---|---|
| | | |

## AS REQUIRED MEDICATION

DRUG ORAMORPH (10 mg/5 mL)

| Dose | Route | Max freq | Start date |
|---|---|---|---|
| 2.5 mg | Oral | 4-hrly | 6/1/15 |

| Signature | Bleep | Review |
|---|---|---|
| A Doctor | 1234 | |

Date / Time / Dose / Route / Given / Check

ADoctor Bleep 1234 7/1/15

Additional instructions
Morphine sulfate immediate release. For breakthrough pain.

DRUG ORAMORPH (10 mg/5 mL)

| Dose | Route | Max freq | Start date |
|---|---|---|---|
| 1 mg | Oral | 4-hrly | 7/1/15 |

| Signature | Bleep | Review |
|---|---|---|
| A.Doctor | 1234 | |

Date / Time / Dose / Route / Given / Check

Additional instructions
Morphine sulfate immediate release. For breakthrough pain.

DRUG

## How do I write the prescription?

The initial prescription for naloxone should be written in the once only section of the drug chart. Usually, you will administer this yourself. Given the urgency of the situation, it is acceptable to administer the drug first then write the prescription afterwards. If you needed to give repeated doses, you can then record the total amount given. In the model chart, for example, we have administered a total of 800 micrograms, in 400 microgram increments.

In administering the drug, do not forget that both you and the nurse should check the vial carefully, and that if you administer it yourself, you will need to sign the administration section of the prescription.

### Further reading
Medical Pharmacology at a Glance. Chapter 29: Opioid analgesics.

## What should I consider when deciding what to prescribe?

Mr Stone is a 58-year-old man who has developed symptomatic hypotension following recent abdominal surgery for colorectal cancer. The key issues in managing his low blood pressure are acute relief of his hypotension and treatment of the underlying cause.

## Acute relief of hypotension

Mr Stone has returned to his bed with the help of the nursing staff. This prompt action, lying him flat with his legs raised, has acted as an internal fluid challenge by increasing venous return to his heart. This has improved his blood pressure. If he remains symptomatic or the blood pressure does not improve on lying flat you could consider an intravenous fluid challenge (see Case 20). However, as Mr Stone's systolic blood pressure is now greater than 100 mmHg and he is peripherally well perfused with a good urine output, this is not currently required.

## Identification and treatment of the underlying cause

Common and important causes of hypotension in the inpatient setting can be divided into the following:

1 *Hypovolaemia*, e.g. 'third space' losses, inadequate fluid replacement, bleeding
2 *Cardiogenic*, e.g. arrhythmia, pulmonary embolus, drug-induced
3 *Vasodilation*, e.g. sepsis, anaphylaxis, drug-induced.

To identify the cause of his hypotension you should fully assess Mr Stone. Using the ABCDE system, we can see that his airway is clear (he is able to talk to you to give you a history) and his breathing appears normal with normal oxygen saturations. Although his blood pressure is low, he appears to be perfusing his vital organs as he is alert with a normal capillary refill, pulse and urine output (>0.5 mL/kg/h). His abdomen is soft, with mild tenderness around his stoma site (which would be expected 5 days postoperatively) and there are no signs of active bleeding.

The cause of his low blood pressure is likely to be multifactorial: first, hypovolaemia due to third space losses and reduced oral intake because of pain and nausea; and, secondly, the vasodilatory effects of amlodipine.

Although regular antihypertensives can be continued perioperatively, in the context of hypotension Mr Stone's amlodipine should be discontinued. His blood pressure should be reviewed before discharge to determine whether it should be restarted. Amlodipine has a long duration of action, around 24 hours, so Mr Stone will be at risk of hypotension for 1–2 days after stopping the drug. You should therefore encourage him to take oral fluids and advise him to avoid sudden changes in posture. Compression stockings, if not already being used for venous thromboembolism prophylaxis, may also be applied to increase venous return from the peripheries.

As his pain is well controlled, you should avoid reducing or stopping his morphine (which is a potential cause of hypotension) for now. It is likely that as Mr Stone's analgesic requirements reduce and his appetite improves his blood pressure will return to its preoperative level.

Beta adrenoceptor blockers, such as bisoprolol, should be continued where possible, particularly in patients taking them for ischaemic heart disease, heart failure and arrhythmias. Abrupt cessation of beta adrenoceptor blockers can lead to dysrhythmias and angina, so it is reasonable to continue it for the time being. However, if his hypotension continues beyond the next 24 hours you should review its on-going need and seek advice from a senior colleague.

| Surname STONE | Hospital number 100018 | Weight 79 kg | Drug intolerances None known |
|---|---|---|---|
| First name THOMAS | Date of birth 11/04/1956 | | |

**REGULAR PRESCRIPTIONS**

Month: January  Year: 2015

| DRUG | Circle/enter times below | 2 | 3 | 4 | 5 | 6 | 7 | | | |
|---|---|---|---|---|---|---|---|---|---|---|
| AMLODIPINE | 06 | | | | | | | | | |
| Dose 5 mg / Route Oral / Freq Daily / Start date 2/1/15 | 08 | | AM | AM | AM | AM | AM | | STOPPED 7/1/15 Due to low BP, consider restarting before discharge | |
| Signature A Doctor / Bleep 1234 / Review | 12 | | | | | | | | | |
| | 16 | | | | | | | | A Doctor 1234 | |
| Additional instructions | 18 | | | | | | | | | |
| | 22 | | | | | | | | | |
| ASPIRIN | 06 | | | | | | | | | |
| Dose 75 mg / Route Oral / Freq Daily / Start date 2/1/15 | 08 | | AM | AM | AM | AM | AM | | | |
| Signature A Doctor / Bleep 1234 / Review | 12 | | | | | | | | | |
| | 16 | | | | | | | | | |
| Additional instructions | 18 | | | | | | | | | |
| | 22 | | | | | | | | | |
| BISOPROLOL | 06 | | | | | | | | | |
| Dose 5 mg / Route Oral / Freq Daily / Start date 2/1/15 | 08 | | AM | AM | AM | AM | AM | | | |
| Signature A Doctor / Bleep 1234 / Review | 12 | | | | | | | | | |
| | 16 | | | | | | | | | |
| Additional instructions | 18 | | | | | | | | | |
| | 22 | | | | | | | | | |
| DALTEPARIN | 06 | | | | | | | | | |
| Dose 5000 units / Route SC / Freq Daily / Start date 2/1/15 | 08 | | | | | | | | | |
| Signature A Doctor / Bleep 1234 / Review | 12 | | | | | | | | | |
| | 16 | | | | | | | | | |
| Additional instructions | 18 | AM | AM | AM | AM | AM | | | | |
| | 22 | | | | | | | | | |
| PARACETAMOL | 06 | | AM | AM | AM | AM | AM | | | |
| Dose 1 g / Route Oral / Freq 4 x daily / Start date 2/1/15 | 08 | | | | | | | | | |
| Signature A Doctor / Bleep 1234 / Review | 12 | | AM | AM | AM | AM | AM | | | |
| | 16 | | | | | | | | | |
| Additional instructions | 18 | | AM | AM | AM | AM | | | | |
| | 22 | AM | AM | AM | AM | AM | | | | |
| MST CONTINUS | 06 | | | AM | AM | AM | AM | | | |
| Dose 10 mg / Route Oral / Freq 12-hrly / Start date 3/1/15 | 08 | | | | | | | | | |
| Signature A Doctor / Bleep 1234 / Review | 12 | | | | | | | | | |
| | 16 | | | | | | | | | |
| Additional instructions Morphine sulfate M/R | 18 | | | AM | AM | AM | AM | | | |
| | 22 | | | | | | | | | |

**ONCE ONLY PRESCRIPTIONS**

| Date | Time to be given | DRUG | Dose | Route | Prescriber Signature | Prescriber Bleep | Administration Date given | Administration Time given | Administration Given by |
|---|---|---|---|---|---|---|---|---|---|
| | | | | | | | | | |
| | | | | | | | | | |
| | | | | | | | | | |

**OXYGEN**

| Target SpO₂ | ○ 94–98% ○ 88–92% |
|---|---|
| Mode of delivery | ○ Continuous ○ As required |
| Starting device | |

| Initials | Bleep | Date |
|---|---|---|
| | | |

**AS REQUIRED MEDICATION**

| DRUG ORAMORPH 10MG/5ML | | | | Date | 2/1 | 3/1 | 3/1 | 4/1 | 5/1 | | | | |
|---|---|---|---|---|---|---|---|---|---|---|---|---|---|
| | | | | Time | 2200 | 0800 | 1600 | 0800 | 1600 | | | | |
| Dose 5 mg | Route Oral | Max freq 4-hrly | Start date 2/1/15 | Dose | 5 mg | 5 mg | 5 mg | 5 mg | 5 mg | | | | |
| | | | | Route | Oral | Oral | Oral | Oral | Oral | | | | |
| Signature A Doctor | Bleep 1234 | Review | | Given | AM | AM | AM | AM | AM | | | | |
| | | | | Check | AD | AD | AD | AD | AD | | | | |
| Additional instructions Morphine sulfate, oral solution, for breakthrough pain | | | | | | | | | | | | | |

| DRUG METOCLOPRAMIDE | | | | Date | 2/1 | 3/1 | | | | | | | |
|---|---|---|---|---|---|---|---|---|---|---|---|---|---|
| | | | | Time | 2300 | 0900 | | | | | | | |
| Dose 10 mg | Route Oral | Max freq 8-hrly | Start date 2/1/15 | Dose | 10 mg | 10 mg | | | | | | | |
| | | | | Route | Oral | Oral | | | | | | | |
| Signature A Doctor | Bleep 1234 | Review | | Given | AM | AM | | | | | | | |
| | | | | Check | AD | AD | | | | | | | |
| Additional instructions For nausea and vomiting | | | | | | | | | | | | | |

| DRUG GLYCERYL TRINITRATE | | | | Date | | | | | | | | | |
|---|---|---|---|---|---|---|---|---|---|---|---|---|---|
| | | | | Time | | | | | | | | | |
| Dose 400 micrograms | Route SL | Max freq 5 min | Start date 2/1/15 | Dose | | | | | | | | | |
| | | | | Route | | | | | | | | | |
| Signature A Doctor | Bleep 1234 | Review | | Given | | | | | | | | | |
| | | | | Check | | | | | | | | | |
| Additional instructions For chest pain. Do not give if systolic BP less than 90 mmHg. | | | | | | | | | | | | | |

| DRUG | | | | Date | | | | | | | | | |
|---|---|---|---|---|---|---|---|---|---|---|---|---|---|
| | | | | Time | | | | | | | | | |
| Dose | Route | Max freq | Start date | Dose | | | | | | | | | |
| | | | | Route | | | | | | | | | |
| Signature | Bleep | Review | | Given | | | | | | | | | |
| | | | | Check | | | | | | | | | |
| Additional instructions | | | | | | | | | | | | | |

**INFUSION PRESCRIPTIONS**

| Date | Time | Fluid | Vol | Drug | Dose | Rate | Doctor initials | Nurse initials | Batch no | Start time | Stop time |
|---|---|---|---|---|---|---|---|---|---|---|---|
| 3/1/15 | 0600 | 0.9% SODIUM CHLORIDE | 1 L | POTASSIUM CHLORIDE | 20 mmol | 125 mL/hour | AD | AM | 01 | 0600 | 1400 |
| | | | | | | | | | | | |
| | | | | | | | | | | | |
| | | | | | | | | | | | |

## Continuing usual treatment

Mr Stone takes aspirin and glyceryl trinitrate for his cardiovascular disease and you should continue these during his admission. It may be useful to add additional instructions for nursing staff on when not to administer the glyceryl trinitrate to avoid unnecessary exacerbation of his hypotension.

## How do I write the prescription?
## Stopping medications

No new medications need to be prescribed for Mr Stone, but changes should be made to his existing medications.

*Amlodipine* should be crossed off the drug chart. You should date and sign the change. It is also helpful to indicate the conditions whereby the drug would need to be reinstated in the medical notes. You should review the need to reinstate the amlodipine before discharging him, or if discontinued you should make a note to his GP in the discharge summary to explain why it was stopped.

*Glyceryl trinitrate* can be continued as he may require it for relief of his angina. However, adding an additional instruction not to give it if his blood pressure is less than 90 mmHg in the context of chest pain will prevent any exacerbation of existing hypotension.

## Further reading

Medical Pharmacology at a Glance. Chapter 15: Drugs used in hypertension.

Prescribing at a Glance. Chapter 5: Reviewing current medicines.

SIGN 77. Principles of postoperative management. Available at: http://www.sign.ac.uk/pdf/qrg77.pdf (accessed 18 January 2014).

## What should I consider when deciding what to prescribe?

The way in which you prescribe fluids depends on what you are trying to achieve. There are two main reasons for prescribing intravenous fluid:

1 Provision of water and/or electrolytes
2 Expansion of intravascular volume.

In this case, there are no features to suggest intravascular volume depletion (see Case 20). Instead, our aim is to provide water and electrolytes. We now need to decide what her water and electrolyte requirements are. These fall under three categories: maintenance requirements, additional ongoing losses and existing deficits.

### Maintenance requirements

We have a baseline requirement for water and electrolytes to serve our physiological needs and to replace normal losses (e.g. through urine, faeces and evaporation). Typical requirements for an average adult are given in Table 19.2. The composition of several commonly-used preparations for fluid and electrolyte replacement is outlined in Table 19.3.

Traditional teaching said that a 'standard' fluid regimen to replace maintenance requirements comprised three bags: 'one salty' (0.9% sodium chloride) and 'two sweet' (5% glucose) – with each 1-L bag administered over 8 hours. We now recognise that this probably provides too much sodium and water for most patients, so our current preferred option is to reduce the volume of 0.9% sodium chloride to 500 mL/day. Assuming that the patient also has normal potassium losses (i.e. their renal function is normal), potassium chloride 20 mmol should be added to each bag. The bags of 5% glucose contain a relatively insignificant amount of glucose, so should be viewed simply as a way of providing water.

If the patient is able to take some, but not all, of their maintenance requirement, this should be taken into account. So, for example, if they can drink 500 mL water per day, then reduce the amount of glucose 5% by the same amount.

### Additional ongoing losses

If there are additional ongoing losses (e.g. from a surgical drain, stoma or through polyuria), these need to be factored in to the replacement regimen. You should replace them at a rate equivalent to the rate at which fluid is being lost (based on the fluid balance chart). Use a fluid preparation that approximates the composition of the fluid being lost:

• Losses from surgical drains, stomas, polyuria and vomiting are electrolyte-rich, and should be replaced by an electrolyte-rich fluid (e.g. Hartmann's solution or sodium chloride 0.9%)
• Losses of free water due to increased evaporation (e.g. in fever and hyperventilation) should usually be replaced with glucose 5%.

| Surname | DE LA CRUZ | Hospital number | 100019 | Weight | 80 kg | Drug intolerances | None known |

**REGULAR PRESCRIPTIONS**

| | | Circle / enter times below ↓ | ↘ Enter dates below | Month: January | Year: 2015 |
| DRUG PARACETAMOL | | 06 | | | |
| Dose 1 g | Route IV | Freq 6-hrly | Start date 7/1/15 | 08 / 12 | |
| Signature A Doctor | Bleep 1234 | Review | | 16 / 18 | |
| Additional instructions | | | | 22 24 | |
| DRUG DALETPARIN | | 06 | | | |
| Dose 2500 units | Route SC | Freq Daily | Start date 7/1/15 | 08 / 12 | |
| Signature A Doctor | Bleep 1234 | Review | | 16 / 18 | |
| Additional instructions | | | | 22 | |
| DRUG METOCLOPRAMIDE | | 06 | | | |
| Dose 10 mg | Route IV | Freq 8-hrly | Start date 7/1/15 | 08 / 12 | |
| Signature A Doctor | Bleep 1234 | Review | | 16 / 18 | |
| Additional instructions | | | | 22 24 | |
| DRUG PATIENT CONTROLLED ANALGESIA | | 06 | | | |
| Dose 1 mg | Route IV | Freq 5 min lockout | Start date 7/1/15 | 08 / 12 | |
| Signature A Doctor | Bleep 1234 | Review | | 16 / 18 | |
| Additional instructions For information only-see PCA chart | | | | 22 | |
| DRUG | | | | | |

**Table 19.2** Typical daily maintenance requirements of water, sodium and potassium, based on recommendations for intravenous fluid therapy in adult patients (see references)

| | Approximate daily requirement |
| --- | --- |
| Water | 30 mL/kg |
| Na$^+$ | 1 mmol/kg |
| K$^+$ | 1 mmol/kg |

**Table 19.3** Electrolyte content and other ingredients in 1 L of the stated crystalloid fluid preparation

| Fluid | Na$^+$ | K$^+$ | Ca$^{2+}$ | Cl$^-$ | Other | pH |
| --- | --- | --- | --- | --- | --- | --- |
| Sodium chloride 0.9% | 154 | – | – | 154 | – | 5.0 |
| Glucose ('dextrose') 5% | – | – | – | – | Glucose 50 g | 4.0 |
| Compound sodium lactate (Hartmann's) | 131 | 5 | 2 | 111 | Lactate 29 g | 6.5 |

## ONCE ONLY PRESCRIPTIONS

| Date | Time to be given | DRUG | Dose | Route | Prescriber | | Administration | | |
|------|------|------|------|------|------|------|------|------|------|
| | | | | | Signature | Bleep | Date given | Time given | Given by |
| | | | | | | | | | |
| | | | | | | | | | |
| | | | | | | | | | |

### OXYGEN

| Target SpO₂ | ○ 94–98% |
|---|---|
| | ○ 88–92% |
| Mode of delivery | ○ Continuous |
| | ○ As required |
| Starting device | |

| Initials | Bleep | Date |
|---|---|---|
| | | |

## AS REQUIRED MEDICATION

| DRUG CYCLIZINE | | | | Date | | | | | | | |
|---|---|---|---|---|---|---|---|---|---|---|---|
| | | | | Time | | | | | | | |
| Dose 50 mg | Route IV | Max freq 8-hrly | Start date 7/1/15 | Dose | | | | | | | |
| | | | | Route | | | | | | | |
| Signature A Doctor | Bleep 1234 | Review | | Given | | | | | | | |
| | | | | Check | | | | | | | |
| Additional instructions | | | | | | | | | | | |

| DRUG | | | | Date | | | | | | | |
|---|---|---|---|---|---|---|---|---|---|---|---|
| | | | | Time | | | | | | | |
| Dose | Route | Max freq | Start date | Dose | | | | | | | |
| | | | | Route | | | | | | | |
| Signature | Bleep | Review | | Given | | | | | | | |
| | | | | Check | | | | | | | |
| Additional instructions | | | | | | | | | | | |

| DRUG | | | | Date | | | | | | | |
|---|---|---|---|---|---|---|---|---|---|---|---|
| | | | | Time | | | | | | | |
| Dose | Route | Max freq | Start date | Dose | | | | | | | |
| | | | | Route | | | | | | | |
| Signature | Bleep | Review | | Given | | | | | | | |
| | | | | Check | | | | | | | |
| Additional instructions | | | | | | | | | | | |

| DRUG | | | | Date | | | | | | | |
|---|---|---|---|---|---|---|---|---|---|---|---|
| | | | | Time | | | | | | | |
| Dose | Route | Max freq | Start date | Dose | | | | | | | |
| | | | | Route | | | | | | | |
| Signature | Bleep | Review | | Given | | | | | | | |
| | | | | Check | | | | | | | |
| Additional instructions | | | | | | | | | | | |

## INFUSION PRESCRIPTIONS

| Date | Time | Fluid | Vol | Drug | Dose | Rate | Doctor initials | Nurse initials | Batch no | Start time | Stop time |
|------|------|------|------|------|------|------|------|------|------|------|------|
| 7/1/15 | 20:00 | GLUCOSE 5% | 1 L | POTASSIUM CHLORIDE | 20 mmol | 8 hr | AD | | | | |
| 7/1/15 | To follow | GLUCOSE 5% | 1 L | POTASSIUM CHLORIDE | 20 mmol | 8 hr | AD | | | | |
| 7/1/15 | To follow | SODIUM CHLORIDE 0.9% | 500 mL | POTASSIUM CHLORIDE | 20 mmol | 8 hr | AD | | | | |

This needs to be added to the maintenance regimen. So, for example, if the patient has the typical maintenance requirement (as detailed in Table 19.1), but is also losing 1.5 L/day from a stoma, the resulting requirement could be met by prescribing 2 L/ day of sodium chloride 0.9% (or Hartmann's solution) and 2 L/day of glucose 5%. Assuming normal renal function and serum potassium concentration, you should also prescribe potassium to cover the patient's maintenance requirement and additional losses. A good starting point would be to prescribe 20 mmol potassium chloride for each 1-L bag, but this should be adjusted according to the individual circumstances, serum potassium concentration and renal function.

Where a relatively large volume of sodium-rich fluid is required, it is often preferable to use Hartmann's solution rather than sodium chloride. The principal advantage of Hartmann's solution is its lower chloride concentration (as chloride, when given in large amounts, can generate a metabolic acidosis). Its disadvantage is that it offers less flexibility in relation to potassium replacement.

### Replacement of existing deficits

If the patient has already lost a significant volume of fluid prior to the institution of replacement therapy (e.g. severe diarrhoea and vomiting before presentation to hospital), the resultant deficits of both water and electrolytes may also need to be replaced. This is potentially complicated, and is heavily dependent on individual circumstances of the case, so you should always seek advice from a senior colleague (see Case 21).

### Putting it together

Mrs de la Cruz is unable to take anything by mouth, so we must replace the whole of her maintenance requirement (19.1). There are no additional on-going losses, and she has no existing deficits.

### How do I write the prescription?

Fluid prescriptions are written in the infusions section of the drug chart. All commonly used fluid preparations (including sodium chloride 0.9%, glucose 5% and Hartmann's solution) should be available in bags of 500 mL or 1 L volume (lower volume bags are also available for other purposes, such as diluting drugs).

When prescribing potassium, it is usually easiest to do this by specifying the amount (in mmol) to be contained in the bag, rather than its concentration. You do this by prescribing it as an additive. The solutions are, in fact, provided in ready-made form – potassium is not actually 'added' on the wards. Sodium chloride 0.9% and glucose 5% are available with potassium chloride in a concentration of 20 or 40 mmol/L. Hartmann's solution (also called compound sodium lactate) already contains a small amount of potassium chloride (5 mmol/L) – this does not need to be prescribed as an additive.

One way to give the 'standard' maintenance regimen is to prescribe two 1-L bags of glucose 5% and one 500-mL bag of sodium chloride 0.9%, each containing potassium chloride 20 mmol/L and administered over 8 hours. This approach will provide 2.5 L water, 77 mmol sodium and 60 mmol potassium per day. It is illustrated on the model chart.

### Further reading

National Institute for Health and Care Excellence. Intravenous fluid therapy in adults in hospital. NICE clinical guideline 174 (2013). Available at: http://guidance.nice.org.uk/CG174 (accessed 14 January 2014).

Powell-Tuck J, Gosling P, Lobo DN, et al. British Consensus Guidelines on Intravenous Fluid Therapy for Adult Surgical Patients. British Association for Parenteral and Enteral Nutrition (2011). Available at: http://www.bapen.org.uk/pdfs/bapen_pubs/giftasup.pdf (accessed 24 January 2014).

## What should I consider when deciding what to prescribe?

The management of a severely ill patient always starts with an ABCDE approach. Mr Hoyles is able to converse with you, suggesting that his airway is patent and his brain is perfused. His normal oxygen saturation while breathing air suggests that oxygenation is satisfactory, although an arterial blood sample will be required to assess the adequacy of ventilation and his acid–base status. However, he has signs of circulatory compromise (hypotension and tachycardia) and impaired tissue perfusion (prolonged capillary refill time and oliguria). Given his admission problem (pyelonephritis), it is most likely that this is due to the development of severe sepsis.

There is much controversy around the finer points of fluid resuscitation in sepsis. However, it is generally accepted that circulatory compromise due to sepsis should initially be assessed and managed by administering a fluid challenge. The aim of the fluid challenge is to bring about a transient expansion of circulating volume and, in turn, increased left ventricular (LV) filling. This serves two main purposes:

1 *Diagnostic.* Shock is often associated with reduced LV filling. The simplest example is haemorrhagic (hypovolaemic) shock, in which there is a reduction in total blood volume and therefore reduced venous return to the heart. In septic shock, reduction in venous return is due to generalised vasodilatation (increasing blood 'pooling' in capacitance vessels) and increased capillary permeability (with resultant diffusion of fluid out of the intravascular compartment). By contrast, in cardiogenic shock, venous return and LV filling may be normal or elevated. If shock is due to hypovolaemia or sepsis and you transiently increase LV filling by administering a fluid challenge, this should bring about favourable changes in physiological variables (e.g. a rise in blood pressure, reduction of tachycardia and improvement in other markers of tissue perfusion). By contrast, if the problem lies with an intrinsic failure of cardiac contractility (cardiogenic shock), the fluid challenge is more likely to cause a transient worsening in physiological variables.

2 *Therapeutic.* If tissue perfusion is compromised as a result of inadequate LV filling, the fluid challenge may (at least temporarily) ameliorate this, and thereby improve cardiac output and tissue oxygen delivery. This may 'buy time' while the underlying cause (e.g. haemorrhage, infection) is treated. It is important to appreciate that fluid resuscitation is not a definitive treatment for any form of shock.

## Principles of administering a fluid challenge

To make best use of a fluid challenge, you need to:
1 Increase LV filling by expanding intravascular (blood) volume
2 Assess the effects of this
3 Respond appropriately to your findings.

| Surname<br>HOYLES | Hospital number<br>100020 | Weight<br>71 kg | Drug intolerances<br>None known |
|---|---|---|---|
| First name<br>EMMANUEL | Date of birth<br>03/02/1955 | | |

**REGULAR PRESCRIPTIONS**

| | | | | Circle / enter times below ↓ | ↘ Enter dates below | Month: January | Year: 2015 |
|---|---|---|---|---|---|---|---|
| | | | | | 7 | | |
| DRUG CO-AMOXICLAV | | | | 06 (00) | An | | |
| | | | | (08) | An | | |
| Dose 1.2 g | Route IV | Freq 8-hrly | Start date 7/1/15 | 12 | | | |
| Signature A Doctor | | Bleep 1234 | Review 48 h | (16) | | | |
| | | | | 18 | | | |
| Additional instructions Pyelonephritis | | | | 22 | | | |
| DRUG DALTEPARIN | | | | 06 | | | |
| | | | | 08 | | | |
| Dose 5000 units | Route SC | Freq Daily | Start date 7/1/15 | 12 | | | |
| Signature A Doctor | | Bleep 1234 | Review | 16 | | | |
| Additional instructions | | | | (18) | | | |
| | | | | 22 | | | |
| DRUG PARACETAMOL | | | | 06 (00) | An | | |
| | | | | 08 (06) | An | | |
| Dose 1 g | Route Oral | Freq 6-hrly | Start date 7/1/15 | (12) | An | | |
| Signature A Doctor | | Bleep 1234 | Review | 16 | | | |
| Additional instructions | | | | (18) | | | |
| | | | | 22 | | | |
| DRUG | | | | | | | |

In order to expand circulating volume, you need to administer an appropriate fluid, in sufficient volume, as fast as possible.

The *fluid choice* may be a sodium-containing crystalloid, or a colloid. This is because the intravascular (blood) volume constitutes only about 10% of total body water (Figure 20.1A). If we use a glucose-based fluid (which will diffuse freely through all body water compartments; Figure 20.1B), we would need to give a large volume to make an appreciable difference to the intravascular volume. By contrast, if we use a sodium-containing crystalloid or a colloid, we can take advantage of natural physiological barriers:

- A *sodium-containing crystalloid* solution will freely diffuse out of the blood vessels, but not into cells (Figure 20.1C). This is because $Na^+/K^+$-ATPase on the cell membranes keeps sodium (and its osmotically-associated water) in the extracellular compartment. As plasma accounts for roughly 25% of extracellular water, about one-quarter of the volume you administer will remain in the intravascular space. The other three-quarters will contribute to the expansion of tissue fluid and the development of oedema.
- The idea behind *colloid* solutions is that they contain large, osmotically-active molecules (e.g. albumin, gelatin or modified starch), which cannot diffuse through the capillary wall. Consequently, in theory, the whole of the administered volume should remain in the intravascular space. This means that less fluid is needed to expand circulating volume and that there should be less oedema. In reality, however, while it is probably true that there is *initially* a greater increase in circulating volume when using a colloid solution, this effect is relatively brief. The mole-

## ONCE ONLY PRESCRIPTIONS

| Date | Time to be given | DRUG | Dose | Route | Prescriber | | Administration | | |
|------|------------------|------|------|-------|-----------|-------|------------|-----------|----------|
| | | | | | Signature | Bleep | Date given | Time given | Given by |
| | | | | | | | | | |
| | | | | | | | | | |
| | | | | | | | | | |

### OXYGEN

| | | |
|---|---|---|
| Target SpO₂ | ○ 94–98% | |
| | ○ 88–92% | |
| Mode of delivery | ○ Continuous | |
| | ○ As required | |
| Starting device | | |

| Initials | Bleep | Date |
|----------|-------|------|
| | | |

## AS REQUIRED MEDICATION

| DRUG CYCLIZINE | | | | Date | 7/1 | 7/1 | | | | | | | |
|---|---|---|---|---|---|---|---|---|---|---|---|---|---|
| | | | | Time | 0200 | 1000 | | | | | | | |
| Dose 50 mg | Route IV/Oral | Max freq 8-hrly | Start date 7/1/15 | Dose | 50mg | 50mg | | | | | | | |
| | | | | Route | IV | IV | | | | | | | |
| Signature A Doctor | Bleep 1234 | Review | | Given | AM | AM | | | | | | | |
| | | | | Check | DA | DA | | | | | | | |
| Additional instructions | | | | | | | | | | | | | |

| DRUG ORAMORPH 10MG/5ML | | | | Date | 7/1 | 7/1 | | | | | | | |
|---|---|---|---|---|---|---|---|---|---|---|---|---|---|
| | | | | Time | 0200 | 0600 | | | | | | | |
| Dose 5mg | Route Oral | Max freq 4-hrly | Start date 7/1/15 | Dose | 5mg | 5mg | | | | | | | |
| | | | | Route | Oral | Oral | | | | | | | |
| Signature A Doctor | Bleep 1234 | Review | | Given | AM | AM | | | | | | | |
| | | | | Check | DA | DA | | | | | | | |
| Additional instructions Morphine sulfate, oral solution, for pain | | | | | | | | | | | | | |

| DRUG | | | | Date | | | | | | | | | |
|---|---|---|---|---|---|---|---|---|---|---|---|---|---|
| | | | | Time | | | | | | | | | |
| Dose | Route | Max freq | Start date | Dose | | | | | | | | | |
| | | | | Route | | | | | | | | | |
| Signature | Bleep | Review | | Given | | | | | | | | | |
| | | | | Check | | | | | | | | | |
| Additional instructions | | | | | | | | | | | | | |

| DRUG | | | | Date | | | | | | | | | |
|---|---|---|---|---|---|---|---|---|---|---|---|---|---|
| | | | | Time | | | | | | | | | |
| Dose | Route | Max freq | Start date | Dose | | | | | | | | | |
| | | | | Route | | | | | | | | | |
| Signature | Bleep | Review | | Given | | | | | | | | | |
| | | | | Check | | | | | | | | | |
| Additional instructions | | | | | | | | | | | | | |

## INFUSION PRESCRIPTIONS

| Date | Time | Fluid | Vol | Drug | Dose | Rate | Doctor initials | Nurse initials | Batch no | Start time | Stop time |
|------|------|-------|-----|------|------|------|-----------------|----------------|----------|-----------|-----------|
| 7/1/15 | 14:00 | 0.9% SODIUM CHLORIDE | 500 mL | - | - | 15 min | AD | | | | |
| | | | | | | | | | | | |
| | | | | | | | | | | | |
| | | | | | | | | | | | |

cule (and its associated water) will eventually leak through the capillary membrane and equilibrate through the extracellular space (Figure 20.1D). Paradoxically, the rate of leak is usually greatest in the most unwell patients – the very patients in whom you would most like the fluid to remain confined to the intravascular space. The other problem with colloids, which is not the case for crystalloids, is that the colloid molecule may incite an anaphylactic reaction in susceptible individuals, or have toxic effects of its own (e.g. modified starches appear to have adverse effects on renal function and coagulation).

The *initial volume* of a fluid challenge depends on the characteristics of the patient and the choice of fluid. For a patient with good physiological reserve (i.e. without significant intrinsic cardiac disease), you would typically prescribe 250–500 mL of a sodium-containing crystalloid. If using a colloid, this volume should be halved (e.g. 125–250 mL). If the patient has poor cardiac reserve, it is prudent to administer a lower volume (say 125–250 mL of a crystalloid).

The *rate of administration* should be as fast as possible. This will maximise the transient volume-expansion effect, and allow you to judge the physiological impact of this. In theory, the rate of administration is governed by the flow characteristics of the cannula, which is dependent on its diameter and length. For example, a

green (18 G) cannula will theoretically allow a maximum flow rate of approximately 100 mL/min (exact figures can be found on the product packaging). In practice, however, there are many other factors that will limit this, such that the quoted maximum is not usually achieved. Prescribing the fluid challenge to be administered over about 15 minutes is reasonable.

### Further assessment

Immediately after administering the fluid challenge it is essential to assess its effects. This should include re-measurement of vital signs, capillary refill time and, where relevant, urine output and serum lactate concentration. Further fluid management must be judged on a case-by-case basis with input from experienced clinicians. The strategies outlined below are broad recommendations only.

- *No response:* Ensure the fluid challenge is optimal (appropriate fluid, sufficient volume, as fast as possible), then repeat and reassess. Seek senior/specialist advice.
- *Improvement in haemodynamic markers:* additional fluid challenges may be needed to achieve and maintain appropriate physiological goals while the underlying cause is being addressed. Prescribe maintenance fluid (see Case 19) if indicated.
- *Deterioration in haemodynamic markers or respiratory function:* seek urgent support from a specialist in the management of critical illness.

### Other aspects of management

This case discussion has focused on fluid resuscitation, but there are several other management strategies that need to be addressed in parallel with this. Foremost amongst these is the need to seek senior support – at F1 level, you should not attempt to manage a severely ill patient such as this on your own.

As noted above, fluid resuscitation is never a definitive treatment for shock; the underlying cause must be identified and addressed. Mr Hoyles probably has severe sepsis due to pyelonephritis, and his antimicrobial treatment may need to be broadened. Imaging (e.g. an ultrasound scan of the urinary tract) may be necessary to exclude urinary tract obstruction: if this is present, drainage will be required to control the infective source. If his condition does not improve promptly with initial management, he may need to be transferred to the high dependency unit. The critical care team should therefore be involved in his care as soon as possible.

### How do I write the prescription?

You should prescribe the fluid challenge in the infusions section of the drug chart. As appropriate, prescribe 0.9% sodium chloride (not 'normal saline', which is a misleading term) or compound sodium lactate (its eponymous name, Hartmann's solution, is also acceptable, but less descriptive). If using a colloid fluid (e.g. Gelofusine®, Volplex®), it is usually best to prescribe it by proprietary name, as approved non-proprietary names do not usually exist. Do *not* prescribe any added drugs (e.g. potassium chloride) in a fluid challenge.

Specify a time period for administration (e.g. 15 min). Do not write 'stat' (meaning 'immediately'), as this is imprecise, leaves an

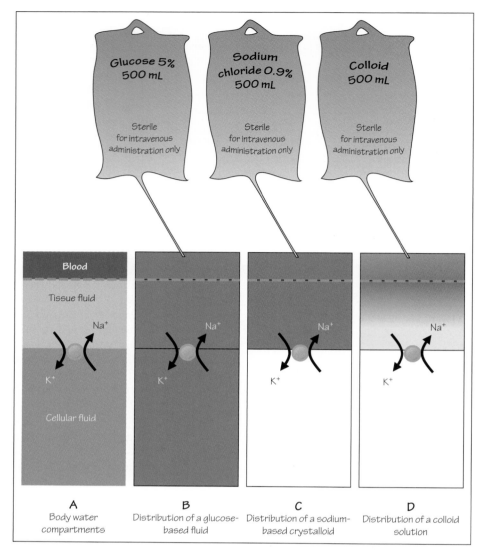

**Figure 20.1** Body water compartments (A) and the distribution of intravenous fluid preparations across these compartments (B–D). The dashed line signifies the capillary membrane.

inadequate audit trail and has various practical interpretations (e.g. 'give at the time prescribed'/'administer over a short time period'/'give as a matter of extreme urgency').

The model prescription chart provides an example of a typical fluid challenge, appropriate for the patient described in the scenario.

### Further reading

National Institute for Health and Care Excellence. Intravenous fluid therapy in adults in hospital. NICE clinical guideline 174 (2013). Available at: http://guidance.nice.org.uk/CG174 (accessed 14 January 2014).

| Surname | Hospital number | Weight | Drug intolerances |
|---|---|---|---|
| JASWAL | 100021 | | None known |
| First name | Date of birth | 12 kg | |
| RANI | 16/10/2013 | | |

**REGULAR PRESCRIPTIONS**

| | | Circle / enter times below ↓ | ⭨ Enter dates below | | | | Month: January | | Year: 2015 | |
|---|---|---|---|---|---|---|---|---|---|---|
| DRUG | | 06 | | | | | | | | |
| | | 08 | | | | | | | | |
| Dose | Route | Freq | Start date | 12 | | | | | | |
| Signature | | Bleep | Review | 16 | | | | | | |
| Additional instructions | | | | 18 | | | | | | |

**INFUSION PRESCRIPTIONS**

| Date | Time | Fluid | Vol | Drug | Dose | Rate | Doctor initials | Nurse initials | Batch no | Start time | Stop time |
|---|---|---|---|---|---|---|---|---|---|---|---|
| 7/1/15 | 17:30 | 0.45% SODIUM CHLORIDE WITH 5% GLUCOSE | 1 L | POTASSIUM CHLORIDE | 20 mmol | 71mL/hr | AD | | | | |
| 7/1/15 | To follow | 0.45% SODIUM CHLORIDE WITH 5% GLUCOSE | 500 mL | POTASSIUM CHLORIDE | 10 mmol | 71 mL/hr | AD | | | | |
| | | | | | | | | | | | |
| | | | | | | | | | | | |

## What should I consider when deciding what to prescribe?

### How much fluid does she need?

As in adults (see Case 19), intravenous fluid prescriptions for children may serve two purposes:
1 Provision of water and electrolytes
2 Expansion of intravascular volume.

Rani has become dehydrated due to viral gastroenteritis, but shows no signs of shock. As such, the focus of this case is on water and electrolyte provision; it does not deal with expansion of intravascular volume (fluid resuscitation; see Case 20).

When determining a child's requirement for water and electrolytes, you should take account of:
• Maintenance requirements (to sustain normal physiological processes)
• Additional ongoing losses (from ongoing pathological processes, e.g. diarrhoea, vomiting)
• Existing deficits (due to fluid loss in excess of intake in the period before presentation).

In contrast to adult practice, however, it is not appropriate to work from 'typical values' when determining a child's fluid needs. Crucially, the fluid requirements of a child depend on body weight, and as such, a calculation is almost always required.

### Maintenance requirement

The method for calculating maintenance fluid requirement is based on dividing the child's body weight into three bands (referred to as A, B and C in Box 21.1). The amount of fluid required per kilogram of body weight is different in each band.

Rani weighs 12 kg, so in her case, only the first two weight bands are relevant. Her maintenance requirement is:

**A** 100 mL/kg/day × 10 kg = 1000 mL/day
**B** 50 mL/kg/day × 2 kg = 100 mL/day
**C** 20 mL/kg/day × 0 kg = 0 mL/day

Maintenance requirement = A + B + C = **1100 mL/day**.

### Additional ongoing losses

The next step is to make an adjustment, if necessary, for any additional ongoing losses. For example, if Rani still had significant vomiting or diarrhoea, the losses associated with this should be added to her maintenance requirement. However, as Rani's gastrointestinal fluid losses have now reduced significantly, no adjustment needs to be made.

### Existing deficits

Finally, you need to replace any existing deficit. Rani is estimated to be 5% dehydrated. Using the formula provided her deficit is:

$$\text{Deficit} = 5 \times 12 \times 10 = 600 \text{ mL}.$$

### Putting it together

The total fluid requirement is the sum of the individual volumes calculated in the steps described above:

Daily fluid requirement = maintenance requirement
+ additional ongoing losses + deficit

This is divided by 24 to give the hourly rate:

Hourly fluid requirement = daily fluid requirement ÷ 24

Applying this in Rani's case gives:

Daily fluid requirement = 1100 mL + 600 mL = 1700 mL
Hourly fluid requirement = 1700 ÷ 24 = 70.8 mL/hr

### Which fluid?

When prescribing for children it is convenient to use a compound fluid preparation that contains both glucose and sodium chloride. Using the same fluid throughout the day avoids the need to stop infusions part way through a bag (because the volumes involved typically do not align with 'standard volume' infusion bags). A common choice for replacement of maintenance fluid and deficits is 0.45% sodium chloride with 5% glucose. Potassium chloride should be included (usually at a concentration of 20 mmol/L) if potassium losses are anticipated (including though normal urine output). Decisions about which fluid to use should always take account of the clinical circumstances and serum electrolyte concentrations. Rani has had gastroenteritis and cannot eat or drink, and her serum potassium concentration is at the lower limit of normal, so she will require potassium replacement.

### Additional considerations
Children receiving IV fluids should be monitored carefully and have daily measurement of the renal profile, particularly to detect hyponatraemia. IV fluids should be stopped and dietary intake resumed as soon as possible.

Prescribing intravenous fluid for children is complex. Remember that you should never prescribe in a situation that goes beyond your level of competence without direct supervision.

### How do I write the prescription?
Write your fluid prescription in the infusions section of the pre-scription chart. When prescribing for children, the rate of admin-istration should always be specified in mL/hour. In the model

prescription, potassium chloride has been prescribed as an additive to the base fluid 0.45% sodium chloride with 5% glucose. Although this is the conventional way of writing the prescription, you should be aware that in practice the fluid is provided ready prepared.

As with adults, fluid comes in set volume bags. We have chosen to prescribe one 1000-mL bag and one 500-mL bag, which will last 21 hours. This is appropriate as Rani's ongoing need for IV fluid replacement may change and should be reviewed within this time period.

### Further reading
Prescribing at a Glance. Chapter 16: Prescribing in children.
Department of Health, Social Services and Public Safety (Northern Ireland). Paediatric parenteral fluid therapy (1 month – 16 years): initial management guideline (2007). Available at: http://www.dhsspsni.gov.uk/hsc__sqsd__20-07_wallchart.pdf (accessed 24 January 2014).

---

## 22 | A 5-year-old boy with a painful right arm

### What should I consider when deciding what to prescribe?
#### How bad is the pain?
It can be difficult to assess severity of pain in children, but there are a variety of tools to help (e.g. the Face, Legs, Activity, Cry, Consolability (FLACC) scale in infants and children aged 2 months to 7 years; or a visual analogue scale for older children). As Charlie is able to describe his pain as 'bad', this is sufficient to indicate the need for analgesia without necessitating reference to a scoring system.

### What measures should be taken?
Thorough clinical assessment of any child in severe pain is very important to ensure the diagnosis is correct and to determine whether any measures other than analgesia are required.

For Charlie, the working diagnosis is postoperative pain. However, it is important to exclude compartment syndrome or other operative complications. Compartment syn-drome occurs when there is swelling, e.g. due to bleeding, within a muscle compartment enclosed by fascial layers. This causes com-pression of vasculature and nerves crossing the compartment and ischaemic damage to muscle, which may result in loss of the limb. Compartment syndrome in the arm can be recognised by pallor, paraesthesia and pulselessness in the hand. Reassuringly, Charlie's hand has normal colour, temperature and sensation, making this diagnosis unlikely. Charlie's vital signs are also normal for a 5-year-old child.

### General approach to analgesia
As in adults, the World Health Organization (WHO) pain ladder can provide a useful reference when prescribing analgesia in chil-dren, with the caveat that this was designed principally to guide the treatment of chronic pain. Nevertheless, it is important to remember that, unless the source of the pain is likely to resolve

| Surname HEWETT | Hospital number 100022 | Weight 22 kg | Drug intolerances None known |
| First name CHARLIE | Date of birth 11/06/2009 | | |

**REGULAR PRESCRIPTIONS**

| | Circle / enter times below ↓ | ↘ Enter dates below | Month: January | Year: 2015 |
|---|---|---|---|---|
| | | 7 | | |
| DRUG PARACETAMOL | 06 | | | |
| Dose 330 mg / Route Oral / Freq 6-hrly / Start date 7/1/15 | 08 | | | |
| | 12 | | | |
| Signature A Doctor / Bleep 1234 / Review 9/1/15 | 16 | | | |
| | 18 | OMIT | | |
| Additional instructions 15mg/kg | 22 | | | |
| DRUG IBUPROFEN | 06 | | | |
| Dose 150 mg / Route Oral / Freq 8-hrly / Start date 7/1/15 | 08 | | | |
| | 12 | | | |
| Signature A Doctor / Bleep 1234 / Review 9/1/15 | ✗ 14 | | | |
| | 18 | | | |
| Additional instructions With meals/food | 22 | | | |
| DRUG | 06 | | | |

imminently, regularly administered analgesia is usually better than as required administration. The WHO pain ladder suggests using paracetamol in the first instance, with non-steroidal anti-inflammatory drugs (NSAIDs) considered as adjuvant therapy in selected cases. So far, Charlie has not been offered any regular analgesia, but has been given intravenous morphine on an as required basis. The prescription of morphine is not necessarily inappropriate, but it would be better if it was supported by regular non-opioid analgesia, and if the adverse effects of morphine were addressed.

### Supplementary prescribing with morphine
#### Anti-emetics
As is commonly the case, morphine has made Charlie vomit. It is important to give an anti-emetic with morphine to prevent this. For children, the choice of anti-emetic is usually a histamine ($H_1$) receptor antagonist, such as cyclizine, or a serotonin ($5HT_3$)

## ONCE ONLY PRESCRIPTIONS

| Date | Time to be given | DRUG | Dose | Route | Prescriber Signature | Prescriber Bleep | Administration Date given | Administration Time given | Administration Given by |
|------|------------------|------|------|-------|-----------|-------|------------|------------|----------|
| 7/1/15 | 16:00 | ONDANSETRON | 2 mg | IV | AD | 1234 | | | |
| 7/1/15 | 16:15 | PARACETAMOL | 440 mg | Oral | AD | 1234 | | | |
| | | | | | | | | | |

## AS REQUIRED MEDICATION

**DRUG** MORPHINE SULFATE

| Dose | Route | Max freq | Start date | | Date | 7/1 | | | | |
|------|-------|----------|-----------|--|------|------|--|--|--|--|
| 2–4 mg | IV | 4-hrly | 7/1/15 | | Time | 14:00 | | | | |
| Signature | | Bleep | Review | | Dose | 4 mg | | | | |
| A Doctor | | 1234 | | | Route | IV | | | | |
| | | | | | Given | AM | | | | |
| | | | | | Check | AM | | | | |

Additional instructions
Titrate to pain.

**DRUG** ONDANSETRON

| Dose | Route | Max freq | Start date | | Date | | | | | |
|------|-------|----------|-----------|--|------|--|--|--|--|--|
| 2 mg | IV | 12-hrly | 7/1/15 | | Time | | | | | |
| Signature | | Bleep | Review | | Dose | | | | | |
| A Doctor | | 1234 | | | Route | | | | | |
| | | | | | Given | | | | | |
| | | | | | Check | | | | | |

Additional instructions
For vomiting caused by morphine

## OXYGEN

| | | |
|--|--|--|
| Target SpO$_2$ | ○ 94–98% | |
| | ○ 88–92% | |
| Mode of delivery | ○ Continuous | |
| | ○ As required | |
| Starting device | | |
| Initials | Bleep | Date |

receptor antagonist, such as ondansetron (for more detail on prescribing anti-emetics, see Case 28). Dopamine (D$_2$) receptor antagonists (e.g. metoclopramide, phenothiazines) should be avoided as they can cause severe dystonic reactions in children and young people. Ondansetron is licensed in children for the treatment of postoperative nausea and vomiting and is a good choice for Charlie.

### Laxatives

If Charlie is likely to need morphine for a few days, it may be worth co-prescribing a laxative. Suitable choices for opioid-induced constipation include osmotic laxatives (e.g. lactulose, macrogols) and stimulant laxatives (e.g. senna). As we do not anticipate an ongoing need for opioids in Charlie's case, we have not prescribed a laxative.

### Other considerations

In children admitted to hospital (unlike in adults) VTE prophylaxis is not routinely required. However, prophylaxis should be considered in children with one or more risk factors for VTE including: central venous access, an inherited predisposition (e.g. factor V Leiden mutation), nephrotic syndrome, severe infection or cancer. None of these apply in Charlie's case.

### How do I write the prescription?
### Weight-based dosing

Dosing information for drugs used in children is provided in the British National Formulary (BNF), but for more detailed information you should ideally refer to the BNF for Children (BNFc). Doses are often specified for the child's weight (e.g. on a mg per kg basis). It is therefore very important that you have an accurate weight for Charlie before writing the prescription. As dose calculations usually use the child's actual body weight, those who are overweight or obese may be at risk of overdosage. To avoid this, you need to refer to the recommended maximum dose for that child's age.

### Route of administration

An important consideration in prescribing for children is the route of administration. Younger children may not be able to swallow tablets, so a liquid formulation of oral medicines is highly desirable. The rectal route is often well tolerated in children, whereas intramuscular injections should generally be avoided.

### Prescribing for Charlie

You should prescribe paracetamol and ibuprofen as regular prescriptions, using dosing guidance from the BNFc. You should check the morphine dose and prescribe ondansetron to be given with morphine in the as-required section of the drug chart.

### Paracetamol

The BNFc states that, for severe postoperative pain, children aged 6–12 years should receive paracetamol 20–30 mg/kg (max 1 g) as a single dose, then 15–20 mg/kg every 4–6 hours (the total daily dose should not exceed 90 mg/kg or 4 g, whichever is lower).

Charlie is 22 kg. On the model prescription we have chosen a regular paracetamol dose of 330 mg 6-hourly (15 mg/kg × 22 kg). This will result in a safe total daily dose of 1320 mg or 60 mg/kg. However, the first regular dose will not be given until 18:00 and it is currently 16:00. You should therefore write up a once only dose for Charlie to take now (or after the anti-emetic when he has stopped vomiting), which could safely be at a slightly higher dose of 440 mg (20 mg/kg). In this situation you should omit the 18:00 dose, as shown.

### Non-steroidal anti-inflammatory drugs

NSAIDs can be used in children, although aspirin should be avoided in those aged <16 years because of the risk of Reye's syndrome. Ibuprofen is a reasonable choice.

The BNFc recommends that children aged 4–7 years should receive ibuprofen at a dose of 150 mg three times daily, preferably after food. This has been prescribed for Charlie on the model prescription.

### Morphine

The BNFc-recommended dose for children aged 6 months–12 years is initially 100 micrograms/kg every 4 hours, adjusted according to response. The prescribed dose for Charlie (2–4 mg) is equivalent to 100–200 micrograms/kg.

### Ondansetron

The BNFc-recommended dose for the treatment of postoperative nausea and vomiting in children aged 1 month–18 years is 100 micrograms/kg (max 4 mg). It is reasonable to give this now, provided it has not already been administered within the last 12 hours, in which case an alternative agent should be used (check the anaesthetic chart to confirm it was not given intra-operatively). At 22 kg, Charlie should receive 2 mg of ondansetron (22 × 100 micrograms = 2200 micrograms = 2.2 mg, rounded down to 2 mg for ease of administration). On the model prescription we have prescribed this to be given as needed at 12-hourly intervals.

### Further reading

Medical Pharmacology at a Glance. Chapter 29: Opioid analgesics; Chapter 32: Non-steroidal anti-inflammatory drugs.
Prescribing at a Glance. Chapter 16: Prescribing in children.
BNF for Children (BNFc). Available at: http://www.bnf.org/bnf/org_450055.htm (accessed 24 January 2014).

## What should I consider when deciding what to prescribe?

Amos Jones is a newborn baby with fever and poor feeding. Although his delivery was uneventful, he is now displaying concerning signs of neonatal sepsis, including respiratory distress. Antibiotics should be started as a matter of urgency while further investigations, particularly microbiological cultures, are being performed as Amos has the potential to deteriorate very quickly.

### Neonatal sepsis

Risk factors for early neonatal sepsis include: maternal group B streptococcal colonisation, invasive group B streptococcal infection in a previous baby, pre-labour rupture of membranes, maternal illness and prematurity (less than 3 weeks' gestational age).

Amos is at high risk of neonatal sepsis because of prolonged rupture of membranes during labour. Neonatal sepsis often presents with non-specific signs, so you should have a high suspicion for it, and a low threshold to start antibiotics.

### Which antibiotics?

NICE guidelines recommend intravenous benzylpenicillin and gentamicin for early neonatal sepsis. Each hospital will have their own antibiotic prescribing guidelines for paediatrics and you should make sure that you refer to these.

Neonates with bacteraemia have potential to go on to develop meningitis, which may also present with non-specific signs. Amos is therefore likely to require a lumbar puncture when it is safe to perform one. If this were to show evidence of meningitis, then the antibiotics would need to be reviewed.

### Oxygen

Amos has oxygen saturations of 92%. Neonates who are unwell are nursed in an incubator where they can receive ambient oxygen. Prescription of this should be by a neonatal specialist. We therefore have not addressed this in this case.

### How do I write the prescription?

### Applying guidelines

For neonatal prescriptions, doses may vary according to postmenstrual (gestational) age. It is therefore very important to know the gestational age of the baby you are prescribing for. Amos was delivered at term, therefore his gestational age is 40 weeks.

### Calculating doses

In neonates it is very important for drug doses to be accurate. You should therefore prescribe to one decimal place. This is because the effect of rounding is proportionately greater when the dose is small.

### Gentamicin

The BNFc dosing guidance indicates that Amos should receive 4–5 mg/kg gentamicin. As he is 4.22 kg, this range would equate to

| Surname | Hospital number | Weight | Drug intolerances |
|---|---|---|---|
| JONES | 100023 | 4.22 kg | None known |
| First name | Date of birth | | |
| AMOS | 06/01/2015 | | |

**REGULAR PRESCRIPTIONS**

**ONCE ONLY PRESCRIPTIONS**

| Date | Time to be given | DRUG | Dose | Route | Prescriber Signature | Prescriber Bleep | Administration Date given | Administration Time given | Administration Given by |
|---|---|---|---|---|---|---|---|---|---|
| 7/1/15 | 10:00 | GENTAMICIN | 21.1 mg | IV | AD | 1234 | | | |
| 7/1/15 | 10:00 | BENZYLPENICILLIN | 211 mg | IV | AD | 1234 | | | |

**OXYGEN**

Target SpO₂: ○ 94–98% ○ 88–92%
Mode of delivery: ○ Continuous ○ As required
Starting device

| Initials | Bleep | Date |
|---|---|---|

**AS REQUIRED MEDICATION**

| DRUG 0.9% SODIUM CHLORIDE | Date | | | | | |
|---|---|---|---|---|---|---|
| | Time | | | | | |
| Dose 0.5–1 mL | Route IV | Max freq As flush | Start date 7/1/15 | Dose | | |
| | | | | Route | | |
| Signature A Doctor | | Bleep 1234 | Review 8/1/15 | Given | | |
| | | | | Check | | |

Additional instructions
To flush cannula as required

16.9–21.1 mg in his case. As Amos is severely unwell we have selected the top of the dose range and prescribed 21.1 mg gentamicin.

### Benzylpenicillin

BNFc dosing guidance indicates that Amos should receive 50 mg/kg as he has severe neonatal sepsis. You should therefore prescribe 211 mg (it is not necessary to write 211.0 mg – indeed, it is preferable to avoid unnecessary use of a decimal point because of the risk of consequent dosing errors).

### Writing the prescription

The task was to prescribe an urgent dose of these antibiotics. We have therefore prescribed them in the once only section of the chart for immediate administration. Both have been written up for intravenous administration. In neonatal medicine, any flush used for the cannula should also be prescribed on the drug chart, as even small repeated volumes of sodium chloride administered for a flush may be significant in altering the fluid balance of a neonate.

### What next?

Amos will need antibiotic treatment for several days depending on how he progresses. You should therefore write the antibiotics up regularly, making sure you include the indication (i.e. what you are treating) as well as a review date. The review date is often initially written as the date when culture results are due (36–48 hours), at which point antibiotics may be altered according to available antimicrobial sensitivities. A further decision can then also be made regarding the duration of treatment.

Where further doses of gentamicin are required, gentamicin levels should be measured (according to local policy) with adjustment of dose and/or frequency according to results. Renal function can be extremely variable in the first few of days of life, which may cause fluctuations in gentamicin levels, with subsequent risk of ototoxicity and nephrotoxicity.

### Further reading
Medical Pharmacology at a Glance. Chapters 38 and 39: Antibacterial drugs.

Prescribing at a Glance. Chapter 16: Prescribing in children.
National Institute for Health and Clinical Excellence. Antibiotics for early-onset neonatal infection. NICE clinical guideline 149 (2012). Available at: http://www.nice.org.uk/nicemedia/live/13867/60633/60633.pdf (accessed 18 January 2014).

## 24  A 60-year-old man who has developed a hot joint

| Surname | Hospital number | Weight | Drug intolerances |
|---|---|---|---|
| GONZALEZ | 100024 | 82 kg | ~~None known~~ |
| First name | Date of birth | | Bendroflumethiazide – acute gout |
| JUAN | 19/10/1954 | | AD 7/1/15 |

**REGULAR PRESCRIPTIONS**

Circle / enter times below ↓ — Enter dates below — Month: January  Year: 2015  Date: 7

| DRUG ALLOPURINOL | | | | 06 / (08) / 12 / 16 / 18 / 22 |
|---|---|---|---|---|
| Dose 100 mg | Route Oral | Freq Daily | Start date 7/1/15 | |
| Signature A Doctor | Bleep 1234 | Review | | |
| Additional instructions | | | | |

| DRUG AMLODIPINE | | | | 06 / (08) / 12 / 16 / 18 / 22 |
|---|---|---|---|---|
| Dose 10 mg | Route Oral | Freq Daily | Start date 7/1/15 | |
| Signature A Doctor | Bleep 1234 | Review | | |
| Additional instructions | | | | |

| DRUG BENDROFLUMETHIAZIDE | | | | (08) / 12 / 16 / 18 / 22 |
|---|---|---|---|---|
| Dose 2.5 mg | Route Oral | Freq Daily | Start date 7/1/15 | STOP 7/1/15 A Doctor Bl 1234 |
| Signature A Doctor | Bleep 1234 | Review | | |
| Additional instructions | | | | |

| DRUG RAMIPRIL | | | | 06 / (08) / 12 / 16 / 18 / 22 |
|---|---|---|---|---|
| Dose 10 mg | Route Oral | Freq Daily | Start date 7/1/15 | |
| Signature A Doctor | Bleep 1234 | Review | | |
| Additional instructions | | | | |

| DRUG DALTEPARIN | | | | 06 / 08 / 12 / 16 / (18) AM / 22 |
|---|---|---|---|---|
| Dose 5000 units | Route SC | Freq Daily | Start date 7/1/15 | |
| Signature A Doctor | Bleep 1234 | Review | | |
| Additional instructions | | | | |

| DRUG NAPROXEN | | | | (06) / 08 / 12 (14) / 16 / 18 / (22) |
|---|---|---|---|---|
| Dose 250 mg | Route Oral | Freq 8-hrly | Start date 7/1/15 | |
| Signature A Doctor | Bleep 1234 | Review 1 week | | |
| Additional instructions With food | | | | |

### What should I consider when deciding what to prescribe?
Mr Gonzalez has an acute monoarthritis of his first metatarsophalangeal joint, without systemic symptoms or signs. He has a history of gout and hypertension, and has recently started taking a new anti-hypertensive medication. In addition, he consumes approximately 35 units a week of alcohol. The key issues in managing his acute monoarthritis are acute relief of his pain and identification and treatment of the underlying cause.

### Identifying the cause and precipitant
Common and important causes of an acute monoarthritis include septic arthritis, crystal arthropathies (e.g. gout and pseudogout), an inflammatory arthritis flare and trauma. In this case, the history and examination findings are suggestive of acute gout. A hot swollen first metatarsophalangeal joint is almost always due to gout and can be diagnosed clinically. However, if there is any diagnostic doubt, particularly regarding the possibility of septic arthritis, you should seek a specialist review and obtain a sample of synovial fluid by needle aspiration. Send this for polarized microscopy, Gram stain and culture.

Precipitants of acute gout include trauma, surgery, dehydration, infection and medications. The likely precipitant here is bendroflumethiazide, which is known to cause hyperuricaemia and gout. This should be stopped and alternative anti-hypertensive therapy considered at a later date.

### Management of acute gout
High-dose non-steroidal anti-inflammatory drugs (NSAIDs) are the first-line treatment for acute gout. You should choose an NSAID which has a rapid onset of action when taken orally. There is no evidence to suggest that any NSAID is more efficacious over another in the treatment of gout. Before starting an NSAID, you should consider any significant cautions or contraindications such as asthma, renal impairment, liver impairment, cardiovascular disease, heart failure and peptic ulcer disease.

In Mr Gonzalez's case, we have selected naproxen. This is because current evidence tends to suggest that, among the various NSAIDs available, naproxen is least likely to precipitate adverse cardiovascular events. Even so, it should be taken for the shortest possible duration.

You should advise Mr Gonzalez that the NSAID should be taken with food, to minimise gastric irritation. You should consider prescribing a gastro-protective medication (e.g. proton pump inhibitor) in high-risk patients (e.g. those with peptic ulcer disease) or when treatment with an NSAID will be prolonged. Where NSAIDs are contraindicated you may consider colchicine (although this may be poorly tolerated due to associated diarrhoea) or intra-articular or oral corticosteroid therapy.

## Continuing usual treatment

Mr Gonzalez already takes allopurinol. Although you should avoid starting allopurinol during acute gout attacks (as it can worsen its severity), patients who are already taking allopurinol should continue to do so, as fluctuations in serum urate levels can make attacks worse. Having stopped his bendroflumethiazide, you should continue his other regular medications as charted.

## Prevention of recurrence

Mr Gonzalez should be seen in a month's time to discuss ways to reduce his risk of further acute attacks. This may include dietary changes, reduced alcohol intake and optimisation of blood pressure control. His renal function and serum urate concentration should be measured to guide allopurinol dosage adjustment.

## How do I write the prescription?
### Starting an NSAID

The standard dosage regimen for naproxen in acute gout starts with 750 mg as an initial dose; this has been prescribed in the once only section of the drug chart. Thereafter, it is given in a dose of 250 mg 8-hourly until the attack abates, and this has been prescribed in the regular section. Like all NSAIDs, naproxen should be taken with food.

## Stopping bendroflumethiazide

Bendroflumethiazide should be stopped by crossing through its prescription clearly on the drug chart, and signing and dating this. Make sure the reason is documented in the clinical notes and the discharge letter, and that a plan is made to review his anti-hypertensive therapy once the acute issues have resolved. You should also note the intolerance in the drug intolerances section of the chart.

## Existing medications

No other changes to his existing medications need to be made.

## Further reading

Medical Pharmacology at a Glance. Chapter 32: Non-steroidal anti-inflammatory drugs (NSAIDs).

Prescribing at a Glance. Chapter 22: Dealing with adverse drug reactions.

Coakley G, Mathews C, Field M, et al. BSR & BHPR, BOA, RCGP and BSAC guidelines for management of the hot swollen joint in adults. Rheumatology (Oxford) 2006;45:1039–41. Available at: http://www.rheumatology.org.uk/includes/documents/cm_docs/2009/m/management_of_hot_swollen_joints_in_adults.pdf (accessed 18 January 2014).

Jordan KM, Cameron JS, Snaith M, et al. British Society for Rheumatology and British Health Professionals in Rheumatology Guideline for the Management of Gout. Rheumatology (Oxford) 2007;46:1372–4. Available at: http://www.rheumatology.org.uk/includes/documents/cm_docs/2009/m/management_of_gout.pdf (accessed 18 January 2014).

**ONCE ONLY PRESCRIPTIONS**

| Date | Time to be given | DRUG | Dose | Route | Prescriber Signature | Prescriber Bleep | Date given | Time given | Given by |
|---|---|---|---|---|---|---|---|---|---|
| 7/1/15 | 20:00 | NAPROXEN | 750 mg | Oral | A Doctor | 1234 | | | |

**OXYGEN**

| Target SpO₂ | ○ 94–98% |
|---|---|
| | ○ 88–92% |
| Mode of delivery | ○ Continuous |
| | ○ As required |

Starting device

| Initials | Bleep | Date |
|---|---|---|
| | | |

**AS REQUIRED MEDICATION**

| DRUG CO-CODAMOL 30/500 | | | | Date | 7/1/15 | | | | | | | | |
|---|---|---|---|---|---|---|---|---|---|---|---|---|---|
| | | | | Time | 1900 | | | | | | | | |
| Dose 1 to 2 tablets | Route Oral | Max freq 4-hrly | Start date 7/1/15 | Dose | 2 tabs | | | | | | | | |
| | | | | Route | Oral | | | | | | | | |
| Signature A Doctor | | Bleep 1234 | Review | Given | AM | | | | | | | | |
| | | | | Check | | | | | | | | | |

Additional instructions
Maximum 8 tablets in 24 hours

**REGULAR PRESCRIPTIONS**

| Surname | Hospital number | Weight | Drug intolerances |
|---|---|---|---|
| MACGEE | 100025 | | None known |
| First name | Date of birth | 82 kg | |
| DEREK | 19/03/1959 | | |

| | Circle / enter times below ↓ | ⇘ Enter dates below | Month: January | | Year: 2015 | | | |
|---|---|---|---|---|---|---|---|---|
| | | 7 | | | | | | |
| DRUG **ASPIRIN** | 06 | | | | | | | |
| | ⑧ | | | | | | | |
| Dose 75 mg / Route Oral / Freq Daily / Start date 7/1/15 | 12 | | | | | | | |
| Signature A Doctor / Bleep 1234 / Review | 16 | | | | | | | |
| | 18 | | | | | | | |
| Additional instructions For atrial fibrillation | 22 | | | | | | | |
| DRUG **AMLODIPINE** | 06 | | | | | | | |
| | ⑧ | | | | | | | |
| Dose 5 mg / Route Oral / Freq Daily / Start date 7/1/15 | 12 | | | | | | | |
| Signature A Doctor / Bleep 1234 / Review | 16 | | | | | | | |
| | 18 | | | | | | | |
| Additional instructions | 22 | | | | | | | |
| DRUG **BISOPROLOL** | 06 | | | | | | | |
| | ⑧ | | | | | | | |
| Dose 10 mg / Route Oral / Freq Daily / Start date 7/1/15 | 12 | | | | | | | |
| Signature A Doctor / Bleep 1234 / Review | 16 | | | | | | | |
| | 18 | | | | | | | |
| Additional instructions | 22 | | | | | | | |
| DRUG **ONDANSETRON** | ⑥ | | | | | | | |
| | 08 | | | | | | | |
| Dose 4 mg / Route IV / Freq 8-hrly / Start date 7/1/15 | 12 ⑭ AM | | | | | | | |
| Signature A Doctor / Bleep 1234 / Review | 16 | | | | | | | |
| | 18 | | | | | | | |
| Additional instructions | ㉒ | | | | | | | |
| DRUG **DALTEPARIN** | 06 | | | | | | | |
| | 08 | | | | | | | |
| Dose 5000 units / Route SC / Freq Daily / Start date 7/1/15 | 12 | | | | | | | |
| Signature A Doctor / Bleep / Review | 16 | | | | | | | |
| | ⑱ | | | | | | | |
| Additional instructions | 22 | | | | | | | |

### What should I consider when deciding what to prescribe?

Hypokalaemia is a potentially dangerous electrolyte abnormality that is usually caused by increased potassium losses from the gut (e.g. diarrhoea, vomiting) or the urinary tract (e.g. thiazide and loop diuretic therapy). Less commonly, it may be the result of redistribution of potassium into cells, due to alkalosis, insulin therapy or other drugs such as theophylline. Hypokalaemia is rarely the result of insufficient dietary potassium intake alone. In Mr MacGee's case, diarrhoea and vomiting are the likely causes.

Symptoms of hypokalaemia are often mild or absent, although muscle weakness and cramps may occur (with muscle necrosis and paralysis in very severe cases). The ECG may show ST-depression, small T-waves and the appearance of U-waves (positive waves that appear after the T-wave). The major risk of hypokalaemia is cardiac arrhythmias. These can take various forms, including ventricular and supraventricular tachyarrhyth-mias, atrioventricular block and ventricular fibrillation. Hypokalaemia also potentiates the effect of digoxin, which may further contribute to the risk of arrhythmias (see Case 47).

### Treatment of hypokalaemia

The treatment of hypokalaemia depends on:
- whether it is symptomatic or causing arrhythmias
- the serum potassium concentration
- other risk factors for arrhythmia (e.g. proarrhythmic drug treatment, particularly with digoxin).

An approach to severity assessment and treatment is outlined in Figure 25.1. Mr MacGee has mild hypokalaemia. Oral therapy would usually be preferred, but IV therapy is likely to be necessary because of his vomiting. The initial aim is to achieve a 'safe' potassium concentration (e.g. around 3.5 mmol/L) as quickly as possible. Thereafter, potassium replacement can be slowed and, as his infective diarrhoea settles, it is to be hoped that it can be discontinued.

All patients with significant hypokalaemia require close monitoring (including cardiac monitoring). The risks of treatment include both: (a) inadequate correction of hypokalaemia and (b) overcorrection with resultant hyperkalaemia. You should therefore re-measure the serum potassium concentration frequently during potassium supplementation. In addition, you should always check the serum magnesium concentration. Hypomagnesaemia and hypokalaemia often co-exist, and where they do, hypokalaemia may not respond to treatment unless magnesium is also replaced (because hypomagnesaemia can increase urinary potassium excretion).

### How do I write the prescription?
#### Oral potassium supplementation

Oral potassium supplementation is usually given as an effervescent tablet containing potassium chloride and potassium bicarbonate (Sando-K®). The dose of Sando-K® is specified by prescribing the number of tablets to be administered – each tablet contains 12 mmol potassium. A typical dosage would be 2 tablets 3 times daily. This should be prescribed in the regular section of the drug chart, with clear instructions that it should be reviewed at least daily, based on the serum potassium concentration.

#### Intravenous potassium supplementation

For patients with severe hypokalaemia or, as in this case, patients unable to tolerate oral therapy, intravenous potassium chloride is required. Potassium chloride is provided in ready mixed solutions with glucose 5% or sodium chloride 0.9%, at concentrations of 20 or 40 mmol/L. Hartmann's solution contains a small amount of potassium (5 mmol/L) but this is insufficient for treatment of hypokalaemia.

A common initial prescription would be for 1 L sodium chloride 0.9% with 40 mmol potassium chloride, administered over 4 hours. This is illustrated in the model answer. In more severe hypokalaemia, it may be administered more rapidly than this, but you should always seek senior advice in these cases.

All patients with severe hypokalaemia, and all patients requiring relatively rapid IV potassium supplementation (like Mr MacGee), should be nursed in a high-visibility area with continuous cardiac rhythm monitoring. You should document a clear plan in Mr MacGee's notes to re-measure his electrolyte profile after administration of this initial therapy, and ensure that this is carried out.

**ONCE ONLY PRESCRIPTIONS**

| Date | Time to be given | DRUG | Dose | Route | Prescriber | | Administration | | |
|------|------|------|------|------|------|------|------|------|------|
| | | | | | Signature | Bleep | Date given | Time given | Given by |
| | | | | | | | | | |
| | | | | | | | | | |

**OXYGEN**

| Target SpO₂ | ○ 94–98% |
| | ○ 88–92% |
| Mode of delivery | ○ Continuous |
| | ○ As required |
| Starting device | |

| Initials | Bleep | Date |
|------|------|------|
| | | |

**AS REQUIRED MEDICATION**

| DRUG CYCLIZINE | | | | Date | | | | | | | | |
|------|------|------|------|------|------|------|------|------|------|------|------|------|
| | | | | Time | | | | | | | | |
| Dose 50 mg | Route ORAL/IV | Max freq 8-hrly | Start date 7/1/15 | Dose | | | | | | | | |
| | | | | Route | | | | | | | | |
| Signature A Doctor | | Bleep 1234 | Review | Given | | | | | | | | |
| | | | | Check | | | | | | | | |
| Additional instructions For nausea/vomiting | | | | | | | | | | | | |

| DRUG | | | | Date | | | | | | | | |
|------|------|------|------|------|------|------|------|------|------|------|------|------|
| | | | | Time | | | | | | | | |
| Dose | Route | Max freq | Start date | Dose | | | | | | | | |
| | | | | Route | | | | | | | | |
| Signature | | Bleep | Review | Given | | | | | | | | |
| | | | | Check | | | | | | | | |
| Additional instructions | | | | | | | | | | | | |

| DRUG | | | | Date | | | | | | | | |
|------|------|------|------|------|------|------|------|------|------|------|------|------|
| | | | | Time | | | | | | | | |
| Dose | Route | Max freq | Start date | Dose | | | | | | | | |
| | | | | Route | | | | | | | | |
| Signature | | Bleep | Review | Given | | | | | | | | |
| | | | | Check | | | | | | | | |
| Additional instructions | | | | | | | | | | | | |

| DRUG | | | | Date | | | | | | | | |
|------|------|------|------|------|------|------|------|------|------|------|------|------|
| | | | | Time | | | | | | | | |
| Dose | Route | Max freq | Start date | Dose | | | | | | | | |
| | | | | Route | | | | | | | | |
| Signature | | Bleep | Review | Given | | | | | | | | |
| | | | | Check | | | | | | | | |
| Additional instructions | | | | | | | | | | | | |

**INFUSION PRESCRIPTIONS**

| Date | Time | Fluid | Vol | Drug | Dose | Rate | Doctor initials | Nurse initials | Batch no | Start time | Stop time |
|------|------|------|------|------|------|------|------|------|------|------|------|
| 7/1/15 | 16:00 | HARTMANN'S SOLUTION | 1 L | | | 4 hr | AD | AN | 001 | 1600 | 2000 |
| 7/1/15 | 20:00 | SODIUM CHLORIDE 0.9% | 1 L | POTASSIUM CHLORIDE | 40 mmol | 4 hr | AD | | | | |
| | | | | | | | | | | | |
| | | | | | | | | | | | |

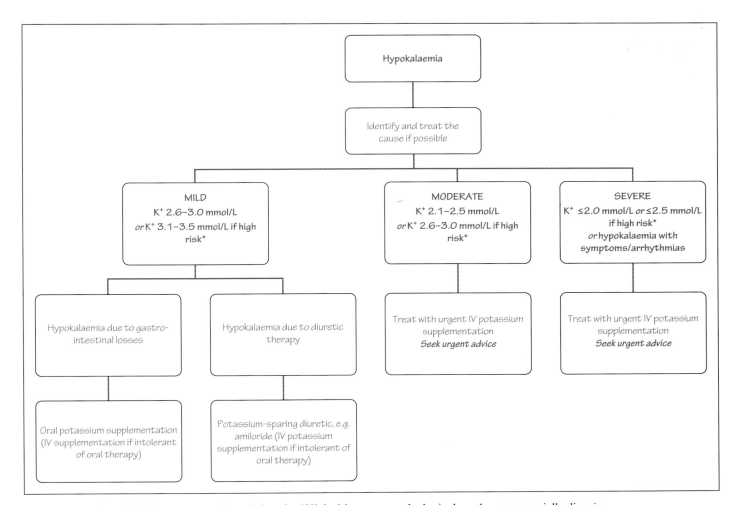

**Figure 25.1** Preferred initial treatment of hypokalaemia. *High risk: e.g. proarrhythmic drug therapy, especially digoxin.

## What should I consider when deciding what to prescribe?

Junior doctors are often called upon to re-dose certain drugs, based on drug concentration data (therapeutic drug monitoring, TDM). Gentamicin is probably the most common example, but other drugs subject to TDM include phenytoin (see Case 41), theophylline and vancomycin. Most hospitals have TDM protocols, which should be followed as applicable. This case illustrates a typical approach that may be taken for gentamicin monitoring and explains its conceptual basis.

## Measuring drug concentrations

As for many drugs subject to TDM, there are two main time points for taking samples for gentamicin concentration measurements (Figure 26.1).

- A *peak level*, taken just after a dose, which is mainly to confirm that a sufficiently high concentration is achieved for antibacterial efficacy
- A *trough level* taken 18–24 hours after a dose (i.e. just before the next anticipated dose), which is mainly to confirm that the drug is being eliminated as expected, to reduce the risk of toxicity.

| Surname HULL | Hospital number 100026 | Weight | Drug intolerances |
|---|---|---|---|
| First name PATRICIA | Date of birth 25/11/1945 | 71 kg | None known |

**REGULAR PRESCRIPTIONS**

Month: January   Year: 2015

| | Circle / enter times below ↓ | Enter dates below 6 | 7 | | |
|---|---|---|---|---|---|
| DRUG TAZOCIN | 06 | | AM | | |
| | 08 | | | | |
| Dose 4.5 g  Route IV  Freq 8-hrly  Start date 6/1/15 | 12 | | | | |
| Signature A Doctor  Bleep 1234  Review 48 hr | 16 (14) | AM | AM | | |
| | 18 | | | | |
| Additional instructions Neutropenic sepsis | (22) | AM | | | |
| **GENTAMICIN** | Level (µg/mL) | N/A | 1.8 | | |
| | Time taken | N/A | 1500 | | |
| Indication Neutropenic sepsis  Start date 6/1/15 | Dose | 300mg OMIT | | | |
| Signature A Doctor  Bleep 1234  Review 48 hr | Dr initials | AD | AD | | |
| Trough levels should be taken 18–24 hours post-dose. The next dose is administered if the level is <1 mg/L. | Time given | 1900 | / | | |
| | Nurse initials | AM | / | | |
| DRUG DALTEPARIN | 06 | | | | |
| | 08 | | | | |
| Dose 5000 units  Route SC  Freq Daily  Start date 6/1/15 | 12 | | | | |
| Signature A Doctor  Bleep 1234  Review | 16 | | | | |
| Additional instructions | (18) | AM | | | |
| | 22 | | | | |
| DRUG | 06 | | | | |

### Once daily gentamicin

In modern practice, gentamicin is usually given once daily. The initial dose is calculated from the patient's body weight (or adjusted body weight in obese patients), modified according to their renal function. In this context, it can usually be assumed that an adequate peak concentration will be achieved, such that it is generally unnecessary to measure peak levels. Much more variable, however, is the rate of gentamicin elimination. Measurement of trough levels is therefore essential to reduce the risk of gentamicin toxicity.

### Gentamicin elimination

The half-life of gentamicin is short: about 2.5 hours if renal function is normal. In other words, 2.5 hours after a dose is administered, only 50% should remain in the body. After 5 hours, 25% should remain, and so on. Twenty hours (eight half-lives) after the dose, almost none should remain (specifically: $0.5^8 \times 100 = 0.4\%$). Therefore, the trough gentamicin level should be very low ($<1\,\mu g/mL$). If not, it implies that the drug is being eliminated more slowly than anticipated. If a further dose was administered at this time (Figure 26.1) the kidneys would be subject to sustained gentamicin exposure. This is thought to increase the risk of nephrotoxicity. Consequently, it is preferable to withhold the second dose until the previous one has been more completely eliminated.

### Re-dosing gentamicin

Most guidelines recommend that gentamicin doses are not administered while the plasma concentration is above $1\,\mu g/mL$. In this situation, you should wait 12 hours then re-measure the concentration (wait 24 hours if the level is $>2\,\mu g/mL$). Once the plasma concentration is below $1\,\mu g/mL$, you can prescribe the next dose. You should recalculate the dose based on the most up-to-date information concerning renal function and body weight.

## How do I write the prescription?

Most hospitals have a dedicated gentamicin prescription, on which the drug concentration data and prescription can both be recorded. Often, this takes the form of a sticker that is attached to the prescription chart, as illustrated in this case. Based on the high trough concentration, the dose has been omitted. The next gentamicin concentration measurement should be made in 12 hours. You should document this in the medical notes and ensure a plan is in place to enact this.

## Further reading

Medical Pharmacology at a Glance. Chapter 39: Antibacterial drugs that inhibit protein synthesis.
Prescribing at a Glance. Chapter 21: Therapeutic drug monitoring.

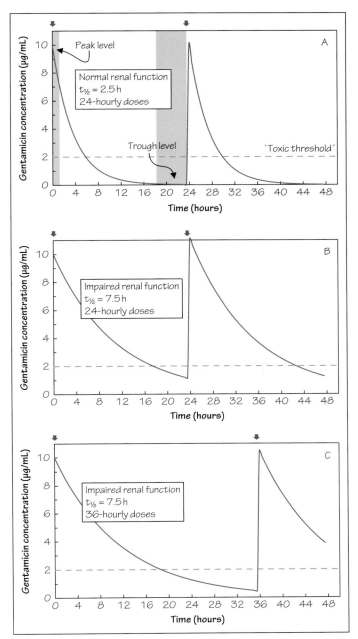

**Figure 26.1** Idealised time–concentration curves representing two IV gentamicin doses (doses are indicated by green arrows). A, The time window for a peak level is up to 1 hour after an IV dose. Peak levels are used to confirm likely antibacterial efficacy, although they are not usually necessary in once daily gentamicin dosing. Trough levels are taken 18–24 hours after a dose and are used to minimise the risk of toxicity. There is a toxic threshold (indicated by the dashed line) at around 2 μg/mL. The amount of time the concentration is above the toxic threshold is understood to predict the risk of nephrotoxicity. When renal function is normal, the half-life ($t_{1/2}$) is approximately 2.5 hours and almost the entire dose is cleared before the next dose is given. B, When renal function is impaired, the half-life increases (to 7.5 hours in this example) and the trough level becomes detectable. If a further dose were administered at this time, the concentration would be above the toxic threshold for most of the dosing interval. C, When renal function is impaired, you need to wait until the concentration falls below 1 μg/mL before administering the next dose. This ensures the concentration is not persistently above the toxic threshold.

## What should I consider when deciding what to prescribe?

Mr Mzimba is 69-year-old man who has been admitted for treatment of pneumonia. As he has a mechanical mitral valve and atrial fibrillation, he takes warfarin to reduce the risk of thromboembolism. You have been asked to prescribe today's dose of warfarin. However, his INR today is 4.6, meaning that his prothrombin time is prolonged by 4.6 times. This is above his INR target of 2.5–3.5.

The key issues to address when managing a high INR in a patient taking warfarin are: why is the INR high; what are the consequences of the high INR (risk or sign of bleeding); and what is the appropriate treatment?

## Why is the INR high?

Alterations in warfarin absorption, plasma protein binding, metabolism and excretion can cause a change in the INR of a patient taking warfarin. Important factors in this case are as follow.

*Drug interactions.* Interactions with warfarin are common. Often this is because of the effect a new drug has on warfarin metabolism. Mr Mzimba started taking clarithromycin 4 days ago. Clarithromycin inhibits the cytochrome P450 enzymes that metabolise warfarin, thereby increasing the anticoagulant effects (also Case 12).

| Surname | Hospital number | Weight | Drug intolerances |
|---|---|---|---|
| MZIMBA | 100027 | 85 kg | None known |
| First name | Date of birth | | |
| FUNSANI | 19/08/1945 | | |

**REGULAR PRESCRIPTIONS**

| | | Circle / enter times below ↓ | ◿ Enter dates below | | | | | Month: January | | Year: 2015 |
|---|---|---|---|---|---|---|---|---|---|---|
| | | | 3 | 4 | 5 | 6 | 7 | | | |
| DRUG AMOXICILLIN | | ⑥ 06 | | AM | AM | AM | AM | | | |
| | | 08 | | | | | | | | |
| Dose 500 mg / Route Oral / Freq 8-hrly / Start date 3/1/15 | | 12 | | | | | | | | |
| Signature A Doctor / Bleep 1234 / Review 10/1/15 | | ✗ ⑭ | AM | AM | AM | AM | AM | | | |
| | | 18 | | | | | | | | |
| Additional instructions Community-acquired pneumonia | | ㉒ 22 | | AM | AM | AM | AM | | | |
| DRUG CLARITHROMYCIN | | 06 | | | | | | | | |
| | | ⑧ 08 | | AM | AM | AM | AM | | | |
| Dose 500 mg / Route Oral / Freq 12-hrly / Start date 3/1/15 | | 12 | | | | | | | | |
| Signature A Doctor / Bleep 1234 / Review 10/1/15 | | 16 | | | | | | | | |
| Additional instructions Community-acquired pneumonia | | ✗ ⑳ 22 | AM | AM | AM | AM | | | | |
| DRUG WARFARIN | | 06 | | | | | | | | |
| | | 08 INR: | 2.2 | 2.3 | x | x | 4.6 | | | |
| Dose Variable / Route Oral / Freq Daily / Start date 3/1/15 | | 12 Dose: | 6mg | 6mg | 5mg | 5mg | 2mg | | | |
| Signature A Doctor / Bleep 1234 / Review Daily | | Doctor: | AD | AD | AD | AD | AD | | | |
| For daily dosing by doctor. To be given at the same time each day – 18:00 | | Nurse: | AM | AM | AM | AM | | | | |
| | | 22 | | Usual dose 5 mg | | | | | | |
| DRUG | | 06 | | | | | | | | |

**ONCE ONLY PRESCRIPTIONS**

| | | | | | Prescriber | | Administration | | | OXYGEN |
|---|---|---|---|---|---|---|---|---|---|---|
| Date | Time to be given | DRUG | Dose | Route | Signature | Bleep | Date given | Time given | Given by | |
| | | | | | | | | | | Target SpO₂: ☑ 94–98%  ☐ 88–92% |
| | | | | | | | | | | Mode of delivery: ☑ Continuous  ☐ As required |
| | | | | | | | | | | Starting device Nasal cannula |
| | | | | | | | | | | Initials AD / Bleep 1234 / Date 3/1/15 |

*Warfarin dosing.* Mr Mzimba was prescribed a slightly higher than normal dose of warfarin at the beginning of his admission because of an INR below his target level. On the two subsequent days, no INR was measured and his standard dose was administered. Given the effects of clarithromycin, it is likely these doses were a little too high.

## What are the consequences of a high INR?

Patients with excessive anticoagulation are at increased risk of bleeding. In managing a high INR you need to look for any sign of bleeding and determine whether other factors, e.g. need for surgery, might impact on their bleeding risk. You also need to consider the reason for anticoagulation and the potential consequences of reversal.

Mr Mzimba has no signs of bleeding. He has been admitted with pneumonia, therefore is not at particular risk of bleeding from his underlying diagnosis. However, his anticoagulation is to prevent intracardiac coagulation relating to a mechanical heart valve. Patients with mechanical mitral valves are at particularly high risk of thromboembolism (4% per year). It is therefore very important that his anticoagulation is maintained to target wherever possible.

## How should I manage the high INR?
### Should I attempt to reverse the anticoagulation?
Warfarin causes anticoagulation by inhibiting production of vitamin K-dependent clotting factors, a process that can be reversed with phytomenadione (vitamin K). However, in the absence of bleeding and in a patient with an INR <8.0, phytomenadione should not routinely be prescribed. Giving a patient phytomenadione prevents warfarin from working effectively and can lead to an undesirably low INR, which is an important consideration for Mr Mzimba. You should not have prescribed phytomenadione in this case. The management of bleeding in a patient taking warfarin is addressed in Case 12.

### What do I do about today's warfarin dose?
There is no one correct answer to this question. You will need to consider the specific situation of your patient: the reasons for anticoagulation; the target INR; the current INR; usual and recent doses. Alongside this, you should consider that warfarin works by inhibiting production of new clotting factors, rather than deactivating clotting factors that have already been made. Today's INR, therefore, does not just directly reflect yesterday's dose, it is a result of the preceding 48–72 hours dosing.

*When selecting a dose.* Avoid making large changes in dose or omitting doses if possible, as this will maintain a smooth change in INR and make subsequent dosing decisions straightforward. Base your decision on INR measurements over the preceding 48–72 hours where available, rather than just on today's level. Importantly, remember to document the reason for a dose change in the notes as it is likely that the subsequent dose will be prescribed by a different healthcare professional and they will need to understand your thought processes.

*Mr Mzimba.* We have selected a warfarin dose of 2 mg for Mr Mzimba today. The reasons for this decision are as follow.

His target INR is 3.0 and, while his INR was low on admission, it is now 4.6, which is too high. Although we do not have INR measurements for the preceding 48–72 hours, the trend is clearly upwards. Omission of warfarin today may cause a pronounced downward swing in his INR over subsequent days, increasing the risk of sub-therapeutic anticoagulation. As his current warfarin dosing has increased his INR excessively, a lower dose is required. Either 2 or 3 mg warfarin would be reasonable, as these doses approximate to half of his previous dose.

You should write the reasons for your choice of dose in his notes. Remember that the next day's INR should be ordered and that owing to how it reflects warfarin therapy, it may be higher than 4.6 despite your dose reduction.

### Should I stop his clarithromycin?

It is going to be difficult to stabilise the warfarin dose while Mr Mzimba is taking clarithromycin. The drug chart indicates that he should continue clarithromycin for the next three days, so you should continue treatment for now. However, clarithromycin is prescribed to treat infection with atypical organisms e.g. *Legionella pneumophila, mycoplasma pneumoniae* (see Case 5). If microbiological investigations have excluded *Legionella* infection (negative urinary antigen) or identified an alternative cause (e.g. *Streptococcus pneumoniae*), it may be possible to stop this macrolide. Advice from a microbiologist will be helpful in making this decision.

### How do I write the prescription?

The practicalities of prescribing warfarin vary from hospital to hospital. Many have a dedicated warfarin prescribing chart which is appended to the main chart, although some hospitals still prescribe warfarin on the main chart. In other hospitals, prescribing is electronic. Make sure you are familiar with the method used at your hospital.

On the model prescription, warfarin is being dosed on the main chart. You should note today's INR in the relevant section and write and sign today's warfarin dose. You should communicate what you have prescribed with the nursing staff and the patient and explain your reasons. Remember that some patients are experts in their own warfarin dosing.

### Further reading

Medical Pharmacology at a Glance. Chapter 19: Drugs used to affect blood coagulation.
Prescribing at a Glance. Chapter 23: Avoiding drug interactions.

---

## 28 A 28-year-old woman with nausea

| Surname BOKHARI | Hospital number 100028 | Weight | Drug intolerances Haloperidol – neuroleptic malignant syndrome |
|---|---|---|---|
| First name AARYA | Date of birth 14/05/1986 | 69 kg | |

**REGULAR PRESCRIPTIONS**

| | | Circle / enter times below ↓ | ↘ Enter dates below | | Month: January | | Year: 2015 |
|---|---|---|---|---|---|---|---|
| | | | 7 | 8 | | | |
| DRUG PARACETAMOL | | 06 | | | | | |
| Dose 1 g | Route IV | Freq 6-hrly | Start date 7/1/15 | 12 | | | |
| Signature A Doctor | Bleep 1234 | Review 48 hr | 16 | | | | |
| Additional instructions | | | 18 | AM | | | |
| | | ✗ 24 | | | | | |
| DRUG IBUPROFEN | | 06 | | | | | |
| Dose 400 mg | Route Oral | Freq 8-hrly | Start date 7/1/15 | 12 | | | |
| Signature A Doctor | Bleep 1234 | Review 48 hr | ✗ 14 | | | | |
| Additional instructions Take with food | | 18 | 22 | | | | |
| DRUG ENOXAPARIN | | 06 | | | | | |
| Dose 20 mg | Route S/C | Freq Daily | Start date 7/1/15 | 12 | | | |
| Signature A Doctor | Bleep 1234 | Review | 16 | | | | |
| Additional instructions VTE prophylaxis | | 18 | AM | | | | |
| | | 22 | | | | | |

### What should I consider when deciding what to prescribe?

Mrs Bokhari is a 28-year-old woman experiencing postoperative nausea, which is most likely a side effect of morphine and anaesthetic drugs. She has a past medical history of schizophrenia and has previously had a severe reaction to haloperidol.

### Nausea

Nausea is a symptom that can be caused by stimuli acting on the gastrointestinal tract (e.g. pharyngeal irritation, infection) or nervous system (e.g. drugs, motion, psychological stimulus). The response is co-ordinated by the chemoreceptor trigger zone (CTZ) in the medulla and the solitary tract nucleus. The CTZ does not have a developed blood–brain barrier (BBB). This is important because it means that anti-emetic drugs do not need to penetrate the BBB to be effective.

### Anti-emetics

There are several classes of anti-emetic and this can make choosing a drug for a nauseated patient feel like a daunting task. Common targets for anti-emetics are serotonin (5HT$_3$) and dopamine (D$_2$) receptors in the CTZ and solitary tract nucleus. In addition, some drugs target histamine (H$_1$) receptors in the solitary tract nucleus. In many situations, there is no one correct drug to choose, although the cause of nausea and contraindications to anti-emetic drugs may help to direct your choice. Table 28.1 outlines some of the properties of commonly used anti-emetics.

### Choosing an anti-emetic for Mrs Bokhari

Most of the classes of anti-emetics can be used for postoperative or drug-induced nausea and vomiting (Table 28.1). However, she was given a dose of an H$_1$-receptor antagonist (cyclizine) only 2.5 hours ago. As this appears not to have been effective and can only be given 8-hourly, a further H$_1$-receptor antagonist would not be appropriate as anti-emetic treatment.

  You should also have noticed that she has had a previous severe adverse reaction to haloperidol (neuroleptic malignant syndrome). Haloperidol is an antipsychotic drug from the butyrophenone class that acts by blocking D$_2$-receptors. In the limbic system, blockade of D$_2$-receptors is effective in controlling the positive symptoms of schizophrenia, such as thought disorders, abnormalities of perception and delusional beliefs. Neuroleptic malignant syndrome is a rare, abnormal response to D$_2$-receptor blockade, resulting in high fever, muscle rigidity and autonomic instability. Neuroleptic malignant syndrome has an estimated 10–20% mortality rate and $\sim$30% risk of recurrence if further D$_2$-receptor antagonists are prescribed. You should therefore avoid prescribing phenothiazines and metoclopramide for Mrs Bokhari.

  We have therefore chosen to prescribe a 5HT$_3$-receptor antagonist, ondansetron, to control Mrs Bokhari's nausea on the model chart.

### Is there anything else to consider?

Mrs Bokhari has been receiving the non-steroidal anti-inflammatory drug ibuprofen. This is a good choice for treatment of bone pain, but has the common side effect of gastrointestinal irritation and could cause nausea. If you have any suspicion that this is contributing to her nausea you should either stop the ibuprofen or prescribe a proton pump inhibitor as gastroprotection.

**ONCE ONLY PRESCRIPTIONS**

| Date | Time to be given | DRUG | Dose | Route | Prescriber Signature | Bleep | Date given | Time given | Given by |
|---|---|---|---|---|---|---|---|---|---|
| 7/1/15 | 17:00 | CYCLIZINE | 50 mg | IV | AD | 1234 | 07/01 | 1700 | AN |
| 7/1/15 | 1700 | MORPHINE | 5 mg | IV | AD | 1234 | 07/01 | 1700 | AN |

**OXYGEN**

Target SpO$_2$: ☑ 94–98% ☐ 88–92%
Mode of delivery: ☑ Continuous ☐ As required
Starting device: Nasal cannula

| Initials | Bleep | Date |
|---|---|---|
| AD | 1234 | 7/1/15 |

**AS REQUIRED MEDICATION**

| DRUG SEVREDOL | | | | Date | 7/1 | | | | |
|---|---|---|---|---|---|---|---|---|---|
| | | | | Time | 1900 | | | | |
| Dose 5-10 mg | Route Oral | Max freq 4-hrly | Start date 7/1/15 | Dose | 10 mg | | | | |
| | | | | Route | Oral | | | | |
| Signature A Doctor | | Bleep 1234 | Review | Given | AN | | | | |
| | | | | Check | BN | | | | |

Additional instructions
Morphine sulfate tablets (immediate release)

| DRUG ONDANSETRON | | | | Date | | | | | |
|---|---|---|---|---|---|---|---|---|---|
| | | | | Time | | | | | |
| Dose 4 mg | Route IV/IM | Max freq 8-hrly | Start date 7/1/15 | Dose | | | | | |
| | | | | Route | | | | | |
| Signature A Doctor | | Bleep 1234 | Review 24 hours | Given | | | | | |
| | | | | Check | | | | | |

Additional instructions
For postoperative nausea and vomiting

### How do I write the prescription?

The BNF recommends that ondansetron should be prescribed at a dose of 4 mg for administration by intramuscular or slow intravenous injection for treatment of postoperative nausea and vomiting. We have therefore prescribed this in the as required section of the chart. The BNF does not provide recommendations for repeat dosing of ondansetron for this indication. As ondansetron is usually given at intervals between 4 and 12 hours for other indications, an interval of 8 hours for repeat doses as charted is reasonable.

  There are many other ways to provide anti-emetic treatment for Mrs Bokhari. For example, you might use a once only dose of ondansetron 4 mg for control of her nausea, followed by regular or as required doses of cyclizine to maintain control.

### Further reading

Medical Pharmacology at a Glance. Chapter 30: Drugs used in nausea and vertigo.
Prescribing at a Glance. Chapter 5: Using drugs for the gastrointestinal system.

**Table 28.1** Properties of some commonly used anti-emetic drugs

| Class (example) | Tips for use | How do they work? | Adverse effects to be aware of |
|---|---|---|---|
| Phenothiazines<br>• Chlorpromazine<br>• Prochlorperazine | Useful for nausea caused by anaesthetic drugs, in patients with cancer or radiation induced nausea | Predominantly $D_2$ antagonists. Chlorpromazine also has $H_1$ antagonist activity | Dystonic reactions<br>Sedation<br>Avoid in the very young and very old |
| Anti-histamines<br>• Cyclizine<br>• Promethazine | Many uses. Used as an over-the-counter treatment for motion sickness | $H_1$-receptor antagonists | Sedation |
| 5HT$_3$-receptor antagonists<br>• Ondansetron<br>• Granisetron | Useful for postoperative nausea and vomiting and nausea from cytotoxic drugs | Central and peripheral 5HT$_3$-receptor antagonists | Associated with QT prolongation |
| Benzamides<br>• Metoclopramide<br>• Domperidone | Useful for nausea and vomiting caused by gastrointestinal disease such as gastroparesis, although should not be used in bowel obstruction. Limited use in postoperative nausea | $D_2$ antagonists (some peripheral 5HT$_3$-receptor antagonism) | Dystonic reactions (particularly young women) although domperidone does not cross the blood–brain barrier so is less likely to cause dystonic reactions<br>Avoid in the very young and very old |

# 29 A 29-year-old man who is in pain following an operation

| Surname BULWER | Hospital number 100029 | Weight | Drug intolerances |
|---|---|---|---|
| First name RORY | Date of birth 12/04/1984 | 75 kg | None known |

**REGULAR PRESCRIPTIONS**

Month: January   Year: 2015

Circle / enter times below — Enter dates below: 5, 6, 7

**DRUG PARACETAMOL**
Dose 1 g | Route Oral | Freq 6-hrly | Start date 5/1/15
Signature A Doctor | Bleep 1234 | Review
Additional instructions
- (06): An An (5,6,7... )
- 08
- (12): An An
- 16
- (18): An An
- ✗ (24): An An

**DRUG IBUPROFEN**
Dose 400 mg | Route Oral | Freq 8-hrly | Start date 5/1/15
Signature A Doctor | Bleep 1234 | Review
Additional instructions: Take with food
- (06): An An
- 08
- ✗ (14): An An
- 16
- 18
- (22): An An

**DRUG DALTEPARIN**
Dose 5000 units | Route SC | Freq Daily | Start date 5/1/15
Signature A Doctor | Bleep 1234 | Review
Additional instructions
- 06
- 08
- 12
- 16
- (18): An An
- 22

**DRUG MST CONTINUS**
Dose 15 mg | Route Oral | Freq 12-hrly | Start date 7/1/15
Signature A Doctor | Bleep 1234 | Review Daily
Additional instructions: Sustained-release morphine sulfate tablets
- 06
- (08)
- 12
- 16
- ✗ (20)
- 22

**DRUG SENNA**
Dose 15 mg | Route Oral | Freq 12-hrly | Start date 7/1/15
Signature A Doctor | Bleep 1234 | Review Daily
Additional instructions: For constipation, review when reducing opioids
- 06
- (08)
- 12
- 16
- ✗ (20)
- 22

## What should I consider when deciding what to prescribe?

Mr Bulwer is a 29-year-old man with significant pain following an operation despite taking analgesics including paracetamol, ibuprofen and Oramorph®.

The key issues in managing his pain relief are as follow.

### Evaluating the cause of the pain

For patients in pain following an operation it is often tempting simply write a prescription for analgesia without a second thought. However, it is important to check that poorly controlled or worsening pain is not being caused by a complication of the procedure, e.g. bleeding or wound infection. In trauma cases, do not forget to think about compartment syndrome (discussed briefly in Case 22), particularly in patients who complain of pain disproportionate to the severity of the injury.

For Mr Bulwer, the operation was uncomplicated and the wound appears normal. Femoral fracture and its subsequent repair are likely to cause considerable pain. It is therefore not unexpected to find that Mr Bulwer's pain is not controlled with the analgesics that are currently prescribed. Poor pain control can increase morbidity in the postoperative period, so adequate pain control is very important.

### Choosing an analgesic

Most hospitals will have a policy for postoperative pain control that may even be specific to the procedure that the patient has undergone and you should familiarise

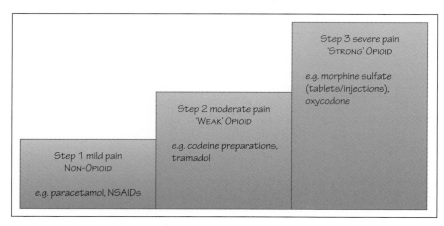

**Figure 29.1** The analgesic ladder. Adapted from the World Health Organization guidelines on treating pain for patients with cancer.

yourself with this. For non-pain specialists, the 'analgesic ladder' (Figure 29.1), originally designed for use in cancer pain, can guide the choice of drugs to prescribe. Analgesia should be prescribed regularly to achieve and maintain control of pain, with as required prescriptions for any pain that breaks through. Importantly, pain control should be reviewed regularly (at least daily) and prescriptions adjusted as necessary.

Mr Bulwer has severe (defined as >6/10) pain that is not controlled by maximal doses of analgesics from step 1 (paracetamol and ibuprofen) and prescription of a strong opioid (Oramorph® – oral morphine sulfate solution) from step 3 of the analgesic ladder. You will therefore need to use further medication from step 3 of the ladder to control his pain.

## Choosing an opioid

Selecting an opioid medication can sometimes feel daunting, as there are a wide variety of preparations available (both synthetic and non-synthetic) and the adverse effects can be life-threatening. However, when prescribed correctly, they are effective and safe. There is usually no single correct way to manage pain with opioids. Whatever you decide to prescribe, it is usual to start at the lowest dose recommended for the type and level of pain and increase as necessary, watching carefully for adverse effects. However, it is important not to leave the patient in pain through taking too cautious an approach. If pain control is difficult to achieve, seek advice from a specialist.

*Weak opioids.* Weak opioids include codeine preparations and tramadol. There is significant variability in the individual response to these drugs. Mr Bulwer still has pain despite taking morphine 2.5 mg every 2 hours. You should not prescribe a weak opioid here as strong opioids, further up the analgesic ladder, are – as prescribed – not sufficient to control his pain.

*Strong opioids.* The most commonly used oral strong opioids are morphine sulfate/hydrochloride and oxycodone hydrochloride. When choosing a strong opioid, it is important to consider the most appropriate route of administration and formulation for the

drug. On a general ward, the oral or intramuscular/subcutaneous route is preferred over intravenous administration, which is usually reserved for settings where there is intensive monitoring (see Cases 3 and 13). Regular subcutaneous or intramuscular injections may be painful and unpleasant and can be avoided if the patient is able to take oral medications. Oral opioids are prepared in tablet and liquid forms and for immediate or continuous/modified release. You must consider carefully which preparation and form to use.

## Increasing analgesia for Mr Bulwer

Mr Bulwer is currently using 2.5 mg oral liquid morphine (Oramorph® 10 mg/5 mL) every 2 hours. Each single dose does not fully control his pain (2.5 mg is a relatively low dose) and the analgesic effect does not last very long. It is therefore important to increase both the dose of morphine and the duration of the effect.

---

**ONCE ONLY PRESCRIPTIONS**

| Date | Time to be given | DRUG | Dose | Route | Prescriber Signature | Prescriber Bleep | Administration Date given | Administration Time given | Administration Given by |
|---|---|---|---|---|---|---|---|---|---|
| | | | | | | | | | |
| | | | | | | | | | |
| | | | | | | | | | |

**OXYGEN**

| Target SpO₂ | ○ 94–98% ○ 88–92% |
| Mode of delivery | ○ Continuous ○ As required |
| Starting device | |

| Initials | Bleep | Date |
|---|---|---|
| | | |

**AS REQUIRED MEDICATION**

DRUG: ORAMORPH 10 MG/5 ML
Dose 2.5 mg | Route Oral | Max freq 2-hrly | Start date 7/1/15
Signature A Doctor | Bleep 1234 | Review
Additional instructions: Oral morphine sulfate solution

| Date | 05/01 | 05/01 | 05/01 | 05/01 | 05/01 | 05/01 | 05/01 | 06/01 | 06/01 | 06/01 | 06/01 | 06/01 | 06/01 | 06/01 |
|---|---|---|---|---|---|---|---|---|---|---|---|---|---|---|
| Time | 1100 | 1300 | 1500 | 1700 | 1900 | 2100 | 2300 | 0100 | 0300 | 0500 | 0700 | 0900 | 1100 | 1300 |
| Dose | 2.5mg | 2.5mg | 2.5mg | 2.5mg | 2.5mg | 2.5mg | 2.5mg | 2.5mg | 2.5mg | 2.5mg | 2.5mg | 2.5mg | 2.5mg | 2.5mg |
| Route | Oral | Oral | Oral | Oral | Oral | Oral | Oral | Oral | Oral | Oral | Oral | Oral | Oral | Oral |
| Given | AM | AM | AM | AM | AM | AM | AM | AM | AM | AM | AM | AM | AM | AM |
| Check | BN | BN | BN | BN | BN | BN | BN | BN | BN | BN | BN | BN | BN | BN |

DRUG: ORAMORPH 10 MG/5 ML
Dose 2.5 mg | Route Oral | Max freq 2-hrly | Start date 7/1/15
Signature A Doctor | Bleep 1234 | Review
Additional instructions: Oral morphine sulfate solution

| Date | 06/01 | 06/01 | 06/01 | 06/01 | 06/01 | 07/01 | 07/01 | 07/01 | 07/01 | |
|---|---|---|---|---|---|---|---|---|---|---|
| Time | 1500 | 1700 | 1900 | 2100 | 2300 | 0100 | 0300 | 0500 | 0700 | STOPPED 7/1/15 as dose increased |
| Dose | 2.5mg | 2.5mg | 2.5mg | 2.5mg | 2.5mg | 2.5mg | 2.5mg | 2.5mg | 2.5mg | A Doctor 1234 |
| Route | Oral | Oral | Oral | Oral | Oral | Oral | Oral | Oral | Oral | |
| Given | AM | AM | AM | AM | AM | AM | AM | AM | AM | |
| Check | BN | BN | BN | BN | BN | BN | BN | BN | BN | |

DRUG: ORAMORPH 10 MG/5 ML
Dose 5 mg | Route Oral | Max freq 2-hrly | Start date 7/1/15
Signature A Doctor | Bleep 1234 | Review 7/1/15
Additional instructions: Oral morphine sulfate solution

| Date | | | | | | | | | |
|---|---|---|---|---|---|---|---|---|---|
| Time | | | | | | | | | |

DRUG: | Date |

*Prescribe sustained release morphine.* Mr Bulwer currently requires 12 doses of short acting oral morphine in 24 hours. Prescription of a sustained-release preparation, e.g. MST Continus® twice daily at a dose equivalent to the total daily dose of immediate release strong opioid can be used to achieve good background pain relief. You should note that Mr Bulwer's pain has not been entirely controlled on this dose of analgesia, so a higher dose of sustained release morphine may eventually be required. Sustained release morphine is suitable for patients like Mr Bulwer, who have had some prior exposure to opioids. They are less suitable for patients with increased sensitivity to opioids, such as the very young or elderly and those with renal impairment. In these patients, sustained release morphine may cause prolonged dangerous side effects such as depression of consciousness and respiration, which can be difficult to treat.

*Immediate release morphine.* Alongside the prescription for sustained release morphine, you should prescribe immediate release morphine as required for breakthrough pain. It may be useful for Mr Bulwer also to receive a dose of immediate release morphine before movement or physiotherapy to aid mobilisation. A general rule is for the dose of the as required prescription to be approximately one-sixth of total regular daily dose.

An alternative strategy for Mr Bulwer would be simply to increase the dose of the immediate release opioid on the as required side of the drug chart and instruct the patient to ask for analgesia when needed. This method probably leads to the lowest possible dose of opioid being given and therefore the lowest risk of side effects. However, the patient must necessarily experience pain before the drug is asked for and may experience a significant period of discomfort while waiting for their medicine. Dispensing opioid medication is a lengthy process, requiring two healthcare professionals to check out the drug from the locked controlled drug cupboard.

### How do I write the prescription?

When prescribing any strong opioid, proprietary (brand) names should be used. You must also specify the form (tablet/liquid) in your prescription. This prescribing strategy is designed to prevent administration errors that might lead to opioid toxicity. For example, an as required prescription for 10 mg morphine sulfate tablets every 2 hours could be interpreted to mean Sevredol®, an immediate release preparation or MST Continus®, a modified release preparation. If MST Continus® was given accidentally instead of Sevredol®, this may not immediately relieve pain. The patient may then request further analgesia, which, added to the slow absorption of MST Continus®, would increase the risk of opioid accumulation and toxicity.

### Regular sustained or modified release opioid prescription

In this case, we have chosen to prescribe regular MST Continus® (morphine sulfate modified release) tablets. The total daily dose of the different oral morphine preparations are equivalent, making conversion straightforward. His current total daily dose of Oramorph® is 30 mg (12 × 2.5 mg), so MST Continus® 15 mg 12-hourly would seem a reasonable starting dose. It is worth noting that he was using the Oramorph® at the maximum dose allowed by the as required prescription and his pain was not fully controlled. It will therefore be important to review his analgesic requirements over the next 24 hours as a higher dose may be necessary. As he continues to heal, his pain will decrease and a dose reduction plan will be important. Finally, note that the first dose is prescribed for 08:00 (the time you are seeing the patient), to allow for a dose to be given immediately.

### As required immediate release opioid prescription

We have increased the as required dose of Oramorph® to 5 mg 2–4-hourly. This is in keeping with the rule that as required prescriptions should be approximately one-sixth of the total daily dose. You should have crossed out the old as required dose and completed a new prescription for this as shown.

### Concomitant laxative prescription

Constipation is a significant problem in patients taking opioids and can lead to some people refusing analgesia despite pain in order to avoid this side effect. You should therefore prescribe a regular laxative alongside any regular opioid to help prevent constipation. A stimulant laxative such as senna is a suitable choice and is prescribed at 15 mg twice daily on the regular section of the drug chart (see Case 37).

### Further reading
Medical Pharmacology at a Glance. Chapter 29: Opioid analgesics.

## What should I consider when deciding what to prescribe?

Variable rate intravenous insulin infusion (VRIII) is the preferred term for what is often colloquially referred to as a 'sliding scale'. This latter term should be avoided, as it is poorly descriptive and – particularly outside the UK – is also used to mean things other than variable rate intravenous insulin infusions.

## General principles for peri-operative glycaemic control

Patients with well-controlled diabetes do not need a VRIII peri-operatively provided the starvation period is short (one missed meal). They should take their usual diabetes treatment (insulin and/or oral anti-hyperglycaemic drugs) up until the day before surgery. On the morning of surgery, doses of oral anti-hyperglycaemic drugs and short-acting insulin should generally be omitted. However, you should familiarise yourself with relevant local protocols and consult with the responsible anaesthetist for more specific instructions.

Patients with diabetes mellitus that is poorly controlled pre-operatively (HbA$_{1c}$ ≥69 mmol/mol [8.5%]) should ideally have their operation deferred to allow their glycaemic control to be optimised. If surgery cannot be deferred, a variable rate intravenous insulin infusion may be required peri-operatively.

## Variable rate intravenous insulin infusions

VRIIIs involve the controlled infusion of insulin via an infusion pump at a rate that is determined by the capillary blood glucose (CBG) concentration. They are indicated for patients with diabetes:
- Who are expected to have a long starvation period (two or more missed meals)
- Who have poor pre-operative glycaemic control and in whom it is not possible to defer surgery to improve this.

The target range for the CBG concentration is usually 6–10 mmol/L. The nursing staff will measure the CBG concentration every hour, and adjust the insulin infusion rate according to the scale specified in the prescription. This scale is usually derived from a hospital protocol. The mock protocol provided on the answer sheet provides two starting scales: one for patients who have received long-acting insulin in the past 12 hours, and one for those who have not. Some hospital protocols will provide a wider range of scales that also take account of, for example, the patient's usual total daily subcutaneous insulin requirement. Whatever scale you prescribe, you should remember that it is just a starting point: if the CBG concentration is persistently outside the target range, the scale should be adjusted.

Intravenous insulin should not be administered without a 'substrate' fluid (one that contains glucose – the term substrate is used because glucose will be consumed by processes driven by insulin). To reduce the risk of inadvertently stopping the glucose infusion while the insulin infusion continues (e.g. due to a blocked cannula), the two infusions should be administered through the same cannula. The rate at which the glucose solution is given should be

| Surname  PATEL | Hospital number  100030 | Weight | Drug intolerances |
|---|---|---|---|
| First name  RANJIT | Date of birth  01/02/1965 | 81 kg | None known |

### Variable rate IV insulin infusion (VRIII) • Daily prescription chart

**Step 1 Subcutaneous long-acting insulin prescription (if required)**

Patients who normally take a long-acting insulin (e.g. glargine, detemir) should usually continue to receive this when receiving a variable rate insulin infusion. Prescribe the long-acting insulin in this section. When starting the insulin infusion, use **Scale A** in the first instance

Once only prescriptions for long-acting insulin (if required)

| Date due | Time due | Insulin (name and device) | Dose (units) | Route | Prescriber sig | Admin time | Nurse sig |
|---|---|---|---|---|---|---|---|
| 7/1/15 | 22:00 | GLARGINE | 18 units | SC | A Doctor | | |

**Step 2 Intravenous insulin prescription**

| Date/time | Prescription | Prescriber sig | Batch no / exp. date | Start time | Nurse sig(s) | Finish time | Nurse sig |
|---|---|---|---|---|---|---|---|
| 7/1/15 | 50 units soluble insulin (Actrapid®) made up to 50 mL with sodium chloride 0.9% | A Doctor | | | | | |
| | 50 units soluble insulin (Actrapid®) made up to 50 mL with sodium chloride 0.9% | | | | | | |
| | 50 units soluble insulin (Actrapid®) made up to 50 mL with sodium chloride 0.9% | | | | | | |

**Step 3 Rate of IV insulin infusion**

| Capillary blood glucose (CBG) concentration (mmol/L) | Initial infusion rate scales | | Adjusted scales | | |
|---|---|---|---|---|---|
| | Scale A  For patients in receiving long-acting insulin concurrent with VRIII | Scale B  All other patients | Use this section to prescribe an adjusted scale if required  Cross-through superseded prescriptions | | |
| <4 (treat) | 0 | 0.5 | | | |
| 4.0–7.0 | 0 | 1 | | | |
| 7.1–9.0 | 1 | 2 | | | |
| 9.1–11.0 | 2 | 3 | | | |
| 11.1–14.0 | 3 | 4 | | | |
| 14.1–17.0 | 4 | 5 | | | |
| 17.1–20.0 | 5 | 6 | | | |
| >20 | 6 and **seek advice** from diabetes/medical team | | | | |
| Prescriber initials and bleep number | A Doctor  Blp 1234 | | | | |
| Date and time | 7/1/15 | | | | |

**Step 4 Intravenous fluid to be administered alongside insulin infusion**

Prescribe the **substrate fluid** in the infusions section of the inpatient prescription chart.

The preferred substrate fluid for administration alongside a variable rate intravenous insulin infusions is **0.45% sodium chloride with 5% glucose**. The fluid should also contain **potassium chloride** in an amount appropriate for the serum potassium concentration:
**40 mmol/L** if serum K⁺ <4.0 mmol/L; **20 mmol/L** if serum K⁺ 4.0–5.5 mmol/L; **no potassium chloride** if serum K⁺ >5.5 mmol/L.

**INFUSION PRESCRIPTIONS**

| Date | Time | Fluid | Vol | Drug | Dose | Rate | Doctor initials | Nurse initials | Batch no | Start time | Stop time |
|---|---|---|---|---|---|---|---|---|---|---|---|
| 7/1/15 | 22:00 | 0.45% SODIUM CHLORIDE WITH 5% GLUCOSE | 1 L | POTASSIUM CHLORIDE | 20 mmol | 100 mL/h | AD | | | | |
| | | | | | | | | | | | |
| | | | | | | | | | | | |
| | | | | | | | | | | | |

determined by the maintenance fluid requirement of the patient, and this rate should then be kept constant so as not to destabilise the patient's insulin requirement. If the patient requires supplementary fluid replacement on top of this (e.g. for rehydration), this should be prescribed and administered separately.

The VRIII should generally be discontinued as soon as the patient is eating and drinking. The transition between IV and SC insulin should be timed to coincide with a meal-related insulin dose. Refer to your local protocol for more detailed guidance on this.

### How do I write the prescription?

Most hospitals have introduced pre-printed VRIII prescription charts, usually accompanied by a protocol to inform its use.

The steps required to initiate a VRIII include the following:

1 *Prescribing the patient's usual dose of long-acting insulin (if applicable).* For patients who usually take long-acting insulin (e.g. glargine, detemir), it is usually best to continue giving this while the patient is on a VRIII. The dose may be prescribed on the dedicated section of the VRIII chart (as illustrated in the model prescription), or, if this is not provided, it should be prescribed on the usual inpatient prescription chart. Mr Patel usually takes 18 units of insulin glargine at bedtime so this has been prescribed for 22:00 as shown.

2 *Prescribing the IV insulin preparation.* The VRIII chart may have this pre-printed for you, in which case you just need to sign against the prescription, as illustrated. If not, you should prescribe it in the infusions section of the drug chart as: Actrapid® 50 units made up to 50 mL with 0.9% sodium chloride.

3 *Prescribing the IV insulin infusion rate scale.* This will be determined by guidance provided in the hospital protocol. Based on the mock protocol provided on the answer sheet, Mr Patel should start on 'Scale A', as a dose of long-acting insulin has also been prescribed.

4 *Prescribing the substrate fluid.* In the example protocol, a solution of 0.45% sodium chloride with 5% glucose is recommended. This should also contain potassium chloride in an amount appropriate for the patient's serum potassium concentration. The fluid should be prescribed at a rate of 83–125 mL/hr to meet the patient's maintenance fluid requirement. The rate of administration selected in this case, 100 mL/hr, will provide Mr Patel with 2.4 L fluid over 24 hours. Potassium 20 mmol/L has also been prescribed, as recommended for his normal serum potassium concentration.

The nursing staff will now administer the VRIII according to your prescription. You should periodically check that Mr Patel's CBG concentration is in the target range. If not, you adjust the infusion rate scale by crossing through the existing scale then prescribing an adjusted one in the space provided. You should ensure his fluid balance and serum electrolyte concentrations are monitored daily, and his fluid therapy adjusted accordingly.

### Further reading

Dhatariya K, Levy N, Kilvert A, et al. NHS Diabetes guideline for the perioperative management of the adult patient with diabetes. Diabet Med. 2012;29(4):420–33. Available at: http://onlinelibrary.wiley.com/doi/10.1111/j.1464-5491.2012.03582.x/pdf (accessed 24 January 2014).

Prescribing at a Glance. Chapters 33 & 34: Using drugs for the endocrine system.

## What should I consider when deciding what to prescribe?

Mrs Harmsworth has an acute kidney injury (AKI). AKI is the preferred term for abrupt onset renal impairment (occurring over hours or days), as it has a broader and more practical definition than acute renal failure (ARF). AKI is usually characterised by an abrupt fall in the urine output (oliguria) and a rising serum creatinine concentration. The estimated glomerular filtration rate (eGFR; which is calculated from the serum creatinine concentration) also falls, although it should be noted that eGFR may not accurately reflect renal function when the creatinine is changing.

The most common cause of AKI is acute tubular necrosis. In hospital inpatients, this is most often due to hypovolaemia, sepsis or nephrotoxic drugs (e.g. non-steroidal anti-inflammatory drugs (NSAIDs), intravenous contrast material).

There are five key steps in the management of AKI.

### 1. Fluid management to maintain euvolaemia

The aim is to maintain adequate renal perfusion, without causing fluid overload. In this case, the clinical examination suggests that Mrs Henderson is euvolaemic, and does not require treatment either to expand her intravascular volume (by fluid challenge; see Case 20) or contract her extracellular fluid volume (by diuresis). However, this may change. You should therefore institute careful fluid balance monitoring and maintain neutral fluid balance. This means her fluid input should match her output (i.e. urine output plus approximately 500 mL/day to account for insensible losses).

### 2. Review the patient's medicines for safety in renal impairment

Look at the prescription chart and check each drug in the BNF for its safety in renal impairment.

### Drugs that cause renal impairment

Common culprit drugs among inpatients are angiotensin converting enzyme (ACE) inhibitors, angiotensin receptor blockers (ARBs) and NSAIDs. These are particularly dangerous in combination, and especially when renal perfusion falls (e.g. in sepsis and hypovolaemia). ACE inhibitors/ARBs and NSAIDs should almost always be suspended in AKI, as they should be in this case (one note of caution is in relation to low-dose aspirin in patients who have recently had a drug-eluting coronary artery stent inserted, which should not usually be stopped unless agreed with the responsible cardiologist; see Case 48).

### Drugs that accumulate in renal impairment

Some drugs are not nephrotoxic but rely on the kidneys for their elimination. These will accumulate if renal function is impaired, and they may need to be stopped or their dose reduced. Again, advice can be found in the BNF.

Mrs Harmsworth is currently being treated with tramadol 100 mg up to 6-hourly. This dose is too high in renal impairment and may cause opioid toxicity. It should be reduced, and she should be monitored carefully for adverse effects if it needs to be administered. Dalteparin is also excreted by the kidneys. The BNF offers two options: to reduce the dosage (e.g. halve it to 2500 units daily), or to replace it with unfractionated heparin (usual dosage 5000 units subcutaneously 12-hourly). Your choice will usually be dictated by local policy.

### 3. Identify and treat reversible causes

One of the most important reversible causes of AKI is nephrotoxic drug treatment – this is dealt with in step 2. Other important

| Surname | Hospital number | Weight | Drug intolerances |
|---|---|---|---|
| HARMSWORTH | 100031 | | |
| First name | Date of birth | 74 kg | None known |
| DOROTHY | 14/04/1935 | | |

**REGULAR PRESCRIPTIONS**

Month: January    Year: 2015

| DRUG ASPIRIN | | | | 06 | | | | | | |
|---|---|---|---|---|---|---|---|---|---|---|
| Dose 75 mg | Route Oral | Freq Daily | Start date 2/1/15 | 08 | AM AM AM AM AM AM | | | | STOPPED 7/1/15 due to AKI | |
| Signature A Doctor | | Bleep 1234 | Review | 12 | | | | | A Doctor 1234 | |
| Additional instructions | | | | 18 / 22 | | | | | | |

| DRUG DALTEPARIN | | | | 06 | | STOPPED 7/1/15 due to AKI A Doctor 1234 |
|---|---|---|---|---|---|---|
| Dose 5000 units | Route SC | Freq Daily | Start date 2/1/15 | 08 / 12 / 16 | | |
| Signature A Doctor | | Bleep 1234 | Review | 18 | AM AM AM AM AM AM | |
| Additional instructions | | | | 22 | | |

| DRUG RAMIPRIL | | | | 06 | | STOPPED 7/1/15 due to AKI A Doctor 1234 |
|---|---|---|---|---|---|---|
| Dose 10 mg | Route Oral | Freq Daily | Start date 2/1/15 | 08 / 12 / 16 | | |
| Signature A Doctor | | Bleep 1234 | Review | 18 | | |
| Additional instructions | | | | 22 | AM AM AM AM AM | |

| DRUG NAPROXEN | | | | 06 | | STOPPED 7/1/15 due to AKI A Doctor 1234 |
|---|---|---|---|---|---|---|
| Dose 250 mg | Route Oral | Freq 8-hrly | Start date 3/1/15 | 08 | AM AM AM AM | |
| Signature A Doctor | | Bleep 1234 | Review | 16 | AM AM AM AM AM AM | |
| Additional instructions | | | | 22 24 | AM AM AM AM | |

| DRUG ATORVASTATIN | | | | 06 / 08 | |
|---|---|---|---|---|---|
| Dose 10 mg | Route Oral | Freq Nightly | Start date 3/1/15 | 12 / 16 / 18 | |
| Signature A Doctor | | Bleep 1234 | Review | 22 | AM AM AM AM |

| DRUG HEPARIN | | | | 06 / 08 | |
|---|---|---|---|---|---|
| Dose 5000 units | Route SC | Freq 12-hrly | Start date 7/1/15 | 12 / 16 | |
| Signature A Doctor | | Bleep 1234 | Review | 18 / 22 | |

**ONCE ONLY PRESCRIPTIONS**

| Date | Time to be given | DRUG | Dose | Route | Prescriber | | Administration | | |
|------|------------------|------|------|-------|------------|--|----------------|--|--|
| | | | | | Signature | Bleep | Date given | Time given | Given by |
| | | | | | | | | | |
| | | | | | | | | | |
| | | | | | | | | | |

**OXYGEN**

| Target SpO₂ | ○ 94–98% ○ 88–92% |
|-------------|--------------------|
| Mode of delivery | ○ Continuous ○ As required |
| Starting device | |

| Initials | Bleep | Date |
|----------|-------|------|
| | | |

**AS REQUIRED MEDICATION**

| DRUG TRAMADOL | | | | Date | 4/1 | 4/1 | 4/1 | 5/1 | 5/1 | 6/1 | 6/1 | 7/1 | | |
|---------------|--|--|--|------|-----|-----|-----|-----|-----|-----|-----|-----|--|--|
| | | | | Time | 08:00 | 14:00 | 22:00 | 08:00 | 20:00 | 10:00 | 22:00 | 18:00 | | |
| Dose 100 mg | Route Oral | Max freq 6-hrly | Start date 3/1/15 | Dose | 100 mg | 100 mg | 100 mg | 100 mg | 100 mg | 100 mg | 100 mg | 100 mg | STOPPED 7/1/15 due to | |
| | | | | Route | Oral | Oral | Oral | Oral | Oral | Oral | Oral | Oral | AKI (dose reduced) | |
| Signature A Doctor | Bleep 1234 | Review 7 days | | Given | AM | AM | AM | AM | AM | AM | AM | AM | A Doctor | |
| | | | | Check | BN | BN | BN | BN | BN | BN | BN | BN | 1234 | |
| Additional instructions Max 400 mg/day | | | | | | | | | | | | | | |

| DRUG TRAMADOL | | | | Date | | | | | | | | | | |
|---------------|--|--|--|------|--|--|--|--|--|--|--|--|--|--|
| | | | | Time | | | | | | | | | | |
| Dose 50 mg | Route Oral | Max freq 8-hrly | Start date 7/1/15 | Dose | | | | | | | | | | |
| | | | | Route | | | | | | | | | | |
| Signature A Doctor | Bleep 1234 | Review | | Given | | | | | | | | | | |
| | | | | Check | | | | | | | | | | |
| Additional instructions Renal dose. Monitor GCS, respiratory rate and pupils hourly for 6 hours after administration. | | | | | | | | | | | | | | |

| DRUG | | | | Date | | | | | | | | | | |

reversible causes include urinary tract obstruction and infection. Always palpate the abdomen for an enlarged bladder and request an urgent ultrasound scan of the urinary tract. If imaging is not immediately available, insert a urinary catheter (this may later be removed if there is no evidence of obstruction and if it is not required for urine output monitoring). Always send a urine microbiology sample for microscopy, culture and sensitivity.

### 4. Identify and treat complications

Key complications of acute kidney injury can be remembered using the mnemonic 'SWEAT' (Table 31.2). This summarises the substances that are usually eliminated by the kidneys. If the kidneys are not working, they will accumulate to generate complications. The initial medical treatment of these complications is outlined in Table 31.2. Mrs Harmsworth does not presently have signs of any complications of AKI.

### 5. Seek specialist advice

AKI is a serious condition that may require specialist investigation and management, including renal replacement therapy (haemodi-alysis or haemofiltration) in some instances. Traditional indications for renal replacement therapy may be recalled using the SWEAT mnemonic (Table 31.2). However, you should not wait for these to occur before seeking specialist advice from a nephrologist or intensive care physician.

### How do I write the prescription?

Discontinue nephrotoxic drugs by crossing through their prescriptions and signing and dating this. Ensure you clearly document in the medical notes why you have stopped the drugs, and under what circumstances you think they might safely be reintroduced.

- Naproxen (and other NSAIDs) should not be reintroduced for the foreseeable future unless there is a compelling reason to do so, and only then under specialist medical advice
- Low-dose aspirin may be reintroduced once her renal function has normalised, provided there are no on-going risk factors for AKI
- Ramipril may be reintroduced cautiously, and with careful monitoring, only once her renal function has normalised, provided there are no on-going risk factors for AKI.

Where you envisage the drugs may be restarted imminently, an alternative and commonly used approach is to endorse the prescription to state that the drug should be, for example, 'reviewed daily' or 'withheld until renal function normalises'. However, this approach tends to generate confusion and inconsistency among both nursing and medical staff, so is best avoided.

To alter the tramadol and dalteparin prescriptions, it is best to stop the existing prescriptions (as above) and rewrite modified prescriptions on a new line. In the model chart, tramadol has been represcribed at a reduced dosage, and dalteparin has been changed to unfractionated heparin.

### Further reading

London Acute Kidney Injury Network. London AKI Network Manual http://www.londonaki.net/downloads/LondonAKInetwork-Manual.pdf (accessed 24 January 2014).
Prescribing at a Glance. Chapter 15: Prescribing in renal disease.

**Table 31.2** A mnemonic to aid recall of the complications of renal impairment, their treatment, and the indications for renal replacement therapy (usually haemodialysis or haemofiltration in the context of acute kidney injury)

| | Substance normally eliminated by the kidneys | Complications associated with accumulation of this substance | Initial medical treatment | Indication for renal replacement therapy |
|--|----------------------------------------------|--------------------------------------------------------------|---------------------------|------------------------------------------|
| S W | Salt Water | Peripheral oedema Pulmonary oedema | Loop diuretic | Pulmonary oedema refractory to medical treatment |
| E | Electrolytes (especially potassium) | Hyperkalaemia | Insulin and glucose | Severe hyperkalaemia refractory to medical therapy |
| A | Acid | Acidosis | Occasionally sodium bicarbonate, but this can be problematic | Severe or progressive metabolic acidosis |
| T | Toxins | Uraemic encephalopathy, neuropathy, and pericarditis | No specific medical treatment | All patients with uraemic complications, if appropriate for the patient |

## What should I consider when deciding what to prescribe?

Mrs Nuttall has developed hospital-acquired pneumonia. Evidence for this includes pyrexia; bronchial breathing and crackles on chest examination; new right lower lobe consolidation on chest X-ray; and markedly elevated white cell count and C-reactive protein. The pneumonia has caused type 1 respiratory failure, with hypoxia, despite 2 L/min of supplemental oxygen administered by nasal cannulae, and compensatory hypocapnoea. She is also tachycardic and her blood pressure has fallen relative to its usual level, consistent with systemic response to infection.

## Urgent management

Hypoxia and severe infection are the two most life-threatening issues for Mrs Nuttall and should be addressed as quickly as possible.

*Hypoxia.* The first thing you should do is make sure that Mrs Nuttall is sitting upright in bed, propped up as necessary with pillows. This allows increased lung expansion and may improve oxygenation. As she has type 1 respiratory failure, you should prescribe oxygen with target saturations of 94–98%. Given the severity of her hypoxia, her nasal cannulae should be replaced by a non-rebreather facemask with reservoir bag, and the oxygen flow rate increased to 15 L/min. This allows delivery of high inhaled oxygen concentrations of 60–80%. If she does not attain oxygen saturations of $\geq$94% using this device, she may need further respiratory support, and you should consult with the critical care team as a matter of urgency.

*Infection.* Pneumonia that develops more than 48 hours after hospital admission is known as hospital-acquired pneumonia. It is distinguished from community-acquired pneumonia as it is often caused by different organisms and requires a different approach to antibiotic treatment.

## Which organisms?

Hospital-acquired pneumonia is most commonly caused by bacteria. Causative bacteria include the following:
- Bacteria causing pneumonia in vulnerable people, including those with acute illness, immunosuppression and chronic chest disease, and/or circulating more commonly in hospitals:
  - Gram-negative organisms, e.g. *Escherichia coli, Klebsiella pneumoniae, Pseudomonas aeruginosa, Acinetobacter* species
  - Antibiotic-resistant organisms e.g. meticillin-resistant *Staphylococcus aureus* (MRSA)
  - Anaerobic organisms (aspiration)
- Bacteria causing pneumonia in the community
  - *Streptococcus pneumoniae*
  - *Haemophilus pneumoniae*
  - Atypical organisms including *Mycoplasma pneumoniae* and *Legionella pneumophila.*

## Which antibiotic?

A broad-spectrum antibiotic regimen should be used as initial treatment for hospital-acquired pneumonia to cover the wide range of potential pathogens. The key distinction with community-acquired pneumonia is that treatment needs to include agents active against Gram-negative organisms. In Mrs Nuttall's case, you should take into account her recent stroke and associated risk of aspiration pneumonia, which means that cover will be needed for anaerobic bacteria. As she has a 50-pack-year smoking history, she may also have undiagnosed chronic lung disease. You should consult and follow local antibiotic guidelines where available, and take advice from a microbiologist as needed.

A reasonable initial antibiotic choice for Mrs Nuttall would be co-amoxiclav, a combination of amoxicillin and clavulanic acid. Amoxicillin is a broad-spectrum penicillin with activity against

| Surname NUTTALL | Hospital number 100032 | Weight 75 kg | Drug intolerances None known |
|---|---|---|---|
| First name DORIS | Date of birth 01/11/1929 | | |

**REGULAR PRESCRIPTIONS**

| | Circle / enter times below ↓ | Enter dates below | Month: January | Year: 2015 |
|---|---|---|---|---|
| | | 4 | 5 | 6 | 7 | 8 | | | | | |

DRUG **AMLODIPINE** — Dose 5 mg | Route Oral | Freq Daily | Start date 4/1/15 — Signature A Doctor | Bleep 1234 | Review — Additional instructions: If systolic >130 mmHg
Times: 06, 08 (circled), 12, 16, 18, 22 — 08 row: AM AM AM AM OMIT

DRUG **CLOPIDOGREL** — Dose 75 mg | Route Oral | Freq Daily | Start date 4/1/15 — Signature A Doctor | Bleep 1234 | Review — Additional instructions
Times: 06, 08 (circled), 12, 16, 18, 22 — 08 row: AM AM AM AM

DRUG **DALTEPARIN** — Dose 5000 units | Route S/C | Freq Daily | Start date 4/1/15 — Signature A Doctor | Bleep 1234 | Review — Additional instructions
Times: 06, 08, 12, 16, 18 (circled), 22 — 18 row: AM AM AM AM

DRUG **RAMIPRIL** — Dose 5 mg | Route Oral | Freq Daily | Start date 4/1/15 — Signature A Doctor | Bleep 1234 | Review — Additional instructions: Review when recovers from sepsis
Times: 06, 08 (circled), 12, 16, 18, 22 — 08 row: AM AM AM AM — STOPPED 7/1/15 A Doctor 1234

DRUG **CO-AMOXICLAV** — Dose 1.2 g | Route IV | Freq 8-hrly | Start date 7/1/15 — Signature A Doctor | Bleep 1234 | Review 7 days — Additional instructions: For hospital-acquired pneumonia, consider oral switch at 48 hr
Times: 06, 08, 14 (circled), 16, 18, 22 — x (14 circled)

## ONCE ONLY PRESCRIPTIONS

| Date | Time to be given | DRUG | Dose | Route | Prescriber Signature | Prescriber Bleep | Administration Date given | Administration Time given | Administration Given by |
|------|------------------|------|------|-------|-----------|-------|------------|------------|----------|
| 7/1/15 | 23:00 | CO-AMOXICLAV | 1.2 g | IV | AD | 1234 | | | |
| | | | | | | | | | |
| | | | | | | | | | |

### OXYGEN

| Target SpO₂ | ✓ 94–98% |
|---|---|
| | ○ 88–92% |
| Mode of delivery | ✓ Continuous |
| | ○ As required |
| Starting device | Non-rebreather mask |

| Initials | Bleep | Date |
|---------|-------|------|
| AD | 1234 | 7/1/15 |

## AS REQUIRED MEDICATION

| DRUG | | | | Date | | | | | | | | |
|------|--|--|--|------|--|--|--|--|--|--|--|--|
| | | | | Time | | | | | | | | |
| Dose | Route | Max freq | Start date | Dose | | | | | | | | |
| | | | | Route | | | | | | | | |
| Signature | Bleep | Review | | Given | | | | | | | | |
| | | | | Check | | | | | | | | |
| Additional instructions | | | | | | | | | | | | |

| DRUG | | | | Date | | | | | | | | |
|------|--|--|--|------|--|--|--|--|--|--|--|--|
| | | | | Time | | | | | | | | |
| Dose | Route | Max freq | Start date | Dose | | | | | | | | |
| | | | | Route | | | | | | | | |
| Signature | Bleep | Review | | Given | | | | | | | | |
| | | | | Check | | | | | | | | |
| Additional instructions | | | | | | | | | | | | |

| DRUG | | | | Date | | | | | | | | |
|------|--|--|--|------|--|--|--|--|--|--|--|--|
| | | | | Time | | | | | | | | |
| Dose | Route | Max freq | Start date | Dose | | | | | | | | |
| | | | | Route | | | | | | | | |
| Signature | Bleep | Review | | Given | | | | | | | | |
| | | | | Check | | | | | | | | |
| Additional instructions | | | | | | | | | | | | |

| DRUG | | | | Date | | | | | | | | |
|------|--|--|--|------|--|--|--|--|--|--|--|--|
| | | | | Time | | | | | | | | |
| Dose | Route | Max freq | Start date | Dose | | | | | | | | |
| | | | | Route | | | | | | | | |
| Signature | Bleep | Review | | Given | | | | | | | | |
| | | | | Check | | | | | | | | |
| Additional instructions | | | | | | | | | | | | |

## INFUSION PRESCRIPTIONS

| Date | Time | Fluid | Vol | Drug | Dose | Rate | Doctor initials | Nurse initials | Batch no | Start time | Stop time |
|------|------|-------|-----|------|------|------|-----------------|----------------|----------|------------|-----------|
| 7/1/15 | 23:00 | 0.9% SODIUM CHLORIDE | 1 L | | | 6 hr | AD | | | | |
| 7/1/15 | To follow | 5% GLUCOSE | 1 L | | | 6 hr | AD | | | | |
| | | | | | | | | | | | |
| | | | | | | | | | | | |

Gram-negative as well as Gram-positive bacteria. Clavulanic acid protects amoxicillin from breakdown by bacterial beta lactamases, which improves its activity against anaerobic bacteria, MRSA, and other bacteria that synthesise beta lactamases.

Before starting antibiotics, blood and (if possible) sputum samples should be taken for microscopy and culture. Results from these tests will usually not be available for about 2 days, but if a particular pathogen is identified, treatment can then be adjusted accordingly.

## Alternatives

You will definitely need microbiological and senior clinical advice when handling any of these alternative situations:
- Antibiotic alternatives to penicillin for hospital-acquired pneumonia include cephalosporins and other beta lactam antibiotics. However, a small proportion of people with penicillin allergy may also be allergic to these agents. Patients with true immunoglobulin E (IgE) mediated penicillin allergy may therefore require an antibiotic from a completely different class, e.g. a quinolone.
- If MRSA is a likely causative organism, vancomycin should be added to treatment.

- If *Pseudomonas aeruginosa* is a likely causative organism, an anti-pseudomonal penicillin (e.g. piperacillin with tazobactam), broad-spectrum cephalosporin (e.g. ceftazidime) or quinolone (e.g. ciprofloxacin) should be prescribed.

## Other treatment
### Nil by mouth
As Mrs Nuttall has a provisional diagnosis of aspiration pneumonia, you should reduce the risk of further aspiration until a more detailed assessment can be made by making her 'nil by mouth'.

### Fluids
As Mrs Nuttall will be 'nil by mouth', her daily fluid and electrolyte requirements must be met by an alternative route of administration. This can be achieved in the middle of the night by administration of intravenous fluid. In the morning, insertion of a nasogastric tube and enteral feeding may be considered.

Doris's fluid and electrolyte requirements include replacement of any deficit, added to normal daily maintenance requirements, adjusted for additional losses (see Case 19).
- *Maintenance.* Approximate daily requirements are 2.5 L water, 75 mmol sodium and 75 mmol potassium
- *Additional losses.* She has a pyrexia and tachypnoea, which will increase her insensible water loss by sweating and evaporation from the respiratory tract
- *Deficit.* She has a mild reduction in blood pressure and elevation of urea, indicating possible reduction in intravascular volume with salt and water deficit.

It is not easy to estimate the exact size of her fluid deficit and additional losses. A reasonable approach over the next 12 hours would be to provide 2 L of fluid, as illustrated, and assess her response to this by monitoring her observations, urine output and biochemistry. As she has sepsis and hypotension, she is at risk of developing acute kidney injury. It would therefore be reasonable to avoid potassium replacement for now, but to monitor serum potassium levels and renal function and review depending on her trajectory.

### Usual medication
As she is 'nil by mouth' she will not receive any medication administered orally. You should review existing medicines and ensure that any essential medicines can be administered by an alternative route.

As Mrs Nuttall has severe sepsis with a rising urea, you need to withhold amlodipine and ramipril as these drugs lower blood pressure and have potential to worsen acute kidney injury.

## How do I write the prescription?
### Oxygen
Oxygen should be prescribed, specifying target saturations of 94–98%, continuous administration and initial delivery via a non-rebreather (reservoir) mask.

### Antibiotics
As Mrs Nuttall is severely unwell and is 'nil by mouth' you should prescribe intravenous antibiotics. The usual intravenous dose of

co-amoxiclav is 1.2 g, which contains 1 g amoxicillin and 200 mg clavulanic acid. As she has a normal eGFR, you should prescribe co-amoxiclav 1.2 g 8-hourly. The dose and/or administration frequency should be reduced in patients with significant renal impairment. It is important that Mrs Nuttall gets her first dose of antibiotics straight away. The first dose has therefore been prescribed in the once only section of the prescription chart.

You should state the indication and duration of treatment for any antibiotics you prescribe, as this facilitates pharmacy and microbiology review and good antibiotic stewardship. In the model prescription a review time of 7 days for antibiotic treatment has been set, with a suggestion to consider a switch from the intravenous to oral route at 48 hours (assuming she can take treatment by mouth or has an enteral tube by this stage).

## Fluids

An initial prescription for 2 L of fluid, based on 0.9% sodium chloride and 5% glucose, has been written in the infusion section. This may be modified depending on her clinical course.

## Existing medications

Amlodipine has been withheld for the next dose. An instruction to give the medication only if systolic blood pressure is >130 mmHg has been added. Ramipril has been stopped for the time being to reduce the risk of this drug worsening acute kidney injury.

## Further reading

Medical Pharmacology at a Glance. Chapters 38 and 39: Antibacterial drugs.
Prescribing at a Glance. Chapter 32: Using drugs for infection.

---

## 33    A 47-year-old man who has developed an abnormal liver profile

### What should I consider when reviewing the drug chart?

Kazim Qureshi has developed an abnormal liver profile during hospital admission. A hepatic ultrasound and other investigations have shown no other cause and suggest that this is due to a drug reaction. You need to review his medications and determine whether any should be stopped or modified to address this problem.

### What drugs cause an abnormal liver profile?

The liver is heavily exposed to circulating drugs, receiving 100% of the portal circulation and 20% of the systemic cardiac output, and being the main site of drug metabolism. Liver toxicity is therefore a common side effect of medicines.

Drug-induced hepatic toxicity can be:

A Dose-related (**A**ugmented). Toxicity relates to the action of the drug and will affect everyone if they take enough of the drug:
  • Example drug: paracetamol.

B Idiosyncratic (**B**izarre). Toxicity is due to an unpredictable interaction between the drug and the individual with underlying mechanisms including immune activation or genetic variation. These reactions affect far fewer people (usually <1%) and are unrelated to the action of the drug:
  • Example drugs: haloperidol, isoniazid, non-steroidal anti-inflammatories, antibiotics, antiepileptics, statins.

C Continued use. Toxicity does not occur with a single dose, but prolonged use of the drug causes chronic inflammation or fibrosis:
  • Example drugs: methotrexate, amiodarone.

There are a variety of patterns of drug-induced liver injury including hepatocellular, biliary (cholestatic) or mixed. These can be distinguished by measurement of plasma liver enzymes. A rise in alanine transaminase (ALT) indicates hepatocyte damage, elevated alkaline

| Surname QURESHI | Hospital number 100033 | Weight 98 kg | Drug intolerances ~~None known~~ Abnormal liver function tests ?haloperidol ?co-amoxiclav |
|---|---|---|---|
| First name KAZIM | Date of birth 01/12/1967 | | |

**REGULAR PRESCRIPTIONS**

Month: Dec/Jan    Year: 2014/2015

| DRUG SIMVASTATIN | Times | 31 | 1 | 2 | 3 | 4 | 5 | 6 | 7 | |
|---|---|---|---|---|---|---|---|---|---|---|
| Dose 40 mg / Route Oral / Freq Daily / Start date 31/12/14 | 06 | | | | | | | | | |
| Signature A Doctor / Bleep 1234 / Review | 08 | | | | | | | | | Withhold for 3 days then review A Doctor 7/1/15 |
| | 12 | | | | | | | | | |
| | 16 | | | | | | | | | |
| Additional instructions | 18 | | | | | | | | | |
| | (22) | | AM | AM | AM | AM | | | | |

| DRUG FOLIC ACID | 06 | | | | | | | | | |
|---|---|---|---|---|---|---|---|---|---|---|
| Dose 5 mg / Route Oral / Freq Daily / Start date 31/12/14 | (08) | | AM | AM | AM | AM | AM | | | |
| Signature A doctor / Bleep 1234 / Review | 12 | | | | | | | | | |
| | 16 | | | | | | | | | |
| Additional instructions | 18 | | | | | | | | | |
| | 22 | | | | | | | | | |

| DRUG CO-AMOXICLAV | (06) | | AM | AM | AM | AM | AM AM | AM | | |
|---|---|---|---|---|---|---|---|---|---|---|
| Dose 1.2 g / Route IV / Freq 8-hrly / Start date 31/12/14 ✗ (14) | 08 | | | | | | | | | STOP 7/1/2015 |
| Signature A Doctor / Bleep 1234 / Review | 14 | | AM | AM | AM | AM | AM AM | | | A Doctor 1234 |
| | 18 | | | | | | | | | |
| Additional instructions | (22) | AM | AM | AM | AM AM | AM AM | | | | |

| DRUG PARACETAMOL | (06) | | AM | AM | AM | AM AM | AM AM | | | |
|---|---|---|---|---|---|---|---|---|---|---|
| Dose 1 g / Route Oral / Freq 6-hrly / Start date 31/12/14 | 08 | | | | | | | | | STOP 7/1/2015 |
| Signature A Doctor / Bleep 1234 / Review | (12) | | AM | AM | AM | AM | AM | | | A Doctor 1234 |
| | (18) | | AM | AM | AM | AM | AM | | | |
| Additional instructions | (22) | | AM | AM | AM | AM AM | AM | | | |

| DRUG DALTEPARIN | 06 | | | | | | | | | |
|---|---|---|---|---|---|---|---|---|---|---|
| Dose 5000 units / Route S/C / Freq Daily / Start date 31/12/14 | 08 | | | | | | | | | |
| Signature A Doctor / Bleep 1234 / Review | 12 | | | | | | | | | |
| | (18) | | AM | AM | AM | AM | AM AM | | | |
| Additional instructions | 22 | | | | | | | | | |

| DRUG METHOTREXATE | 06 | | | | | | | | | |
|---|---|---|---|---|---|---|---|---|---|---|
| Dose 15 mg / Route Oral / Freq Weekly / Start date 31/12/14 | (12) | | | | | | | | Omit | |
| Signature A Doctor / Bleep 1234 / Review | 16 | | | | | | | | | A Doctor 7/1/15 |
| | 18 | | | | | | | | | |
| Additional instructions | 22 | | | | | | | | | |

## ONCE ONLY PRESCRIPTIONS

| Date | Time to be given | DRUG | Dose | Route | Prescriber Signature | Prescriber Bleep | Administration Date given | Administration Time given | Administration Given by |
|------|------|------|------|-------|------|------|------|------|------|
| 31/12/14 | 22:00 | GENTAMICIN | 500 mg | IV | AD | 1234 | 31/12/14 | 2200 | AN |
| 31/12/14 | 22:00 | COAMOXICLAV | 1.2 g | IV | AD | 1234 | 31/12/14 | 2200 | AN |

**OXYGEN**

Target SpO₂: ✓ 94–98%  ○ 88–92%
Mode of delivery: ✓ Continuous  ○ As required
Starting device: Face mask

| Initials | Bleep | Date |
|------|------|------|
| AD | 1234 | 1/1/15 |

## AS REQUIRED MEDICATION

**DRUG** MORPHINE

Dose 10 mg | Route S/C | Max freq 4 hrly | Start date 31/12/14
Signature A Doctor | Bleep 1234 | Review
Additional instructions

| Date | 1/1 | 1/1 | 1/1 | 1/1 | 2/1 | 3/1 | 3/1 | 3/1 | 4/1 | 4/1 | 5/1 | STOP |
|------|------|------|------|------|------|------|------|------|------|------|------|------|
| Time | 06 | 12 | 18 | 24 | 06 | 10 | 18 | 22 | 08 | 14 | 06 | 7/1/2015 |
| Dose | 10mg | 10mg | 10mg | 10mg | 10mg | 10mg | 10mg | 10mg | 10mg | 10mg | 10mg | A Doctor |
| Route | SC | SC | SC | SC | SC | SC | SC | SC | SC | SC | SC | 1234 |
| Given | AN | AN | AN | AN | AN | AN | AN | AN | AN | AN | AN | |
| Check | AN | AN | AN | AN | AN | AN | AN | AN | AN | AN | AN | |

**DRUG** CODEINE PHOSPHATE

Dose 30–60mg | Route Oral | Max freq 4 hrly | Start date 31/12/14
Signature A Doctor | Bleep 1234 | Review
Additional instructions

| Date | 2/1 | 2/1 | 2/1 | 3/1 | 3/1 | 4/1 | 4/1 |
|------|------|------|------|------|------|------|------|
| Time | 12 | 18 | 24 | 06 | 18 | 08 | 22 |
| Dose | 30mg | 30mg | 30mg | 30mg | 30mg | 30mg | 30mg |
| Route | Oral | Oral | Oral | Oral | Oral | Oral | Oral |
| Given | AN | AN | AN | AN | AN | AN | AN |
| Check | AN | AN | AN | AN | AN | AN | AN |

**DRUG** HALOPERIDOL

Dose 2mg | Route Oral/IM | Max freq 8 hrly | Start date 27/1/15
Signature A Doctor | Bleep 1234 | Review
Additional instructions

| Date | 2/1 | 3/1 | 3/1 | 4/1 | 4/1 | 5/1 | 5/1 | STOP |
|------|------|------|------|------|------|------|------|------|
| Time | 22 | 12 | 24 | 10 | 22 | 08 | 22 | 7/1/2015 |
| Dose | 2mg | 2mg | 2mg | 2mg | 2mg | 2mg | 2mg | A Doctor |
| Route | IM | IM | IM | IM | IM | IM | IM | 1234 |
| Given | AN | AN | AN | AN | AN | AN | AN | |
| Check | AN | AN | AN | AN | AN | AN | AN | |

**DRUG** PARACETAMOL

Dose 1 g | Route Oral | Max freq 8 hrly | Start date 7/1/15
Signature A Doctor | Bleep 1234 | Review
Additional instructions: Maximum 3 g per day

| Date | |
|------|------|
| Time | |
| Dose | |
| Route | |
| Given | |
| Check | |

---

phosphatase (ALP) indicates biliary canalicular cell damage and elevated gamma glutamyl transferase (GGT), being released from all hepatic mitochondria, indicates liver damage without specific indication of site. Liver function can be assessed by the excretion of bilirubin and synthesis of albumin and clotting factors. Impairment of liver function indicates severe drug-induced liver damage and is a poor prognostic sign.

### How do you interpret Mr Qureshi's liver tests?

Mr Qureshi's liver function tests were actually abnormal in October, before his acute illness. At this time, elevated ALT and GGT, with normal ALP, albumin and bilirubin, indicated a mild hepatitis. Simvastatin causes a mild elevation of transaminases in approximately 5% of patients and serious liver injury more rarely. Methotrexate causes hepatic abnormalities ranging from mild fatty liver to more serious fibrosis, necrosis and cirrhosis.

At admission, his liver function tests remained abnormal but were stable. A falling albumin could be the result of sepsis. Following surgery, he has an acute rise in GGT and ALP with a smaller rise in ALT. This indicates an acute cholestatic reaction and indicates that one of the new drugs he has received during hospital admission has caused this new abnormality. Haloperidol and co-amoxiclav are the most likely culprit drugs.

### What action should you take?

Liver injury usually recovers when the culprit drug is removed and the chances of recovery are greatest if the drug is stopped promptly. Stopping drugs can be difficult if the drug is still required for treatment or if there are several drugs that could have caused the adverse drug reaction. If in doubt, drugs used for chronic disease can be withheld for 24–48 hours until more senior decision-makers are available. Drugs for acute illness can be stopped if the acute illness has resolved.

Drugs metabolised by the liver may accumulate in patients with acute liver injury. You should consider stopping these drugs or reducing the dose or dose interval.

### How do I write the prescription?

You should review each of the drugs on the chart and consider whether they should be continued, stopped or substituted, or whether a dose reduction is required. You should record likely new drug intolerances in the appropriate section of the chart.

### Drugs

*Simvastatin* is used for chronic management of hypercholesterolaemia. It would therefore be reasonable for you to withhold simvastatin until the acute liver injury has resolved. In the longer term, it may be the cause of the chronic elevation in ALT and may need to be stopped or substituted. In the model chart, a T-bar and additional information have been used to indicate that simvastatin has been withheld and when it should restart.

*Folic acid* does not cause liver injury and does not accumulate in hepatic failure so can be continued.

*Co-amoxiclav* is an essential life-saving treatment for intra-abdominal sepsis, but is also a likely cause of Mr Qureshi's acute liver injury. You need to decide whether it can be stopped or changed. After 7 days of intravenous antibiotics, Mr Qureshi is well with normal observations and abdominal examination, good wound healing and resolving inflammatory markers. It would be reasonable to stop the intravenous antibiotics at this stage and either observe for clinical deterioration or continue antibiotic treatment orally with an alternative drug. However, you should discuss further need for antibiotics with your senior colleagues or local microbiologist and consult local antibiotic guidelines. In the model chart a decision has been made to stop antibiotics and observe the patient.

*Paracetamol* is metabolised by the liver to a toxic metabolite which could potentially accumulate in and worsen liver injury. As Mr Qureshi is not currently in pain, you could stop regular paracetamol and write up paracetamol as required as shown. However, it is important to ensure that pain control is maintained.

*Dalteparin* (a low molecular weight heparin) does not cause liver toxicity and is not metabolised by the liver. However, as an anticoagulant it can add to the risk of bleeding in patients with liver disease who have impaired clotting. In the model prescription it has been decided to keep Mr Qureshi – who has normal clotting – on dalteparin until discharge from hospital as he has had sepsis, reduced mobility and abdominal surgery which are all risk factors for venous thromboembolism.

*Methotrexate* is due tomorrow for treatment of psoriasis. It would be reasonable for you to withhold tomorrow's dose both because of the acute liver injury and because of the recent sepsis (methotrexate causes immunosuppression).

*Opioid analgesia.* Mr Qureshi is no longer requiring opioid analgesia. At this stage it is reasonable for you to stop the morphine to reduce the risk of further administration if his liver injury deteriorates (opioids can cause coma and precipitate encephalopathy in patients with hepatic failure). It is also reasonable to leave a prescription for a more moderate opioid analgesic (codeine phosphate) in case he still has some postoperative pain.

*Haloperidol* is a strong candidate for the cause of acute liver injury and is no longer required for delirium. It should therefore be stopped.

### Additional considerations

Mr Qureshi should have his liver profile monitored until it returns to baseline. If this does not occur he may need further review by a hepatologist. As he appears to have had an idiosyncratic reaction to co-amoxiclav or haloperidol he is at risk of recurrence and should be warned of this. It should also be documented on his drug chart in the intolerances section. His simvastatin and methotrexate treatment need review in light of his chronic elevation of ALT. One option would be to stop the simvastatin and see if his liver function returns to normal. His psoriasis is now well controlled and on-going methotrexate treatment should also be reviewed. Due to the severity of this suspected drug reaction, it should be reported to the medicines regulator by completing a Yellow Card (yellowcard.mhra.gov. uk). It does not matter that the exact cause of the reaction is uncertain, or that he has not yet completely recovered from it.

### Further reading

Medical Pharmacology at a Glance. Chapter 27: Antipsychotic drugs (neuroleptics).
Prescribing at a Glance. Chapter 14: Prescribing in liver disease.

---

## 34    An 83-year-old man who develops diarrhoea

### What should I consider when reviewing Mr George's treatment?

#### Causes of hospital-acquired diarrhoea

Mr George has developed diarrhoea during a 6-day hospital stay. Hospital-acquired diarrhoea is most commonly related to medication. Other causes include infection, particularly with *Clostridium difficile* or norovirus; overflow diarrhoea secondary to faecal impaction; dietary, e.g. relating to enteric feeding; and new-onset or flare of underlying bowel disease such as diverticular, inflammatory bowel or coeliac disease.

#### Medications

As most medicines are taken orally, the gastrointestinal (GI) tract is heavily exposed to drugs and GI side effects are very common. Over 700 different drugs have been described as causing diarrhoea. Among the most common are the following:

- Antibiotics
- Cancer chemotherapy
- Colchicine
- Digoxin
- Laxatives
- Magnesium-containing antacids
- Metformin
- Non-steroidal anti-inflammatory drugs
- Proton pump inhibitors (PPIs)
- Thiazide diuretics.

#### Infection

Risk factors for acquiring infective diarrhoea in hospital include poor hand hygiene of potential carriers (staff and visitors) and patients, circulating organisms in the hospital environment, and use of broad-spectrum antibiotics. After seeing a patient with diarrhoea you should always wash your hands with soap and water. Do not rely solely on alcohol hand gels as these do not kill all the organisms that cause diarrhoea.

CHART 2 OF 2

| Surname | Hospital number | Weight | Drug intolerances |
|---|---|---|---|
| GEORGE | 100034 | 55 kg | None known |
| First name | Date of birth | | |
| FREDERICK | 21/10/1931 | | |

## REGULAR PRESCRIPTIONS

Month: **January**  Year: **2015**

Enter dates below: 1 2 3 4 5 6 7 8 9 10

| DRUG | Circle/enter times | 1 | 2 | 3 | 4 | 5 | 6 | 7 | 8 | 9 | 10 |
|---|---|---|---|---|---|---|---|---|---|---|---|
| **LANSOPRAZOLE** — Dose 30 mg, Route Oral, Freq Daily, Start date 1/1/15. Signature A Doctor, Bleep 1234. Additional instructions: Review once diarrhoea settling | 06 | | | | | | | | | | |
| | (08) | AM | AM | AM | AM | AM | AM | AM | Omit | Omit | Omit |
| | 12 | | | | | | | | | | |
| | 16 | | | | | | | | | | |
| | 18 | | | | | | | | | | |
| | 22 | | | | | | | | | | |
| **SERTRALINE** — Dose 50 mg, Route Oral, Freq Daily, Start date 1/1/15. Signature A Doctor, Bleep 1234. | 06 | | | | | | | | | | |
| | (08) | AM | AM | AM | AM | AM | AM | AM | | | |
| | 12 | | | | | | | | | | |
| | 16 | | | | | | | | | | |
| | 18 | | | | | | | | | | |
| | 22 | | | | | | | | | | |
| **SIMVASTATIN** — Dose 40 mg, Route Oral, Freq Daily, Start date 1/1/15. Signature A Doctor, Bleep 1234. | 06 | | | | | | | | | | |
| | 08 | | | | | | | | | | |
| | 12 | | | | | | | | | | |
| | 16 | | | | | | | | | | |
| | 18 | | | | | | | | | | |
| | (22) | AM | AM | AM | AM | AM | AM | | | | |
| **DALTEPARIN** — Dose 5000 units, Route S/C, Freq Daily, Start date 1/1/15. Signature A Doctor, Bleep 1234. | 06 | | | | | | | | | | |
| | 08 | | | | | | | | | | |
| | 12 | | | | | | | | | | |
| | 16 | | | | | | | | | | |
| | (18) | AM | AM | AM | AM | AM | AM | AM | | | |
| | 22 | | | | | | | | | | |
| **METRONIDAZOLE** — Dose 400 mg, Route Oral, Freq 8-hrly, Start date 7/1/15. Signature A Doctor, Bleep 1234, Review 10 days. Additional instructions: For ?C. diff – stop if toxin negative | (06) | | | | | | | | | | |
| | 08 | | | | | | | | | | |
| | ✗ (14) | | | | | | | | | | |
| | 16 | | | | | | | | | | |
| | 18 | | | | | | | | | | |
| | (22) | | | | | | | | | | |
| **SANDO-K** — Dose 2 tabs, Route Oral, Freq 8-hrly, Start date 7/1/15. Signature A Doctor, Bleep 1234, Review 48 hrs. Additional instructions: Stop when serum K⁺ >3.8 mmol/L | 06 | | | | | | | | | REVIEW | |
| | (08) | | | | | | | | | | |
| | (12) | | | | | | | | | | |
| | 16 | | | | | | | | | | |
| | (18) | | | | | | | | | | |
| | 22 | | | | | | | | | | |

## ONCE ONLY PRESCRIPTIONS

| Date | Time to be given | DRUG | Dose | Route | Prescriber Signature | Bleep | Date given | Time given | Given by |
|---|---|---|---|---|---|---|---|---|---|
| 7/1/15 | 20:00 | SANDO K | 2 tabs | Oral | AD | 1234 | | | |

## OXYGEN

| Target SpO₂ | ✔ 94–98% |
|---|---|
| | ☐ 88–92% |
| Mode of delivery | ✔ Continuous |
| | ☐ As required |
| Starting device | Face mask |
| Initials | Bleep | Date |
| AD | 1234 | 1/1/15 |

*Clostridium difficile* is an organism normally found in the GI tract of up to 3% of adults, where it is a harmless commensal. However, some forms of *C. difficile* produce enterotoxins, which cause colonic inflammation. Enterotoxin-producing *C. difficile* persists in the hospital environment as spores, which can survive on inanimate objects such as curtains and bedside lockers (fomites). Patients may then transfer these spores on their hands and ingest them. Where patients are also taking broad-spectrum antibiotics, these kill normal gut flora, reducing bacterial competition and allowing *C. difficile* to proliferate and produce enterotoxin. Patients with *C. difficile* infection experience profuse diarrhoea and may develop pseudomembranous colitis with the rare complications of toxic megacolon (colonic dilatation) and perforation.

### Why does Mr George have diarrhoea?

The nursing staff suspect that Mr George has *C. difficile* infection. In your assessment you should note that he has risk factors for *C. difficile* infection, i.e. he has received broad-spectrum antibiotics administered over a 6-day hospital stay. You also note that he has abdominal pain as well as a new elevation in temperature, white cell count and C-reactive protein (CRP), despite complete recovery of his chest symptoms and signs. Taken together, these make *C. difficile* infection a likely diagnosis. However, you also note that he is taking two laxatives (bisacodyl and ispaghula husk) and a PPI, all of which can cause diarrhoea. Of note, diarrhoea is also a recognised side effect of statins (e.g. simvastatin) and serotonin-specific reuptake inhibitors (e.g. sertraline).

### How should you treat his diarrhoea?

As you have a strong suspicion that Mr George has *C. difficile* infection, it would be reasonable to start an antibiotic to treat this. In many hospitals, the first-line antibiotic is metronidazole, although others recommend vancomycin. You should consult local antibiotic guidelines. A stool sample should be sent to test for *C. difficile* toxin to confirm the diagnosis, and the antibiotic treatment should be reviewed when results are available. In addition, you should review his existing medication and stop laxatives and any non-essential drugs that may be contributing to the diarrhoea.

### What other issues should you consider?

#### Stopping broad-spectrum antibiotics

In patients with *C. difficile* infection, you should stop broad-spectrum antibiotics where possible to facilitate recovery. Mr George has received almost 7 days of treatment with high-dose intravenous broad-spectrum antibiotics (amoxicillin) for community-acquired pneumonia. The usual duration of antibiotic treatment for pneumonia is 7–10 days. Mr George has no further chest symptoms, normal oxygen saturations while breathing room air, normal chest examination and considerable improvement in inflammatory markers on 05/01/2015, indicating resolution of his pneumonia. You could therefore reasonably stop the amoxicillin.

It is worth noting that Mr George's antibiotics could have been switched from intravenous to oral administration several days ago. Intravenous antibiotics are required when patients are severely ill or unable to take anything by mouth. They can be changed to oral antibiotics when signs of severe and/or systemic infection (e.g. fever, tachycardia) have resolved and patients are able to take and absorb medicines orally. Prompt switching of antibiotics from intravenous to the oral route can facilitate earlier discharge, reduce the risk of hospital complications such as *C. difficile* infection and reduce costs.

### Proton pump inhibitors

Mr George is taking aspirin, for secondary prevention of myocardial infarction, and lansoprazole, a PPI, for gastroprotection. There is some evidence that PPIs may be associated with an increased risk of *C. difficile* infection, possibly because of reduced killing of *C. difficile* spores in the stomach at more alkaline pH. In Mr George's case, it would be reasonable to withhold lansoprazole for a few days while treatment for *C. difficile* is initiated, with review of gastroprotection once the infection is controlled.

### Fluid and electrolytes

Mr George has the triple challenges for fluid and electrolyte balance of underlying heart failure, furosemide treatment and diarrhoea.

*Volume status.* In your assessment you note that he does not have volume overload (no oedema, normal JVP) and may be slightly volume depleted (rising urea). As he is on a beta blocker (bisoprolol), this may mask any rise in pulse expected with volume depletion.

*Electrolytes.* His serum potassium concentration has been dropping during admission. This may be due to gastrointestinal losses from diarrhoea, urinary losses from diuretic treatment or a combination of the two.

You should replace Mr George's fluid and electrolyte deficits and minimise further losses. As Mr George is taking fluids freely, you could replace fluid and electrolytes orally. Make sure he has access to and drinks plenty of fluids and prescribe oral potassium supplements. If he is unable to drink sufficiently, then intravenous fluids may be required. However, you should prescribe and monitor these carefully to avoid exacerbating his heart failure. Further fluid and electrolyte losses can be reduced by omitting the next dose of furosemide. You should *not* prescribe anti-motility drugs, such as loperamide, as these may slow rate of clearance of intestinal toxins.

### How do I write the prescription?
### New drugs

*Antibiotics.* You should prescribe oral antibiotics for *C. difficile* infection, as the site of action is in the intestine. We have chosen to prescribe metronidazole.

The timing of antibiotic review is difficult to encapsulate on the chart. The results of the stool test should be reviewed and metronidazole stopped if *C. difficile* infection is not confirmed. If the diagnosis is confirmed, response to treatment should be assessed daily. If the patient is deteriorating or has not responded to metronidazole after 5 days, then you should seek microbiology advice about changing treatment to an alternative antibiotic (oral vancomycin or fidaxomicin). Duration of treatment is usually 10–14 days, with stop date decided by response to treatment and discharge from hospital.

*Potassium supplements.* On the model chart we have elected to replace potassium using oral supplements. Options for oral potassium administration include effervescent tablets, syrup or modified release tablets. Effervescent tablets or syrup are preferred, as modified release tablets have potential to cause gastrointestinal obstruction, ulceration and bleeding.

Sando-K® (effervescent potassium bicarbonate and chloride) tablets are taken dissolved in water. Each Sando-K® tablet contains 12 mmol $K^+$. If Mr George is able to take the six tablets per day prescribed, he will receive 72 mmol $K^+$ per 24 hours. As usual $K^+$ requirements are approximately 1 mmol/kg/day, this supplementation may be sufficient to meet his needs and restore normal serum $K^+$ concentrations. Careful monitoring is required to ensure that Mr George can tolerate treatment (as it can cause GI side effects) and that target serum $K^+$ concentrations are reached. On the model chart, we have prescribed the Sando-K® at mealtimes to try to minimise GI side effects. As it is now 20:00, we have prescribed the first dose tonight on the once only section of the chart to ensure he gets it.

### Modifying existing medication

Mr George is on multiple medications, which need careful review. You should stop the amoxicillin, bisacodyl (stimulant laxative) and ispaghula husk (bulk laxative).

You should make it clear that you would like the next dose of furosemide to be omitted. On the model chart, this has been indicated by the word OMIT in the box where the next dose would be signed for. Good communication is essential to support this action. You need to advise the staff administering the drugs as to the need to omit the drug, document the decision and reasons in the notes and make a plan for when and how this decision should be reviewed the next day. Similar measures should be taken to ensure that lansoprazole is omitted. On the model chart this has been done initially for the next 3 days, after which the conflicting priorities of *C. difficile* infection and the need for gastroprotection should again be weighed up.

### Further reading

Medical Pharmacology at a Glance. Chapter 37: Antibacterial drugs.
Prescribing at a Glance. Chapter 32: Using drugs for infection.

| Surname | Hospital number | Weight | Drug intolerances |
|---|---|---|---|
| ALBERICI | 100035 | 79 kg | None known |
| First name | Date of birth | | |
| MARCO | 12/01/1926 | | |

**REGULAR PRESCRIPTIONS**

| | Circle / enter times below ↓ | ▷ Enter dates below | 2 | 3 | 4 | 5 | 6 | 7 | Month: **January** | Year: **2015** |
|---|---|---|---|---|---|---|---|---|---|---|
| **DRUG** BISOPROLOL | 06 | | | | | | | | | |
| Dose 5 mg / Route Oral / Freq Daily / Start date 2/1/15 | (08) | | AM | AM | AM | AM | AM | | | |
| Signature A Doctor / Bleep 1234 / Review | 12 16 18 | | | | | | | | | |
| Additional instructions | 22 | | | | | | | | | |
| **DRUG** FUROSEMIDE | 06 | | | | | | | | | |
| Dose 20 mg / Route Oral / Freq Daily / Start date 2/1/15 | (08) | | AM | AM | AM | AM | AM | | | |
| Signature A Doctor / Bleep 1234 / Review | 12 16 18 | | | | | | | | | |
| Additional instructions | 22 | | | | | | | | | |
| **DRUG** RAMIPRIL | 06 08 | | | | | | | | | |
| Dose 10 mg / Route Oral / Freq Daily / Start date 2/1/15 | 12 | | | | | | | | | |
| Signature A Doctor / Bleep 1234 / Review | 16 18 | | | | | | | | | |
| Additional instructions Review plasma potassium | (22) | AM | AM | AM | AM | AM | OMIT | | | |
| **DRUG** SIMVASTATIN | 06 08 | | | | | | | | | |
| Dose 40 mg / Route Oral / Freq Daily / Start date 2/1/15 | 12 | | | | | | | | | |
| Signature A Doctor / Bleep 1234 / Review | 16 18 | | | | | | | | | |
| Additional instructions | (22) | AM | AM | AM | AM | AM | | | | |
| **DRUG** TRIMETHOPRIM | (06) 08 | AM | AM | AM | AM | AM | | STOPPED 7/1/15 A Doctor 1234 | |
| Dose 200 mg / Route Oral / Freq 12-hrly / Start date 2/1/15 | 12 | | | | | | | | | |
| Signature A Doctor / Bleep 1234 / Review 5-7 days | 16 (18) | AM | AM | AM | AM | AM | | | |
| Additional instructions Urinary tract infection | 22 | | | | | | | | | |

## What should I consider when deciding what to prescribe?

Mr Alberici has hyperkalaemia associated with serious ECG abnormalities. This indicates a high risk of potentially lethal cardiac arrhythmias, so treatment must be administered as a matter of urgency. There are three key steps in the management of hyperkalaemia, listed below in the order in which they should be considered.

### 1. Stabilise the myocardium

If, as in this case, there are serious hyperkalaemic changes on the ECG (e.g. prolonged PR interval, broad QRS complex, arrhythmias), your first priority is to stabilise the myocardium.

You do this by administering intravenous calcium, usually in the form of calcium gluconate. This raises the threshold potential in myocardial cells, making them less excitable and more resistant to the effects of hyperkalaemia. It acts within a few minutes and lasts

for about an hour. Importantly, calcium has no effect on the serum potassium concentration.

### 2. Shift potassium into cells

If the hyperkalaemia is severe (e.g. >6.5 mmol/L and/or associated with any ECG changes – the earliest of which is usually the development of tall T-waves), the serum potassium concentration needs to be lowered urgently.

The quickest way to do this is to move potassium into cells by administering insulin and glucose intravenously. Insulin activates the $Na^+/K^+$-ATPase pump on cell membranes, causing extracellular potassium to be exchanged for intracellular sodium. Glucose is administered just to counteract the hypoglycaemic effect of insulin.

Salbutamol, which can be given by nebuliser, has a similar effect but is less reliable – it may be a useful adjunct if you have difficulty obtaining IV access. If hyperkalaemia is accompanied by metabolic acidosis (not the case here), it may respond to IV sodium bicarbonate, but this should only be done under senior guidance.

All these measures have a relatively quick effect on serum potassium concentration (acting within about 30 minutes), but this is transient. The total-body potassium load is unchanged – you have just forced more of it inside cells, where it will do less harm. It will leak back out again over the next few hours.

### 3. Lower total body potassium load

Steps 1 and 2 just 'buy time'. To produce a durable effect on serum potassium concentration, you need to lower the total body potassium load. The best way to do this is by correcting the factors that are causing hyperkalaemia. Always check that there are no potassium-containing infusions running – if there are, stop them immediately. Then review the patient's prescription chart for drugs that may cause or worsen hyperkalaemia. Advise the patient to avoid foodstuffs with high potassium content, such as fruit juices, biscuits, coffee and salt substitutes.

In Mr Alberici's case, several drugs are potential contributors to hyperkalaemia:

- *Ramipril.* ACE inhibitors are a common and important cause of hyperkalaemia. You should therefore consider withholding Mr Alberici's ramipril until his potassium concentration has normalised.
- *Bisoprolol.* Beta adrenoceptor blockers may elevate the serum potassium concentration principally through their effects on the $Na/K^+$-ATPase pump on cell membranes, reducing cellular potassium uptake (i.e. the opposite effect of salbutamol, a beta adrenoceptor agonist); they also reduce renin secretion. However, a significant hyperkalaemic effect is more likely with a non-selective beta adrenoceptor blocker (e.g. propranolol, labetalol).

- *Trimethoprim* often causes a rise in serum potassium and creatinine concentrations (due to altered tubular potassium handling) – this may be important in individuals with other risk factors for hyperkalaemia, as is the case here. Given that Mr Alberici has had 5 days' treatment for his urinary tract infection and is now asymptomatic, the best course of action is probably just to stop his antibiotic treatment then monitor his symptoms.
- *Other drugs* that may elevate serum potassium concentration, but which are not relevant in this case, include potassium-sparing diuretics (e.g. amiloride, spironolactone), potassium-containing laxatives (e.g. Movicol®, Klean-Prep®), digoxin and non-steroidal anti-inflammatory drugs.

Another method of lowering total-body potassium load is to increase its excretion through the gut. This can be achieved by administering calcium polystyrene sulfonate (commonly referred to by its tradename, Calcium Resonium®). This takes several days to work and invariably causes constipation (which, in turn, impairs its potassium-lowering effect), so co-administration of a laxative is almost always required. For these reasons, it is used less commonly now than it was in the past, but it still retains a role in selected cases. Ultimately, if medical options are insufficient, renal replacement therapy (by haemodialysis or haemofiltration) may be required.

Always seek senior advice in the management of severe hyperkalaemia, as it is a dangerous condition requiring urgent and sometimes complex management.

### How do I write the prescription?
### Calcium gluconate

Calcium gluconate is administered by slow IV injection over about 5 minutes, typically at an initial dose of 10 mL calcium gluconate 10%. You should prescribe this in the once only section of the chart and, ideally, administer it yourself. Use the biggest vein you can find, and check that the cannula is correctly sited first (e.g. by flushing it with 10 mL 0.9% sodium chloride, which should flow freely and any not cause any local tissue swelling). This is because if calcium extravasates (leaks out of the vein) it can cause tissue necrosis, and will not be delivered to the heart. Have a cardiac monitor attached and/or record an ECG before and after administration. Your aim is to suppress the serious ECG changes – in this case, to shorten the PR interval and QRS duration. If these persist despite calcium administration, you should administer more (to a maximum of 40 mL, after checking again that there is no problem with the cannula).

### Insulin–glucose infusion

While you are stabilising the myocardium with calcium, ask a nurse colleague to prepare the insulin–glucose infusion. Prescribe this in the infusion section of the chart. A typical dose is 10 units soluble insulin (e.g. Actrapid®) added to 50 mL glucose 50%, infused over 15 minutes. Many hospitals now prefer lower-concentration glucose solutions, as these are less irritating to veins (e.g. 10 units soluble insulin in 250 mL glucose 20%, infused over 30 minutes).

**ONCE ONLY PRESCRIPTIONS**

| Date | Time to be given | DRUG | Dose | Route | Prescriber Signature | Prescriber Bleep | Administration Date given | Administration Time given | Administration Given by |
|---|---|---|---|---|---|---|---|---|---|
| 7/1/15 | 13:15 | 10% CALCIUM GLUCONATE | 10 mL | Slow IV | A Doctor | 1234 | | | |
| | | | | | | | | | |
| | | | | | | | | | |

**OXYGEN**

| Target SpO₂ | ○ 94–98% ○ 88–92% |
|---|---|
| Mode of delivery | ○ Continuous ○ As required |
| Starting device | |

| Initials | Bleep | Date |
|---|---|---|
| | | |

**AS REQUIRED MEDICATION**

| DRUG | | | | Date | |
|---|---|---|---|---|---|
| | | | | Time | |
| Dose | Route | Max freq | Start date | Dose | |
| | | | | Route | |
| Signature | | Bleep | Review | Given | |
| | | | | Check | |
| Additional instructions | | | | | |

| DRUG | | | | Date | |
|---|---|---|---|---|---|
| | | | | Time | |
| Dose | Route | Max freq | Start date | Dose | |
| | | | | Route | |
| Signature | | Bleep | Review | Given | |
| | | | | Check | |
| Additional instructions | | | | | |

| DRUG | | | | Date | |
|---|---|---|---|---|---|
| | | | | Time | |
| Dose | Route | Max freq | Start date | Dose | |
| | | | | Route | |
| Signature | | Bleep | Review | Given | |
| | | | | Check | |
| Additional instructions | | | | | |

| DRUG | | | | Date | |
|---|---|---|---|---|---|
| | | | | Time | |
| Dose | Route | Max freq | Start date | Dose | |
| | | | | Route | |
| Signature | | Bleep | Review | Given | |
| | | | | Check | |
| Additional instructions | | | | | |

**INFUSION PRESCRIPTIONS**

| Date | Time | Fluid | Vol | Drug | Dose | Rate | Doctor initials | Nurse initials | Batch no | Start time | Stop time |
|---|---|---|---|---|---|---|---|---|---|---|---|
| 7/1/15 | 13:15 | 50% GLUCOSE | 50 mL | ACTRAPID | 10 units | Over 15 min | AD | | | | |
| | | | | | | | | | | | |
| | | | | | | | | | | | |
| | | | | | | | | | | | |

### Stopping precipitant drugs

As trimethoprim is a potential precipitant of hyperkalaemia, stop this by crossing through the prescription and signing and dating this. To withhold his next dose of ramipril, write OMIT in the administration box corresponding to the next dose (or follow local policies on the use of coding systems), and record this in the medical notes.

### Other measures

If you are advised by a senior colleague to start calcium polystyrene sulfonate, ensure you also prescribe a laxative (e.g. lactulose, provided the patient has adequate fluid intake) to prevent constipation. You must not prescribe magnesium-containing laxatives, as these may interact with calcium polystyrene sulfonate. If you are advised to administer sodium bicarbonate, ensure this is *not* allowed to mix with calcium gluconate (either in the giving set or the vein), as they can react to form calcium carbonate, which precipitates.

### Further reading

London Acute Kidney Injury Network. London AKI Network Manual (2012). http://www.londonaki.net/downloads/LondonAKI network-Manual.pdf (accessed 24 January 2014).

| Surname BEATTY | Hospital number 100036 | Weight | Drug intolerances |
|---|---|---|---|
| First name MAUREEN | Date of birth 12/09/1945 | 54 kg | None known |

**REGULAR PRESCRIPTIONS**

| | Circle / enter times below ↓ | ↘ Enter dates below | | | Month: January | | Year: 2015 |
|---|---|---|---|---|---|---|---|
| | | 5 | 6 | 7 | | | |
| DRUG DALTEPARIN | 06 | | | | | | |
| Dose 5000 units / Route SC / Freq Daily / Start date 5/1/15 | 08 | | | | | | |
| | 12 | | | | | | |
| | 16 | | | | | | |
| Signature A Doctor / Bleep 1234 / Review | ⑱ | — | A11 | | | | |
| Additional instructions | 22 | | | | | | |
| DRUG CO-CODAMOL 30/500 | ⑥ | — | A11 | | | | |
| Dose 2 tabs / Route ORAL / Freq 6-hrly / Start date 5/1/15 | 08 | | | | | | |
| | ⑫ | — | A11 | | | | |
| Signature A Doctor / Bleep 1234 / Review | 16 | | | | | | |
| | ⑱ | — | A11 | | | | |
| Additional instructions | 22 ㉔ | A11 | A11 | | | | |
| DRUG LACTULOSE | ⑥ | — | A11 | | | | |
| Dose 10 mL / Route ORAL / Freq 12-hrly / Start date 5/1/15 | 08 | | | | | | |
| | 12 | | | | | | |
| Signature A Doctor / Bleep 1234 / Review | 16 | | | | | | |
| | ⑱ | — | A11 | | | | |
| Additional instructions | 22 | | | | | | |
| DRUG PABRINEX | ⑥ | | | | | | |
| Dose 2 pairs / Route IV / Freq 8-hrly / Start date 7/1/15 | 08 | | | | | | |
| | ⑫ | | | | | | |
| Signature A Doctor / Bleep 1234 / Review 2 days | 16 | | | | | | |
| | 16 ㉔ | | | | | | |
| Additional instructions | 22 | | | | | | |
| DRUG | 06 | | | | | | |

**ONCE ONLY PRESCRIPTIONS**

| Date | Time to be given | DRUG | Dose | Route | Prescriber Signature | Prescriber Bleep | Administration Date given | Administration Time given | Administration Given by |
|---|---|---|---|---|---|---|---|---|---|
| 7/1/15 | 03:40 | PABRINEX | 2 pairs | IV | A Doctor | 1234 | | | |
| | | | | | | | | | |
| | | | | | | | | | |

**OXYGEN**

| Target SpO₂ | ○ 94–98% ○ 88–92% |
|---|---|
| Mode of delivery | ○ Continuous ○ As required |
| Starting device | |

| Initials | Bleep | Date |
|---|---|---|
| | | |

**AS REQUIRED MEDICATION**

| DRUG CHLORDIAZEPOXIDE | Date | | | | | |
|---|---|---|---|---|---|---|
| | Time | | | | | |
| Dose 25-50mg / Route ORAL / Max freq 2-hrly / Start date 7/1/15 | Dose | | | | | |
| | Route | | | | | |
| Signature A Doctor / Bleep 1234 / Review 24 hr | Given | | | | | |
| | Check | | | | | |
| Additional instructions If CIWA-Ar score 10–14 give 25 mg; if score ≥15 give 50 mg. Seek medical review if dose >300 mg in 24 hr. | | | | | | |
| DRUG | Date | | | | | |

## What should I consider when deciding what to prescribe?

### Acute alcohol withdrawal

Alcohol (ethanol) enhances the actions of the inhibitory neurotransmitter, gamma-aminobutyric acid (GABA) and inhibits the excitatory N-methyl-D-aspartate (NMDA) receptor. Chronic alcohol intake causes downregulation of the inhibitory receptors and increases neuroexcitatory tone. Thus, when chronic alcohol intake ceases suddenly, e.g. at hospital admission, increased neuroexcitation is unopposed by inhibitory pathways, causing with-

drawal symptoms. Alcohol withdrawal effects include features of autonomic stimulation (sweating, tremor, tachycardia), anxiety and insomnia, hallucinations and seizures. Delirium tremens is an extreme and life-threatening form of alcohol withdrawal.

You should take an alcohol history in all patients you admit, and consider the possibility of withdrawal in those with a high alcohol intake or a history suggestive of alcohol dependence (e.g. past withdrawal symptoms). Mrs Beatty has drunk 700 mL vodka every day for the past 5 years. Assuming an alcohol content of 40%, this equates to 28 units/day or approximately 200 units/week. Against this background, her presentation now – just over 24 hours into the admission – with tremor, agitation and probable delirium is highly suggestive of acute alcohol withdrawal. It would have been easier and safer to have started appropriate management on admission, rather than allow her withdrawal symptoms to progress unchecked.

### Prevention and treatment

#### Benzodiazepines

Benzodiazepines are used to prevent and treat alcohol withdrawal. Like alcohol, they potentiate the action of GABA and thereby help to restore its neuroinhibitory effects. They are most effective in preventing seizures, but also reduce other withdrawal symptoms. Benzodiazepines with a long duration of action and active metabolites (e.g. chlordiazepoxide, diazepam) are generally preferred, because their sustained effect reduces the risk of breakthrough seizures. In advanced cirrhosis, lorazepam may be preferred as its clearance is less affected by hepatic impairment, and it is therefore less likely to cause over-sedation.

Mrs Beatty has a mild elevation of liver enzymes, but normal clotting and albumin, indicating that her liver function is intact. Chlordiazepoxide would therefore be a reasonable first choice for her treatment.

#### Route of administration

Chlordiazepoxide is only available as an oral preparation. In patients who are fitting, severely agitated (posing risk to themselves and others) or are delirious and refusing oral treatment, intravenous diazepam or lorazepam is most appropriate. If intravenous access cannot be obtained, intramuscular midazolam can be used temporarily. The management of agitated delirium is complex and you should not hesitate to seek anaesthetic support.

#### Dosage regimens

Administration of benzodiazepines for alcohol withdrawal may either be scheduled or symptom triggered. In the case of scheduled administration, recurrent doses are prescribed for administration at predetermined times of the day. The dose is gradually reduced, usually over a period of around a week. In addition, an as required prescription is written to allow additional doses to be given for breakthrough symptoms. In the symptom triggered approach, the patient is assessed regularly using a scoring system such as the revised Clinical Institute Withdrawal Assessment for Alcohol scale (CIWA-Ar; Figure 36.1). Treatment is administered according to a protocol if the score exceeds certain threshold levels. In order to avoid generating unnecessary complexity, you should refer to local guidelines when determining which management approach to use.

Whichever system is used, the aim is to reduce the benzodiazepine dosage gradually, usually over the course of about a week. The patient should be free from withdrawal symptoms off benzodiazepines before they are discharged from hospital, as benzodiazepines themselves carry a risk of dependency.

## What other treatment does she need?

*Thiamine.* In view of her history of longstanding alcohol dependence, Mrs Beatty is likely to be severely deficient in thiamine (vitamin B1) and is at risk of Wernicke's encephalopathy – a complication of thiamine deficiency classically characterised by ataxia, ophthalmoplegia and confusion, although not all features are present in all patients. Left untreated, this may progress to Korsakoff's syndrome, a devastating and largely irreversible neuropsychiatric condition characterised by marked impairment of short-term memory. Both conditions may be prevented by giving high dose thiamine, which is usually administered intravenously in the form of Pabrinex® (a combination preparation of B and C vitamins). This should be started urgently.

*Supportive care.* Fluid and electrolyte balance should be monitored and abnormalities corrected. Intravenous fluids may be needed if the patient is not drinking, but oral intake is preferable. In patients with ischaemic heart disease, autonomic activation may cause arrhythmias or angina and hypertension. If these occur, a beta blocker may be added to benzodiazepine therapy.

*Review of other treatment.* Her treatment with co-codamol for abdominal pain is not unreasonable, but consideration should be given to whether inadequate pain control might be contributing to her agitation.

## How do I write the prescription?
### Chlordiazepoxide

The model prescription illustrates a symptom triggered treatment approach. Chlordiazepoxide has been prescribed in the as required section at a dose of 25–50 mg up to 2-hourly. The symptom triggered approach should ideally be used in conjunction with a vali-

dated instrument such as the CIWA-Ar score alongside a local protocol. Typically, this protocol will advise that CIWA-Ar assessment (and other routine observations) be performed every 2 hours initially, and chlordiazepoxide administered according to the CIWA-Ar score. For example, we illustrate a prescription for chlordiazepoxide based on a protocol that specifies that 25 mg should be given if the CIWA-Ar score is 10–14, and 50 mg if the score is ≥15 (the maximum score on the CIWA-Ar scale is 67). The total dosage of chlordiazepoxide required in the first 24 hours may then be used to inform the prescription of chlordiazepoxide in the next few days.

If a scheduled treatment approach is used, chlordiazepoxide would be prescribed for regular administration (e.g. 6-hourly initially). Selection of the initial dose should take account of her usual alcohol intake. Given her small body size, an appropriate starting dose might be 30 mg 6-hourly, modified as appropriate according to response. The dosage should then be gradually decreased to stop over the following week.

## Intravenous high dose thiamine

Pabrinex® IV high potency injection contains high dose vitamins from B and C groups, including thiamine, nicotinamide, pyridoxine, riboflavin and ascorbic acid. Pabrinex® is presented as two 5-mL ampoules, which are mixed, diluted with either sodium chloride 0.9% or glucose 5% solutions, then infused immediately over 30 minutes. Pabrinex® is therefore prescribed in 'pairs of ampoules' as shown.

As Mrs Beatty has incipient Wernicke's encephalopathy (thiamine deficiency with confusion), you should prescribe 2–3 pairs of ampoules three times daily for 2 days, as indicated in the BNF. Treatment should continue at one pair once daily for up to 5 further days if she has a good initial response.

Pabrinex® infusion can cause anaphylaxis, although this is rare. As sensitisation may occur with early infusions, the risk is likely to still be present or even greater during later infusions. Mrs Beatty therefore should be monitored during all Pabrinex® infusions and resuscitation facilities should be available to treat anaphylaxis if it occurs. Once Pabrinex® treatment is complete, patients are commonly advised to take oral thiamine 100–200 mg/day.

## Further reading

Medical Pharmacology at a Glance. Chapter 24: Anxiolytics and hypnotics.

Prescribing at a Glance. Chapter 15: Prescribing in liver disease.

Sullivan JT, Sykora K, Schneiderman J, Naranjo CA & Sellers EM. Assessment of alcohol withdrawal: The revised Clinical Institute Withdrawal Instrument for Alcohol Scale (CIWA-Ar). British Journal of Addiction 1989;84:1353–7. Available at: http://onlinelibrary.wiley.com/doi/10.1111/j.1360-0443.1989.tb00737.x/pdf (accessed 24 January 2014).

NAUSEA AND VOMITING—Ask 'Do you feel sick to your stomach? Have you vomited?'

0 no nausea and no vomiting
1 mild nausea with no vomiting
2
3
4 intermittent nausea with dry heaves
5
6
7 constant nausea, frequent dry heaves and vomiting

TREMOR—Arms extended and fingers spread apart. Observation.

0 no tremor
1 not visible, but can be felt fingertip to fingertip
2
3
4 moderate with patient's arms extended
5
6
7 severe, even with arms not extended

PAROXYSMAL SWEATS—Observation.

0 no sweat visible
1 barely perceptible sweating, palms moist
2
3
4 beads of sweat obvious on forehead
5
6
7 drenching sweats

ANXIETY—Ask 'Do you feel nervous?'

0 no anxiety, at ease
1 mildly anxious
2
3
4 moderately anxious, or guarded, so anxiety is inferred
5
6
7 equivalent to acute panic states as seen in severe delirium or acute schizophrenic reactions

AGITATION—Observation.

0 normal activity
1 somewhat more than normal activity
2
3
4 moderately fidgety and restless
5
6
7 paces back and forth during most of the interview, or constantly thrashes about

TACTILE DISTURBANCES—Ask 'Do you have any itching, pins and needles sensations, burning, numbness or do you feel bugs crawling on/under your skin?'

0 none
1 very mild itching, pins and needles, burning or numbness
2 mild itching, pins and needles, burning or numbness
3 moderate itching, pins and needles, burning or numbness
4 moderately severe hallucinations
5 severe hallucinations
6 extremely severe hallucinations
7 continuous hallucinations

AUDITORY DISTURBANCES—Ask 'Are you aware of sounds around you? Are they harsh? Do they frighten you? Are you hearing anything that is disturbing to you? Are you hearing things you know are not there?'

0 not present
1 very mild harshness or ability to frighten
2 mild harshness or ability to frighten
3 moderate harshness or ability to frighten
4 moderately severe hallucinations
5 severe hallucinations
6 extremely severe hallucinations
7 continuous hallucinations

VISUAL DISTURBANCE—Ask 'Does the light appear to be too bright? Is its color different? Does it hurt your eyes? Are you seeing anything that is disturbing to you? Are you seeing things you know are not there?'

0 not present
1 very mild sensitivity
2 mild sensitivity
3 moderate sensitivity
4 moderately severe hallucinations
5 severe hallucinations
6 extremely severe hallucinations
7 continuous hallucinations

HEADACHE, FULLNESS IN HEAD—Ask 'Does your head feel different? Does it feel like there is a band around your head?' Do not rate for dizziness or lightheadedness. Otherwise, rate severity.

0 not present
1 very mild
2 mild
3 moderate
4 moderately severe
5 severe
6 very severe
7 extremely severe

ORIENTATION AND CLOUDING OF SENSORIUM—Ask 'What day is this? Where are you? Who am I?'

0 oriented and can do serial additions
1 cannot do serial additions or is uncertain about date
2 disoriented for date by no more than 2 calendar days
3 disoriented for date by more than 2 calendar days
4 disoriented for place and/or person

**Figure 36.1** Addiction Research Foundation Clinical Institute Withdrawal Assessment for Alcohol (CIWA-Ar); from Sullivan JT, et al. (1989).

# Section 3: Routine inpatient review

# Cases

## 37 A 69-year-old woman with constipation

| | |
|---|---|
| **Patient name:** | Felicity Aldridge |
| **ID number:** | 100037 |
| **Date of birth:** | 24/02/1955 |
| **Age:** | 69 years |
| **Weight:** | 75 kg |
| **Admission date:** | 05/01/2015 |
| **Date/time seen:** | 07/01/2015 1900 |

### History

**Problem**    Mrs Aldridge has not opened her bowels for 3 days.

**History**    She underwent elective knee replacement surgery 2 days ago. Her recovery has been good and the physiotherapists think that she will be ready to go home in 3–4 days' time. Her pain is well controlled, although she needs doses of extra pain relief prior to physiotherapy. Normally, she opens her bowels every morning but since the operation she has not opened them at all. She does, however, say that she has been 'passing wind'.

**PMH**    None.

**DH**    Paracetamol 1 g 6-hourly, dihydrocodeine 30 mg 6-hourly, Sevredol® (morphine sulfate tablets) 5 mg 4-hourly as required.
Intolerances: none known.

### Examination

**General**    She looks well.

**Obs**    T 36.8°C, HR 80 beats/min, BP 126/83 mmHg, RR 17 breaths/min, SpO$_2$ 97% breathing air.

**Systems**    Normal other than for expected postoperative findings. Digital rectal examination reveals an empty rectum.

### Investigations

Postoperative blood tests were unremarkable; electrolytes, including calcium, are normal.

### Task

Prescribe appropriate medication for Mrs Aldridge's constipation.

## 38 A 71-year-old man who has developed a tremor

| | |
|---|---|
| **Patient name:** | Josiah Roach |
| **ID number:** | 100038 |
| **Date of birth:** | 06/06/1943 |
| **Age:** | 71 years |
| **Weight:** | 68 kg |
| **Admission date:** | 06/01/2015 |
| **Date/time seen:** | 07/01/2015 14:30 |

### History

**Problem**    Tremor.

**History**    Mr Roach was admitted to the acute medical unit yesterday following a fall. The admitting doctor noted he has a symmetrical tremor. He has been reviewed on the post-take ward round, and a series of investigations to identify the cause for his fall have been requested.

**PMH**    Schizophrenia. At his last psychiatric outpatient review 3 months ago his psychotic symptoms were noted to be well controlled with quetiapine; on review of side effects he complained of nausea and occasional vomiting, so metoclopramide was started.

**DH**    Quetiapine 150 mg 12-hourly, which he has been taking for the past 5 years. Metoclopramide 10 mg 8-hourly for the past 3 months.
Intolerances: none known.

**SH**    He works as a tyre fitter in a garage. He does not smoke and does not drink alcohol.

### Examination

**General**    Appears well.

**Obs**    T 37.0°C, HR 88 beats/min, BP 118/68 mmHg, RR 14 breaths/min, SpO$_2$ 98% breathing air.

**NS**    He has a mild chin tremor and a symmetrical resting tremor affecting his hands with some cogwheeling. There is no discernible bradykinesia. He has a normal gait and postural reflexes, and motor, sensory and cerebellar examinations are otherwise normal.

### Task

Your consultant has reviewed Mr Roach on her post-take ward round. She has asked you to review his medications to look for a drug cause for his tremor and modify his treatment if appropriate.

*Prescribing Scenarios at a Glance*, First Edition. Emma Baker, Daniel Burrage, Dagan Lonsdale, and Andrew Hitchings.

**128** © 2014 John Wiley & Sons, Ltd. Published 2014 by John Wiley & Sons, Ltd. Companion website: www.ataglanceseries.com/prescribingscenarios

## 39 An 81-year-old woman at risk of fragility fractures

Patient name: Alice Pellow
ID number: 100039
Date of birth: 02/11/1933
Age: 81 years
Weight: 58 kg
Admission date: 27/12/2014
Date/time seen: 07/01/2015 13:00

### History

Problem At risk of further fragility fractures.

History Ms Pellow was admitted following a fall having tripped on a rug while trying to answer her phone. She injured her left hip and was diagnosed with a displaced intracapsular fracture of her left neck of femur. She underwent a total hip replacement on the day of her admission. She is now recovering well, mobilising with a frame on the ward, and will be discharged tomorrow with community physiotherapy follow-up.

PMH None.

DH None.
Intolerances: none known.

SH She lives in sheltered accommodation and was previously independent for all activities of daily living. She does not smoke and drinks one brandy a week on Sundays.

### Examination

General She appears well. Her teeth and mouth appear healthy.

Obs T 36.5°C, HR 82 beats/min, BP 110/68 mmHg, RR 14 breaths/min, SpO$_2$ 96% breathing air.

### Investigations

For results of investigations, see Table 39.1.

### Task

Your registrar has asked you to make sure Ms Pellow is on the right medications to reduce the risk of a further fragility fracture.

Table 39.1 Case 39 investigation results

| Test | Value | Normal range |
| --- | --- | --- |
| Hb | 124 g/L | 120–160 |
| MCV | 86 fL | 78–97 |
| WCC | 6.8 × 10⁹/L | 4.0–11.0 |
| Plt | 248 × 10⁹/L | 150–400 |
| Na$^+$ | 138 mmol/L | 135–145 |
| K$^+$ | 4.4 mmol/L | 3.5–4.7 |
| Ur | 3.0 mmol/L | 2.5–8.0 |
| Creat | 62 µmol/L | 60–110 |
| eGFR | >60 mL/min/1.73 m² | >60 |
| Alb | 35 g/L | 35–48 |
| Adj Ca$^{2+}$ | 2.20 mmol/L | 2.20–2.50 |
| PO$_4^{2-}$ | 0.8 mmol/L | 0.75–1.50 |
| Vit D | 75 nmol/L | 75–200 |

## 40 A 23-year-old pregnant woman with pulmonary embolism

Patient name: Sathya Srikanth
ID number: 100040
Date of birth: 14/08/1991
Age: 23 years
Weight: 75 kg
Admission date: 07/01/2015 09:00
Date/time seen: 07/01/2015 18:30

### History

Problem Pulmonary embolism.

History Mrs Srikanth was admitted this morning with chest pain and shortness of breath. She is 29 weeks pregnant and, for the past 2 weeks, has become increasingly short of breath on exertion. She has had intermittent fevers but has had no cough. The admitting doctor started treatment for a lower respiratory tract infection while waiting for the results of investigations. You have just been called with the result of the CT pulmonary angiogram (CTPA).

PMH No significant medical history. Her pregnancy has been normal until now. Of note, from her maternal notes, her booking weight was 65 kg.

DH Nil.
Intolerances: none known.

### Examination

General She appears breathless.

Obs T 37.5°C, HR 105 beats/min, BP 115/75 mmHg, RR 24 breaths/min, SpO$_2$ 93% breathing air.

Systems Normal examination other than for the presence of tachypnoea.

### Investigations

For results of investigations, see Table 40.1.

### Task

Review Mrs Srikanth's drug chart and prescribe appropriate therapy to treat pulmonary embolus.

Table 40.1 Case 40 investigation results

| Test | Value | Normal range |
| --- | --- | --- |
| Hb | 125 g/L | 120–160 |
| WCC | 8.9 x 10⁹/L | 4.0–11.0 |
| Neutr | 6.3 x 10⁹/L | 1.7–8.0 |
| CRP | 15 mg/L | <10 |
| eGFR | >60 mL/min/1.73 m² | >60 |
| INR | 1.0 | 0.8–1.1 |
| APTT ratio | 1.06 | 0.85–1.15 |
| ECG | Sinus tachycardia at 115 beats/min; normal axis and morphology | |
| CXR | Normal | |
| CTPA | Multiple small pulmonary emboli | |

## 41  A 31-year-old man with increased seizure frequency

| | |
|---|---|
| Patient name: | Abdul Raffiq |
| ID number: | 100041 |
| Date of birth: | 25/02/1983 |
| Age: | 31 years |
| Weight: | 68 kg |
| Admission date: | 01/01/2015 10:00 |
| Date/time seen: | 07/01/2015 13:00 |

### History

Problem  You are asked to review and act on a serum phenytoin concentration result.

History  Mr Raffiq was admitted 6 days ago with recurrent complex partial seizures. He has epilepsy and usually experiences 1–2 short-lived seizures per week. On presentation, the type of seizure had not changed, but their frequency had increased to more than 20 per day. He did not always recover to baseline in between. Phenytoin was started with an initial intravenous loading dose and oral maintenance therapy thereafter.

His seizures are now occurring at a frequency of about 5–10 per day, with full recovery in between. No cause for the increased seizure activity has yet been found. The neurology team have advised that you should 'aim to achieve a serum phenytoin concentration in the upper half of the target range'.

PMH  Focal epilepsy due to a cerebral arteriovenous malformation.

DH  Phenytoin 300 mg daily, levetiracetam 1.5 g 12-hourly.
Intolerances: none known.

SH  Non-smoker; no alcohol consumption; independent.

### Examination

General  Normal.

Obs  T 37.0°C, HR 65 beats/min, BP 122/86 mmHg, RR 16 breaths/min, SpO$_2$ 99% breathing air.

Systems  Normal.

### Investigations

For results of investigations, see Table 41.1.

### Task

Adjust his phenytoin dosage in light of the drug concentration data and neurology advice.

**Table 41.1** Case 41 investigation results

| Test | Value | Normal range |
|---|---|---|
| Creat | 82 μmol/L | 60–110 |
| eGFR | >60 mL/min/1.73 m$^2$ | >60 |
| Alb | 38 g/L | 35–48 |
| Serum phenytoin: | | |
| 02/01/2015 12:00 | 14.5 μg/mL | 10–20 |
| 07/01/2015 07:30 | 12.9 μg/mL | 10–20 |

## 42  A 58-year-old man with diabetes mellitus treated with insulin

| | |
|---|---|
| Patient name: | Gareth Edwards |
| ID number: | 100042 |
| Date of birth: | 14/01/1956 |
| Age: | 58 years |
| Weight: | 95 kg |
| Admission date: | 05/01/2015 |
| Date/time seen: | 07/01/2015, 17:00 |

### History

Problem  Mr Edwards is a patient on your ward. Before going home one evening, you are asked by the nursing staff to prescribe his insulin for the next day.

History  Mr Edwards was admitted 2 days ago, in the early hours of the morning, for treatment of cellulitis.

PMH  Type 2 diabetes mellitus.

DH  Metformin 1 g twice daily, aspirin 75 mg daily, Humalog® Mix 25: usual doses, 23 units am, 21 units pm; flucloxacillin 1 g IV 6-hourly, new on this admission.
Intolerances: none known.

### Examination

General  Resolving cellulitis around right ankle.

Obs  T 37.2°C, HR 89 beats/min, BP 118/86 mmHg, RR 12 breaths/min, SpO$_2$ 98% breathing room air.

### Investigations

For results of capillary glucose readings, see Table 42.1. In addition, an HbA$_{1c}$ reading taken on 21/11/2012 was 78 mmol/mol.

### Task

Review the insulin that Mr Edwards has received during this admission and prescribe doses for as many days as you see fit.

**Table 42.1** Recent capillary glucose readings (mmol/L)

| Date | 06:00 | 12:00 | 18:00 | 22:00 |
|---|---|---|---|---|
| 05/01/2015 | 12.1 | 14.9 | 13.6 | 13.8 |
| 06/01/2015 | 7.9 | 13.2 | 14.7 | 8.4 |
| 07/01/2015 | 8.5 | 13.5 | | |

**A 53-year-old man who wants to stop smoking**

| Patient name: | Malcolm Hines |
|---|---|
| ID number: | 100043 |
| Date of birth: | 26/05/1961 |
| Weight: | 101 kg |
| Admission date: | 06/01/2015 |
| Date/time seen: | 07/01/2015 11:00 |

### History

Problem   Malcolm Hines wants to stop smoking.

History   Mr Hines was admitted 24 hours ago with a non-ST elevation acute coronary syndrome and has been strongly advised to stop smoking. He is very anxious, as his father died of a heart attack aged 55 years and Mr Hines is worried that this will happen to him. Mr Hines knows that he should not smoke, but the anxiety is making him need a cigarette and he has already been outside three times this morning 'for a smoke'.

Mr Hines has smoked since the age of 10 years and currently smokes 30 cigarettes per day. He mostly smokes out of habit and through boredom, but gets a strong urge to smoke if he has been without a cigarette for more than an hour. He has tried to stop smoking once in the past using willpower, but became very irritable and cranky and restarted at his partner's request. He now wants to stop smoking as he thinks that if he does not he will die of a heart attack.

PMH   Inguinal hernia repair 5 years ago.

DH   Aspirin 75 mg daily, atorvastatin 40 mg daily, clopidogrel 75 mg daily, fondaparinux 2.5 mg daily, metoprolol 12.5 mg three times daily.
Intolerances: none known.

SH   He lives with his partner and two children in a third floor flat. He does not drink alcohol.

### Examination

General   He has nicotine-stained fingers and smells of cigarette smoke.

Obs   T 36.5°C, HR 64 beats/min (regular), BP 134/78 mmHg, RR 13 breaths/min, SpO$_2$ 98% breathing air.

CVS   JVP 2 cm above the sternal angle, HS I + II + 0, no oedema.

### Task

Review Mr Hines's inpatient prescription chart and prescribe appropriate treatment to support his smoking cessation attempt.

---

**A 90-year-old woman on numerous medications**

| Patient name: | Rachel Dennis |
|---|---|
| ID number: | 100044 |
| Date of birth: | 09/03/1924 |
| Weight: | 56 kg |
| Admission date: | 05/01/2015 |
| Date/time seen: | 07/01/2015 13:00 |

### History

Problem   A complete review of her medication is required.

History   Mrs Dennis was admitted following a fall. She felt lightheaded after getting up quickly to answer the door and fell, losing consciousness for a few seconds. She bruised her right hip. Although a pelvic X-ray excluded a fracture, she is still in pain, rated at 2/10 (improved from 7/10 on admission). She is now able to walk with a stick.
Concerns are not having opened her bowels for 3 days and poor sleep due to a noisy ward at night.

PMH   Hypothyroidism, hypertension, hypercholesterolaemia, myocardial infarction with drug-eluting stent inserted 18 months ago, stage 3 chronic kidney disease, folate-deficiency megaloblastic anaemia diagnosed 6 months ago.

DH   Mrs Dennis did not bring a list of medications with her to hospital, so an old discharge summary was used to prescribe at admission. The pharmacist has now contacted Mrs Dennis's GP and documented her current medications: aspirin 75 mg daily, atorvastatin 40 mg daily, bisoprolol 2.5 mg daily, folic acid 5 mg daily, levothyroxine 100 micrograms daily, ramipril 5 mg daily.
Intolerances: penicillin, which causes a rash.

SH   She lives with her husband, and is normally independent in her activities of daily living. She is a lifelong non-smoker and only drinks alcohol on special occasions.

### Examination

General   She appears well.

Obs   T 36.8°C, HR 68 beats/min, BP (lying) 124/68 mmHg, BP (standing) 98/56 mmHg, RR 16 breaths/min, SpO$_2$ 96% breathing air.

### Investigations

For results of investigations, see Table 44.1.

### Task

Correct any errors on Mrs Dennis's drug chart and make any further changes you feel necessary in light of her fall and recent blood test results.

---

**Table 44.1** Case 44 investigation results

| Test | Value | Normal range | Test | Value | Normal range |
|---|---|---|---|---|---|
| Hb | 124 g/L | 120–160 | Ur | 7.9 mmol/L | 2.5–8.0 |
| MCV | 93 fL | 78–97 | Creat | 118 μmol/L | 60–110 |
| WCC | 4.2 × 10$^9$/L | 4.0–11.0 | eGFR | 40 mL/min/1.73 m$^2$ | >60 |
| Plt | 360 × 10$^9$/L | 150–400 | TSH | 2.4 mU/L | 0.4–5.0 |
| Na$^+$ | 136 mmol/L | 135–145 | Folate | 38.0 mg/L | 5.0–10.0 |
| K$^+$ | 4.7 mmol/L | 3.5–4.7 | Vit B12 | 420 ng/L | 180–1000 |

## 45 A 54-year-old woman with a peptic ulcer

| | |
|---|---|
| **Patient name:** | Sheila McKinnon |
| **ID number:** | 100045 |
| **Date of birth:** | 03/03/1960 |
| **Age:** | 54 years |
| **Weight:** | 71 kg |
| **Admission date:** | 04/01/2015 |
| **Date/time seen:** | 07/01/2015 10:00 |

### History

**Problem**  Routine review before discharge.

**History**  Sheila McKinnon was admitted 3 days ago after vomiting up blood. Over the past 3 months she has had intermittent epigastric pain relieved by eating and indigestion tablets. Her weight has been steady and she has had no change in bowel habit. On the day of admission she felt nauseated for several hours, before vomiting up a large amount of bright red blood and passing black tarry stools.

On admission to hospital she received a blood transfusion and underwent urgent endoscopy, at which bleeding from a duodenal ulcer was controlled.

She now feels well with a good appetite and no abdominal discomfort. Her bowel motions are a normal colour. Her energy levels are good, she has no shortness of breath and she is keen to get home as soon as possible.

**PMH**  Pre-eclampsia, hypertension.

**DH**  At admission: amlodipine 5 mg daily, ramipril 5 mg daily (both withheld during the admission).

Started during the admission: 72-hour IV infusion of high-dose omeprazole completed this morning, cyclizine 50 mg IV/IM 8-hourly as required (last dose 3 days ago).

Intolerances: erythromycin causes itching and a rash.

**SH**  She smokes 20 cigarettes and drinks 2 glasses of wine per day.

### Examination

**General**  She looks well.

**Obs**  T 36.7°C, HR 72 beats/min, BP 168/96 mmHg, RR 13 breaths/min, SpO$_2$ 98% breathing air.

**Abdo**  Soft, non-tender.

### Investigations

Endoscopy report 04/01/2015:
- Normal oesophagus and stomach.
- Moderate-sized ulcer in duodenum, visible vessel in base, injected with adrenaline. Good haemostasis achieved.
- Campylobacter-like organism (CLO) test positive for *Helicobacter pylori*.

### Task

Mrs McKinnon is now ready for discharge. Review her treatment and prescribe her discharge medication as appropriate.

## 46 A 64-year-old woman with chronic kidney disease

| | |
|---|---|
| **Patient name:** | Janet Morris |
| **ID number:** | 100046 |
| **Date of birth:** | 16/01/1950 |
| **Admission date:** | 06/01/2015 16:00 |
| **Date/time seen:** | 07/01/2015 14:00 |

### History

**Problem**  Chronic kidney disease (CKD).

**History**  Mrs Morris presented to her GP yesterday with malaise. He performed some blood tests which showed significant renal impairment. He noted that mild renal impairment was evident 1 year ago, and referred her to hospital for full assessment.

Baseline investigations have now been completed and the impression is that of CKD due to diabetic nephropathy. She is to be discharged tomorrow and seen in the nephrology clinic next week.

**PMH**  Type 2 diabetes mellitus, obesity.

**DH**  Atorvastatin 10 mg nightly, metformin 1 g twice daily, NovoMix® 30 24 units morning and 18 units evening subcutaneously.

Intolerances: none known.

**SH**  Non-smoker; no alcohol; independent.

### Examination

**General**  Central obesity.

**Obs**  T 36.8°C, HR 90 beats/min, BP 154/92 mmHg, RR 18 breaths/min, SpO2 96% breathing air.

**Systems**  Normal JVP and skin turgor. Mild ankle oedema.

### Investigations

For results of investigations, see Table 46.1.

### Task

Adjust her treatment regimen in light of her renal function.

**Table 46.1** Case 46 investigation results

| Test | Value | Normal range |
|---|---|---|
| Hb | 101 g/L | 120–160 |
| MCV | 85 fL | 78–97 |
| WCC | $9.6 \times 10^9$/L | 4.0–11.0 |
| Plt | $344 \times 10^9$/L | 150–400 |
| ESR | 16 mm/hour | <20 |
| Na$^+$ | 135 mmol/L | 135–145 |
| K$^+$ | 4.4 mmol/L | 3.5–4.7 |
| Ur | 17.9 mmol/L | 2.5–8.0 |
| Creat | 259 μmol/L | 60–110 |
| eGFR | 18 mL/min/1.73 m$^2$ | >60 |
| Adj Ca$^{2+}$ | 2.33 mmol/L | 2.20–2.50 |
| PO$_4{}^{2-}$ | 1.56 mmol/L | 0.75–1.50 |
| Urine MC&S | Inactive sediment, no organisms | |
| Urine albumin: creat ratio | 18.3 mg/mmol | |
| USS KUB | Mildly enlarged kidneys with increased cortical echogenicity in keeping with diabetic nephropathy. No obstruction. | |

## 47 A 66-year-old man with palpitations

| | |
|---|---|
| **Patient name:** | David Edwards |
| **ID number:** | 100047 |
| **Date of birth:** | 13/12/1948 |
| **Weight:** | 74 kg |
| **Admission date:** | 06/01/2015 |
| **Date/time seen:** | 07/01/2015 14:00 |

### History
| | |
|---|---|
| Problem | Palpitations. |
| History | Mr Edwards was admitted with a 4-day history of diarrhoea secondary to viral gastroenteritis, complicated by pre-renal acute kidney injury. Treatment with intravenous fluids has improved his creatinine from 184 to 144 µmol/L. However he now feels nauseated and is experiencing palpitations. |
| PMH | Atrial fibrillation, asthma. Renal function was normal 1 month ago. |
| DH | Digoxin 125 micrograms daily, salbutamol 100 micrograms inhaled as required, warfarin 4 mg daily. Intolerances: beta blockers cause bronchospasm. |
| SH | He is a retired football coach. |

### Examination
| | |
|---|---|
| General | Dry mucous membranes. |
| Obs | T 36.4°C, HR 48 beats/min, BP 110/68 mmHg, RR 18 breaths/min, SpO$_2$ 97% breathing air. |
| Fluid bal | Total input 3000 mL in past 26 hours; output 1040 mL of urine in 26 hours plus eight episodes of loose stool of estimated volume 3000 mL. |
| CVS | He has an irregular pulse, capillary refill time 3 seconds, JVP not visible while sitting, and normal heart sounds. |

### Investigations
For results of investigations, see Table 47.1.

### Task
Review Mr Edwards' drug chart and make any necessary changes to address his deterioration.

**Table 47.1** Case 47 investigation results

| Test | Value | Normal range |
|---|---|---|
| Na$^+$ | 138 mmol/L | 135–145 |
| K$^+$ | 3.3 mmol/L | 3.5–4.7 |
| Ur | 13.4 mmol/L | 2.5–8.0 |
| Creat | 144 µmol/L | 60–110 |
| Mg$^{2+}$ | 0.8 mmol/L | 0.7–1.0 |
| Digoxin level 6 h post dose | 2 µg/L | 0.5–0.9 |
| ECG | Sinus bradycardia with premature ventricular complexes. The ST segments are depressed with a 'reverse-tick' configuration | |

## 48 A 70-year-old man with ST-elevation acute coronary syndrome

| | |
|---|---|
| **Patient name:** | Ben Hawkins |
| **ID number:** | 100048 |
| **Date of birth:** | 25/11/1944 |
| **Weight:** | 80 kg |
| **Admission date:** | 06/01/2015 |
| **Date/time seen:** | 07/01/2015 14:00 |

### History
| | |
|---|---|
| Problem | ST-elevation acute coronary syndrome (ACS). |
| History | Mr Hawkins was admitted yesterday following an ST-elevation ACS. Coronary angiography identified occlusion of the left anterior descending coronary artery and a drug-eluting stent was inserted. Currently, he is symptom-free. |
| PMH | Diet-controlled type 2 diabetes mellitus 5 years. |
| DH | New since admission: aspirin 75 mg daily, clopidogrel 75 mg daily, fondaparinux 2.5 mg daily, lansoprazole 30 mg daily. Intolerances: none known. |
| SH | He has never smoked. |

### Examination
| | |
|---|---|
| General | Appears well. |
| Obs | T 35.5°C, HR 80 beats/min, BP 146/70 mmHg, RR 16 breaths/min, SpO$_2$ 96% breathing air. |

### Investigations
For results of investigations, see Tables 48.1 and 48.2.

### Task
The cardiology registrar has asked you to make sure Mr Hawkins is on appropriate medications following an ACS. She recommends that aspirin 75 mg daily should be continued life-long and clopidogrel 75 mg daily should be continued for 1 year and it should not be stopped without prior discussion. She also recommends that you start eplerenone in view of Mr Hawkins's echocardiogram result.

**Table 48.1** Case 48 investigation results

| Test | Value | Normal range |
|---|---|---|
| Na$^+$ | 135 mmol/L | 135–145 |
| K$^+$ | 4.0 mmol/L | 3.5–4.7 |
| Ur | 6.8 mmol/L | 2.5–8.0 |
| Creat | 84 µmol/L | 60–110 |
| CBG | 6.8 mmol/L | |

**Table 48.2** Case 48 results of echocardiogram

Normal left ventricle cavity size with increased wall thickness. Overall systolic function is severely impaired with a left ventricular ejection fraction of 30%. Hypokinetic apical anterior wall. Right ventricle appears normal size and function. No significant valvular abnormality

## 49 A 49-year-old woman with chronic liver disease complaining of pain

**Patient name:** Angela Morrison
**ID number:** 100049
**Date of birth:** 13/12/1965
**Weight:** 55 kg
**Admission date:** 05/01/2015
**Date/time seen:** 07/01/2015 14:00

### History
Problem | Right arm pain following a fall.
History | Mrs Morrison was admitted with ascites secondary to decompensated liver disease.
PMH | Cirrhosis of the liver, oesophageal varices, previous bleed.
DH | Furosemide 40 mg daily, propranolol 20 mg 12-hourly, spironolactone 100 mg daily, thiamine 100 mg daily.
| Intolerances: none known.
SH | She stopped drinking alcohol 1 year ago. She currently smokes 10 cigarettes per day.

### Examination
General | She is mildly jaundiced with spider naevi and purpura. Throughout the assessment she is irritable and inattentive.
Obs | T 36.4°C, HR 56 beats/min, BP 138/76 mmHg, RR 14 breaths/min, SpO$_2$ 95% breathing air.
NS | Abbreviated mental test score 6/10.
MSS | Her right arm is bruised and tender.

### Investigations
For results of investigations, see Table 49.1.

A diagnosis of soft tissue injury of the right arm is made.

### Task
Prescribe suitable analgesia and make any other changes to her treatment that you consider appropriate.

**Table 49.1** Case 49 investigation results

| Test | Value | Normal range |
|---|---|---|
| Hb | 118 g/L | 120–160 |
| MCV | 104 fL | 78–97 |
| WCC | 9.8 x 10$^9$/L | 4.0–11.0 |
| Plt | 126 x 10$^9$/L | 150–400 |
| INR | 1.8 | 0.8–1.1 |
| Ur | 2.9 mmol/L | 2.5–8.0 |
| Creat | 48 μmol/L | 60–110 |
| Alb | 24 g/L | 35–48 |
| Bil | 52 μmol/L | <17 |
| ALT | 216 U/L | <40 |
| ALP | 142 U/L | 35–120 |
| GGT | 290 U/L | <38 |
| X-ray right humerus and shoulder | Normal appearance of shoulder joint. No fracture identified | |

## 50 An 89-year-old man approaching the end of life

**Patient name:** Terry Smith
**ID number:** 100050
**Date of birth:** 27/01/1925
**Age:** 89 years
**Weight:** 64 kg
**Admission date:** 04/01/2013 17:00
**Date/time seen:** 07/01/2013 14:00

### History
Problem | You are asked to write a syringe driver prescription.
History | Mr Smith has advanced non-small cell lung cancer, and was admitted 3 days ago with severe pain and debility. He has since deteriorated further, and is now only semi-conscious. Following a careful discussion between Mr Smith's family, his doctors and the palliative care team, it has been decided that his treatment should now focus on relief of symptoms rather than extending his life. Arrangements will be made to transfer him to a local hospice for end-of-life care. As he is no longer able to take medicines orally, you have been asked to convert his current oral analgesic regimen to an equivalent subcutaneous infusion.
PMH | Non-small cell lung cancer (squamous cell type) with bulky mediastinal nodes and multiple bone metastases.
DH | Haloperidol 1.5 mg nightly (for nausea), MST Continus® (morphine sulfate modified release) 30 mg 12-hourly, Oramorph® (morphine sulfate oral solution) 10 mg 2-hourly as required, senna 15 mg nightly, simvastatin 40 mg nightly, Symbicort® 400/12 (budesonide with formoterol) two puffs inhaled 12-hourly.
| Intolerances: none known.
SH | Ex-smoker of 60 pack-years.

### Examination
General | Cachexia. Squeezes hand in response to voice. Pupils 4 mm and reactive.
Obs | T 36.9°C, HR 80 beats/min, BP 119/88 mmHg, RR 24 breaths/min, SpO$_2$ 92% on air.
Systems | No findings of relevance to the current task.

### Investigations
None of relevance.

### Task
Convert his oral analgesic regimen to an equivalent subcutaneous infusion.

# Answers

| Surname ALDRIDGE | Hospital number 100037 | Weight | Drug intolerances |
|---|---|---|---|
| First name FELICITY | Date of birth 24/02/1955 | 75 kg | None known |

**REGULAR PRESCRIPTIONS**

| | Circle / enter times below ↓ | ↘ Enter dates below | | | Month: January | Year: 2015 |
|---|---|---|---|---|---|---|
| | | 5 | 6 | 7 | | |
| DRUG **DIHYDROCODEINE** | 06 | AM | AM | AM | | |
| | 08 | | | | | |
| Dose 30 mg / Route ORAL / Freq 6-hrly / Start date 5/1/15 | 12 | AM | AM | | | |
| Signature A Doctor / Bleep 1234 / Review | 16 | | | | | |
| | 18 | AM | AM | | | |
| Additional instructions For postoperative pain | 24 | AM | AM | | | |
| DRUG **PARACETAMOL** | 06 | AM | AM | AM | | |
| | 08 | | | | | |
| Dose 1 g / Route ORAL / Freq 6-hrly / Start date 5/1/15 | 12 | AM | AM | | | |
| Signature A Doctor / Bleep 1234 / Review | 16 | | | | | |
| | 18 | AM | AM | | | |
| Additional instructions For postoperative pain | 24 | AM | AM | | | |
| DRUG **DABIGATRAN** | 06 | | | | | |
| | 08 | | | | | |
| Dose 220 mg / Route Oral / Freq Daily / Start date 5/1/15 | 12 | | | | | |
| Signature A Doctor / Bleep 1234 / Review | 16 | | | | | |
| | 18 | ⊢ | AM | | | |
| Additional instructions Total 10 days treatment | 22 | | | | | |
| DRUG **SENNA** | 06 | | | | | |
| | 08 | | | | | |
| Dose 15 mg / Route ORAL / Freq Daily / Start date 7/1/15 | 12 | | | | | |
| Signature A Doctor / Bleep 1234 / R Every 48 hours | 16 | | | | | |
| | 18 | | | | | |
| Additional instructions For opioid-induced constipation | 22 | ⊢ | | | | |

**ONCE ONLY PRESCRIPTIONS**

| Date | Time to be given | DRUG | Dose | Route | Prescriber Signature | Prescriber Bleep | Administration Date given | Administration Time given | Administration Given by |
|---|---|---|---|---|---|---|---|---|---|
| 5/1/15 | 1800 | DABIGATRAN | 110 mg | ORAL | A Doctor | | 5/1/15 | 1800 | AN |
| | | | | | | | | | |

**OXYGEN**

| Target SpO₂ | ○ 94–98% ○ 88–92% |
|---|---|
| Mode of delivery | ○ Continuous ○ As required |
| Starting device | |

| Initials | Bleep | Date |
|---|---|---|

**AS REQUIRED MEDICATION**

| DRUG **SEVREDOL** | Date | 5/1 | 5/1 | 6/1 | 7/1 | | | |
|---|---|---|---|---|---|---|---|---|
| | Time | 1400 | 2000 | 1300 | 1545 | | | |
| Dose 5 mg / Route ORAL / Max freq 4-hrly / Start date 5/1/15 | Dose | 5 mg | 5 mg | 5 mg | 5 mg | | | |
| | Route | ORAL | ORAL | ORAL | ORAL | | | |
| Signature A Doctor / Bleep 1234 / Review 8/1/14 | Given | AM | AM | AM | AM | | | |
| | Check | AD | AD | AD | AD | | | |
| Additional instructions Morphine sulfate immediate release tablets. For break through pain relief. Inform doctor if insufficient. | | | | | | | | |
| DRUG | Date | | | | | | | |

## What should I consider when deciding what to prescribe?

Constipation is a common side effect of therapy with opioid analgesics. In Mrs Aldridge's case, the regularly administered dihydrocodeine is most likely to be the culprit, although the as required doses of morphine sulfate may also be contributing. Patients complain of the discomfort that results from constipation, and com-

plications such as haemorrhoids and anal fissures are not uncommon. In elderly patients, constipation is recognised as a cause of acute confusion. It should therefore not be ignored and ideal practice would be to offer patients a regular laxative prescription whenever you prescribe opioid medications.

Laxatives can be divided into four broad groups: stimulant, bulk forming and osmotic laxatives, and faecal softeners.

*Stimulant laxatives* (e.g. senna, docusate sodium) induce peristalsis by direct irritation of large bowel mucosa. Side effects include abdominal cramping and they should not be used in intestinal obstruction. Excessive use can lead to diarrhoea and subsequent complications with electrolyte imbalance.

*Bulk forming laxatives* (e.g. ispaghula husk, methylcellulose) improve transit by increasing faecal mass and thereby induce peristalsis. It is important that patients taking such agents drink plenty of water to prevent bowel obstruction. Side effects include abdominal distension, obstruction or impaction and flatulence.

*Osmotic laxatives* (e.g. lactulose, macrogols) increase the water content of the large intestine, thereby easing passage of stool through lubrication and increasing faecal bulk (in turn inducing peristalsis). Macrogols (e.g. Movicol®) are licensed only for use in chronic constipation. Again, it is particularly important to advise patients to drink plenty of water, which is necessary for the action of this drug class and may help to reduce side effects. Such side effects include nausea, flatulence and abdominal cramps.

*Faecal softeners* (e.g. paraffin, arachis oil). All of the above laxative classes have some softening action. The role of oral paraffin is generally limited to patients with haemorrhoids or anal fissure. The major side effect is anal irritation. Rectal arachis oil is useful in faecal impaction. Arachis oil is a peanut oil so *must not* be used in patients with peanut allergy.

For patients experiencing constipation as a result of the side effects of analgesia, you should first assess the on-going need for the culprit medication. In Mrs Aldridge's case, you are told that, while her pain is generally well controlled, she still needs an occasional dose of morphine. It would therefore be inappropriate to discontinue any of her current analgesic medications although you should regularly review the need for them.

As with many prescribing situations, there is no one perfect solution to treating constipation resulting from opioid analgesia.

*Prescribing Scenarios at a Glance*, First Edition. Emma Baker, Daniel Burrage, Dagan Lonsdale, and Andrew Hitchings.
© 2014 John Wiley & Sons, Ltd. Published 2014 by John Wiley & Sons, Ltd. Companion website: www.ataglanceseries.com/prescribingscenarios

We have chosen to prescribe a stimulant laxative as their presentation in the form of small tablets makes them generally more palatable than bulk-forming laxatives and their side effect profile is potentially more tolerable than that of lactulose. Of note, as her rectum was empty, a suppository or enema would not be useful.

### How do I write the prescription?
Senna is given at a dose of 7.5–15 mg orally, usually at night (maximum dose 30 mg/day). Docusate sodium is a reasonable alternative, which would be prescribed at a dose of 100–200 mg orally 8- or 12-hourly (maximum daily dose 500 mg).

Remember that laxative prescriptions should be regularly reviewed, particularly in the postoperative phase where analgesic requirements, mobility and dietary intake all change rapidly and will affect bowel transit. It is worth noting a regular review date on the drug chart.

### Further reading
Medical Pharmacology at a Glance. Chapter 13: Drugs acting on the gastrointestinal tract II.
Prescribing at a Glance. Chapter 25: Using drugs for the gastrointestinal system.

---

## 38 A 71-year-old man who has developed a tremor

### What should I consider when deciding what to prescribe?
Mr Roach is a 71-year-old man who has been admitted with a fall. He has a background of schizophrenia, which has been well controlled on quetiapine for 5 years. He has been noted to have a tremor that is Parkinson-like (present at rest, associated cogwheeling). This is symmetrical and he has no other demonstrable features of parkinsonism (such as rigidity or bradykinesia), although it is notable that he has just had a fall. Your consultant has raised the suspicion of a drug-induced parkinsonism.

### Drug-induced parkinsonism
Drug-induced parkinsonism is an example of a 'continued use' adverse drug reaction: where prolonged use over weeks to months (i.e. the cumulative dose) leads to an adverse effect. Drugs are a common cause of secondary parkinsonism. Features to suggest drug-induced parkinsonism include symptoms that relate to the timing of drug administration, symmetrical tremor (as opposed to unilateral) and associated abnormal oral–buccal movements. Patients particularly at risk include the elderly and women. Once the offending drug has been stopped, symptoms tend to fade over a period of months depending on the length of treatment, although some patients may require treatment with anti-muscarinic drugs or even levodopa or a dopamine agonist.

### Which drugs?
Common drug causes of parkinsonism include drugs with central and peripheral anti-dopaminergic effects including first-generation anti-psychotic drugs (e.g. prochlorperazine, chlorpromazine and haloperidol) which block dopamine $D_2$-receptors, anti-emetics (e.g. metoclopramide) and other drugs with non-dopaminergic effects such as anti-histamines (e.g. cinnarazine). The possible drug causes of Mr Roach's parkinsonism include metoclopramide and quetiapine.

*Metoclopramide* is a dopamine $D_2$-receptor antagonist, which is commonly used as an anti-emetic. Although the risk of extrapyramidal side effects such as tardive dyskinesia and parkinsonism is rare, this risk increases with prolonged use. It is therefore recommended that long-term treatment (>3 months) is avoided where possible and patients are regularly reviewed.

*Quetiapine* is an atypical anti-psychotic with similar properties to clozapine. It antagonises various neurotransmitters in the brain,

**Surname:** ROACH
**Hospital number:** 100038
**Weight:** 68 kg
**First name:** JOSIAH
**Date of birth:** 06/06/1943
**Drug intolerances:** None known / Metoclopramide – Suspected drug-induced parkinsonism AD 7/1/15

**REGULAR PRESCRIPTIONS**

Month: January   Year: 2015

| DRUG QUETIAPINE | Circle/enter times below | 6 | 7 | | | | | | |
|---|---|---|---|---|---|---|---|---|---|
| | 06 | | | | | | | | |
| Dose 150 mg  Route Oral  Freq 12-hrly  Start date 6/1/15 | (08) | AM | | | | | | | |
| | 12 | | | | | | | | |
| Signature A Doctor  Bleep 1234  Review | 16 | | | | | | | | |
| | 18 | | | | | | | | |
| Additional instructions | (22) | AM | | | | | | | |
| DRUG | 06 | | | | | | | | |

**ONCE ONLY PRESCRIPTIONS**

| Date | Time to be given | DRUG | Dose | Route | Prescriber Signature | Prescriber Bleep | Administration Date given | Administration Time given | Administration Given by |
|---|---|---|---|---|---|---|---|---|---|
| | | | | | | | | | |
| | | | | | | | | | |
| | | | | | | | | | |

**OXYGEN**

Target SpO₂: ○ 94–98%  ○ 88–92%
Mode of delivery: ○ Continuous  ○ As required
Starting device:

| Initials | Bleep | Date |
|---|---|---|

**AS REQUIRED MEDICATION**

| DRUG METOCLOPRAMIDE | Date | 6/1 | 6/1 | 7/1 | | | | STOPPED 7/1/15 |
|---|---|---|---|---|---|---|---|---|
| | Time | 1600 | 2200 | 0800 | | | | |
| Dose 10 mg  Route Oral  Max freq 6-hrly  Start date 6/1/15 | Dose | 10mg | 10mg | 10mg | | | | |
| | Route | Oral | Oral | Oral | | | | |
| Signature A Doctor  Bleep 1234  Review | Given | AM | AM | AM | | | | A Doctor 1234 |
| | Check | | | | | | | |
| Additional instructions  Maximum 3 doses in 24 hours | | | | | | | | |
| DRUG CYCLIZINE | Date | | | | | | | |
| | Time | | | | | | | |
| Dose 50 mg  Route Oral  Max freq 6-hrly  Start date 7/1/15 | Dose | | | | | | | |
| | Route | | | | | | | |
| Signature A Doctor  Bleep 1234  Review | Given | | | | | | | |
| | Check | | | | | | | |
| Additional instructions  Maximum 3 doses in 24 hours | | | | | | | | |
| DRUG | Date | | | | | | | |

notably via the serotonin and dopamine $D_2$ receptors. It is used in the management of schizophrenia, bipolar affective disorder and depression. In schizophrenia it has been shown to be effective at treating both 'positive' and 'negative' psychotic symptoms, and is at least as effective as typical anti-psychotics. Unlike most other anti-psychotics it has a low incidence of extrapyramidal side effects, similar to placebo. In fact, studies have demonstrated quetiapine to be a useful anti-psychotic agent in patients with Parkinson's disease who have psychotic symptoms. However, although extrapyramidal side effects are less common with second-generation anti-psychotic drugs, they do still occur with appreciable frequency (incidence quoted in the quetiapine summary of product characteristics 1–10%).

**What action should I take?**

The first thing to do in Mr Roach's case is to stop the metoclopramide and replace it with an anti-emetic that does not interfere with dopaminergic transmission. Regarding the on-going use of quetiapine, your options are:

1 Continue quetiapine and wait to see if his symptoms subside after stopping metoclopramide

2 Continue quetiapine and consider adding an anticholinergic drug to control his tremor, or

3 Consider an alternative antipsychotic regimen, e.g. lower dose quetiapine, or switching to an alternative anti-psychotic such as clozapine.

The decision is a balance between minimising side effects while continuing to manage his schizophrenia. The simplest and probably best approach would be to stop the metoclopramide, continue quetiapine and wait to see if this leads to resolution of his tremor. If the parkinsonian symptoms do not resolve over the coming days to weeks, you may then need to reconsider whether it is appropriate to continue quetiapine. Adding in an anti-cholinergic drug to control his tremor is best avoided, as quetiapine has anti-cholinergic effects too, and it is good practice to avoid treating drug problems with more drugs where possible (see Case 44). Switching to an alternative agent would probably not be the best option in view of the fact that his schizophrenia appears to have been well controlled on quetiapine for the past 5 years. Any decision that could impact on the treatment of his schizophrenia should be guided by expert psychiatric advice.

**How do I write the prescription?**
**Stopping medications**

Metoclopramide should be discontinued by crossing through the prescribing and signing and dating this. Be sure to record your assessment in the notes, making clear the reason for stopping metoclopramide, and add this to Mr Roach's list of intolerances. If he still has nausea, you should consider prescribing an alternative anti-emetic that does not act on dopamine receptors. A reasonable choice would be cyclizine.

**Existing medications**

He should continue to take quetiapine while we wait to see if withdrawing metoclopramide improves his tremor.

**Further reading**

Medical Pharmacology at a Glance. Chapter 27: Antipsychotic drugs (neuroleptics); Chapter 30: Drugs used in nausea and vomiting (antiemetics).

Prescribing at a Glance. Chapter 22: Dealing with adverse drug reactions.

## What should I consider when deciding what to prescribe?

Ms Pellow is an 81-year-old post-menopausal woman who has sustained a fragility fracture. A fragility fracture is one that occurs due to mechanical forces that should not normally lead to bone fracture, such as a fall from standing height. Fragility fractures confer an increased risk of further fractures in the future and an increased risk of death. So, although Ms Pellow has recovered well from her total hip replacement, you now need to consider how to prevent further fractures.

Fragility fractures in a post-menopausal woman are highly suggestive of osteoporosis. Osteoporosis is a reduction in bone mass and organised structure. There are many risk factors for osteoporosis: female sex, menopause, older age, family history of maternal hip fracture, previous fragility fracture, low body mass index (BMI), smoking, corticosteroid use, alcohol excess, prolonged immobilisation, low calcium intake and vitamin D deficiency. A diagnosis of osteoporosis can be assumed in a woman aged over 75 years who has sustained a fragility fracture. A dual-energy X-ray absorptiometry (DXA) scan can be used to measure bone density in other people where there is a suspicion of osteoporosis.

## What drugs reduce the risk of recurrent osteoporotic fractures in post-menopausal women?

Bisphosphonates can reduce the risk of recurrent fracture in people with osteoporosis by around 50%. Bisphosphonates accumulate in osteoclasts where they cause apoptosis. This reduces the rate of bone turnover and resorption. According to current NICE guidance, alendronic acid is the first-line bisphosphonate for secondary prevention of osteoporotic fragility fractures. Second-line bisphosphonates for prevention of osteoporotic fractures include risedronate and etidronate. Strontium ranelate, raloxifene and teriparatide are alternative drugs with different mechanisms of action, currently reserved for patients who cannot tolerate a bisphosphonate.

## What should I check before prescribing a bisphosphonate?

*Able to take and tolerate medication.* Oral bisphosphonates are poorly absorbed and can cause oesophageal irritation, ulceration, erosion and stricture. You should therefore check if Ms Pellow has any history of gastro-oesophageal disease, ulcers, bleeding or gastrointestinal surgery. You should also check if she is able to swallow the tablet safely and sit upright for at least 30 minutes after taking it. Parenteral preparations are available for patients who cannot tolerate an oral bisphosphonate.

*Renal function.* Bisphosphonates are renally excreted, so you should check the renal profile before starting one, and avoid prescribing one if there is significant renal impairment (e.g. eGFR $<35\,\text{mL/minute/}1.73\,\text{m}^2$ for alendronic acid). Ms Pellow has normal renal function.

*Calcium and vitamin D.* You should check serum calcium and vitamin D levels. In Ms Pellow's case her values are at the lower

| Surname PELLOW | Hospital number 100039 | Weight 58 kg | Drug intolerances None known |
| --- | --- | --- | --- |
| First name ALICE | Date of birth 02/11/1933 | | |

**REGULAR PRESCRIPTIONS**     Chart rewritten 6/1/15

Month: January    Year: 2015

| DRUG PARACETAMOL | Circle/enter times below | 6 | 7 |
| --- | --- | --- | --- |
| Dose 1 gram / Route Oral / Freq 6-hrly / Start date 27/12/14 | 06 | AM | AM |
| | 08 | | |
| | 12 | AM | AM |
| Signature A Doctor / Bleep 1234 / Review | 16 | | |
| Additional instructions | 18 | AM | |
| | 22 (24) | AM | |

| DRUG DABIGATRAN | 06 | | |
| --- | --- | --- | --- |
| Dose 150 mg / Route Oral / Freq Daily / Start date 27/12/14 | 08 | | |
| | 12 | | |
| Signature A Doctor / Bleep 1234 / Review 27 days | 16 | | |
| Additional instructions VTE prophylaxis Continue for 27-34 days | 18 | AM | |
| | 22 | | |

| DRUG ADCAL D₃ ® | 06 | | |
| --- | --- | --- | --- |
| Dose Two tablets / Route Oral / Freq Daily / Start date 7/1/15 | 08 | | |
| | 12 | | |
| Signature A Doctor / Bleep 1234 / Review | 16 | | |
| Additional instructions | 18 | | |
| | 22 | | |

| DRUG ALENDRONIC ACID | 06 (07) | | |
| --- | --- | --- | --- |
| Dose 70 mg / Route Oral / Freq Once weekly / Start date 7/1/15 | 08 | | |
| | 12 | | |
| Signature A Doctor / Bleep 1234 / Review | 16 | | |
| Additional instructions | 18 | | |

Swallow whole, while sitting, with plenty of water and on empty stomach. Take 30 min before breakfast. Sit upright for ≥30 min after taking tablet.

**ONCE ONLY PRESCRIPTIONS**

| Date | Time to be given | DRUG | Dose | Route | Prescriber Signature | Prescriber Bleep | Administration Date given | Administration Time given | Administration Given by |
| --- | --- | --- | --- | --- | --- | --- | --- | --- | --- |
| | | | | | | | | | |
| | | | | | | | | | |
| | | | | | | | | | |

**OXYGEN**

| Target SpO₂ | ○ 94–98% |
| --- | --- |
| | ○ 88–92% |
| Mode of delivery | ○ Continuous |
| | ○ As required |
| Starting device | |

| Initials | Bleep | Date |
| --- | --- | --- |

**AS REQUIRED MEDICATION**

| DRUG CODEINE PHOSPHATE | Date | |
| --- | --- | --- |
| | Time | |
| Dose 30-60 mg / Route Oral / Max freq 4-hrly / Start date 27/12/14 | Dose | |
| | Route | |
| Signature A Doctor / Bleep 1234 / Review | Given | |
| Additional instructions | Check | |

limits of the normal range. Elderly patients often have poor dietary intake of calcium and vitamin D and those who are housebound may get little sun exposure for vitamin D synthesis. It is therefore good practice to prescribe calcium and vitamin D supplements alongside a bisphosphonate in this group. There is some evidence to suggest that this reduces fracture risk too. A combined preparation of calcium with colecalciferol (vitamin $D_3$) is preferable here to treat the combined calcium and vitamin D deficiency, and also to reduce tablet burden. You should aim to supplement dietary intake with 1–1.2 g calcium and 800 international units/day vitamin D. There are not (at present) approved non-proprietary names for combined preparations of calcium and vitamin D, so here it is acceptable to prescribe using the proprietary (brand) name. Various preparations are available, so your choice should be based on your local formulary. It is often simpler to specify the dose as the number of tablets to be taken rather than doses of calcium and vitamin D, provided the tablets do not come in different strengths.

*Risk of drug interactions.* Bisphosphonates bind calcium. If they do this in the gut they will not be absorbed. The absorption of bisphosphonates is therefore reduced if taken at the same time as calcium salts, oral iron or antacids. You therefore need to make sure that alendronic acid is prescribed to be taken on an empty stomach 30 minutes before any other medication or meal is taken.

*Dentition.* A rare but serious adverse effect of bisphosphonates is osteonecrosis of the jaw. Patients most at risk include smokers and those with a history of dental disease. Ms Pellow is a non-smoker with good dentition.

## What should I advise my patient?

You should have a discussion with Ms Pellow about the benefits and risks of taking a bisphosphonate. You should emphasise the dose of alendronic acid and how frequently you want her to take it (normally 70 mg once weekly) to avoid any overdosing errors.

Due to the risk of oesophageal irritation you should advise Ms Pellow to swallow the alendronic acid tablets whole, with plenty of water while sitting or standing. She should take the alendronic acid on an empty stomach 30 minutes before breakfast, and remain upright (sitting or standing) for 30 minutes after taking it. You should advise her to report any difficulties swallowing or symptoms of oesophageal irritation.

You should ask her to arrange a dental appointment before (or soon after starting) and during bisphosphonate treatment to minimise the risk of osteonecrosis of the jaw.

## Other prophylaxis

Patients undergoing major orthopaedic surgery are high risk for venous thromboembolism (VTE). In this case, Ms Pellow has been started on a direct thrombin inhibitor, dabigatran, by the admitting team to reduce her risk of VTE. Dabigatran is given orally for 27–34 days following hip or knee replacement surgery to prevent VTE. This extended prophylaxis against VTE is required as the risk continues for several weeks beyond the initial surgery. It is given at a reduced dose in elderly patients over 75 years. Alternatives to dabigatran include rivaroxaban (an inhibitor of activated factor X), fondaparinux and low molecular weight heparins.

## How do I write the prescription?
### Calcium and vitamin D supplementation

Adcal $D_3$® is prescribed here. One tablet would provide 600 mg calcium and 400 units colecalciferol, so two tablets are required. This has been prescribed as a single daily dose, but could be given in divided doses depending on Ms Pellow's preference.

### Alendronic acid

Alendronic acid should be prescribed at a dose of 70 mg once weekly. When prescribing a medication on a weekly basis it is good practice to use 'T-bars' to score off the 6 days in between dosing to reduce the chance of accidental daily administration. You should also note in the 'additional instructions' box that the tablet should be given at least 30 minutes before breakfast, taken with plenty of water and the patient should remain upright for 30 minutes after.

### Further reading

Medical Pharmacology at a Glance. Chapter 33: Corticosteroids.
Prescribing at a Glance. Chapter 17: Prescribing in the elderly.
NICE technology appraisal guidance 161. Alendronate, etidronate, risedronate, raloxifene, strontium ranelate and teriparatide for the secondary prevention of osteoporotic fragility fractures in postmenopausal women (2008). http://www.nice.org.uk/nicemedia/live/11748/42508/42508.pdf (accessed 18 January 2014).

## What should I consider when deciding what to prescribe?

Mrs Srikanth is a 23-year-old woman in the third trimester of pregnancy. She has been found to have a pulmonary embolus (PE) and is hypoxic. She has no immediate life-threatening features (systolic BP <90 mmHg, reduced level of consciousness) and so emergency thrombolytic therapy is not indicated.

## Key issues in managing her current problems

### Relief of hypoxia and breathlessness

*Oxygen.* Her oxygen saturation is 93%. This is sub-optimal for her and the fetus. You should prescribe oxygen therapy targeting $SpO_2$ 94–98%.

### Anti-coagulation

*Low molecular weight heparin (LMWH).* Anti-coagulation in venous thromboembolic (VTE) disease prevents clot propagation, allowing degradation of the clot through the normal fibrinolytic process. LMWH (e.g. dalteparin, enoxaparin) is the preferred treatment option in pregnancy because it does not cross the placenta (unlike warfarin) and because of its relatively predictable anti-coagulant effect. However, because LMWH is eliminated more rapidly in pregnancy than in the non-pregnant state, LMWH should be administered 12-hourly rather than daily, and its anti-coagulant effect monitored to guide dosage adjustment.

*Monitoring therapy.* Normally, the anti-coagulant effect of LMWH is not monitored with laboratory tests. However, when treating PE in pregnancy anti-Xa assays are used to ensure that the desired anti-coagulant effect is achieved. You should seek advice from a haematology specialist early in the management of such cases to guide you in this process.

*Hospital discharge.* Patients can be discharged from hospital once therapy has commenced, provided there is no haemodynamic instability, no on-going need for supplementary oxygen or significant hypoxia on exertion and any pain is adequately controlled. In the case of a pregnant patient, the obstetric team should be involved throughout the admission.

*Duration of therapy.* LMHW therapy should be discontinued prior to delivery and restarted afterwards; specialist advice from the responsible haematology and obstetric specialists should be sought on exact timings.

## Other anti-coagulants in pregnancy

Intravenous unfractionated heparin is occasionally used in unstable patients or in those at high risk of bleeding as it has a shorter half-life than that of LMWH and can be reversed, if necessary, with protamine. In stable patients, however, LMWH is generally safer and more convenient.

Warfarin should be avoided throughout pregnancy: it is teratogenic in the first trimester and there is a risk of fetal haemorrhage in the last trimester. The newer oral anti-coagulants such as direct thrombin inhibitors (e.g. dabigatran) and anti-Xa inhibitors (e.g. rivaroxaban, fondaparinux) are also not currently recommended in pregnancy.

## How do I write the prescription?

*Oxygen.* Prescribe oxygen to target saturations of 94–98%. Nasal cannulae are the preferred means of administration in non-critically ill patients.

Surname: SRIKANTH | Hospital number: 100040 | Weight: 75 kg (booking weight: 65 kg) | Drug intolerances: No known intolerances
First name: SATHYA | Date of birth: 14/08/1991

**REGULAR PRESCRIPTIONS** — Month: July, Year: 2013

AMOXICILLIN — Dose 500 mg, Route ORAL, Freq 8-hrly, Start date 07/01, Signature A Doctor, Bleep 1234, Review 48 hr. Additional instructions: For lower respiratory tract infection. STOP 7/1/15 1830 A Doctor 1234

ENOXAPARIN — Dose 60 mg, Route S/C, Freq Twice daily, Start date 07/01, Signature A Doctor, Bleep 1234. Additional instructions: For PE. Check anti-Xa assay after 48 hr.

**ONCE ONLY PRESCRIPTIONS**

| Date | Time to be given | DRUG | Dose | Route | Signature | Bleep | Date given | Time given | Given by |
|------|------------------|------|------|-------|-----------|-------|-----------|-----------|----------|
| 7/1/15 | 1830 | ENOXAPARIN | 60 mg | S/C | A Doctor | 1234 | | | |

**OXYGEN**
Target $SpO_2$: ✓ 94–98%, ○ 88–92%
Mode of delivery: ✓ Continuous, ○ As required
Starting device: Nasal cannula
Initials AD, Bleep 1234, Date 7/1/15

**AS REQUIRED MEDICATION**

PARACETAMOL — Dose 1g, Route ORAL, Max freq 4-6 hrly, Start date 7/1/15, Signature A Doctor, Bleep 1234. Additional instructions: For chest pain. Max 4 g/day

LMWH. We have chosen to prescribe enoxaparin, the initial dose of which is 60 mg 12-hourly. Whichever agent you have selected, it is important that you have prescribed a dose appropriate to her booking weight rather than her current weight. The first anti-Xa assay should be performed 6 hours after the third or fourth dose, and it is useful to note this on the drug chart. You should have prescribed her first dose at 18:30 (the time of this encounter) to avoid any delays in administration. We have elected to prescribe the first dose as a once only prescription.

*Other issues.* As a diagnosis of PE rather than lower respiratory tract infection has now been made, you should stop the antibiotic prescription. Do this by crossing through the prescription and signing and dating this action.

### Further reading
Medical Pharmacology at a Glance. Chapter 19: Drugs used to affect blood coagulation.
Prescribing at a Glance. Chapter 18: Prescribing in pregnancy and breast feeding.

---

## 41  A 31-year-old man with increased seizure frequency

| Surname RAFFIQ | Hospital number 100041 | Weight 68 kg | Drug intolerances None known |
|---|---|---|---|
| First name ABDUL | Date of birth 25/02/1983 | | |

**REGULAR PRESCRIPTIONS**

Month: January  Year: 2015

| DRUG LEVETIRACETAM | Circle/enter times below | 1 | 2 | 3 | 4 | 5 | 6 | 7 | | | |
|---|---|---|---|---|---|---|---|---|---|---|---|
| Dose 1.5 g  Route Oral  Freq 12-hrly  Start date 1/1/15 | 06 | | AN | AN | AN | AN | AN | AN | | | |
| Signature A Doctor  Bleep 1234  Review | 08 | | | | | | | | | | |
| Additional instructions | 12 | | | | | | | | | | |
| | 16 | | | | | | | | | | |
| | 18 | | AN | AN | AN | AN | AN | AN | | | |
| | 22 | | | | | | | | | | |

| DRUG PHENYTOIN (TABLETS) | 06 | | | | | | | | | | |
|---|---|---|---|---|---|---|---|---|---|---|---|
| Dose 300 mg  Route Oral  Freq Daily  Start date 1/1/15 | 08 | | AN | AN | AN | AN | AN | AN | | STOP 7/1/15 AD 1234 | |
| Signature A Doctor  Bleep 1234  Review | 12 | | | | | | | | | | |
| Additional instructions New this admission | 16 | | | | | | | | | | |
| | 18 | | | | | | | | | | |
| | 22 | | | | | | | | | | |

| DRUG PHENYTOIN (TABLETS) | 06 | | | | | | | | | | |
|---|---|---|---|---|---|---|---|---|---|---|---|
| Dose 350 mg  Route Oral  Freq Daily  Start date 7/1/15 | 08 | | | | | | | | | | |
| Signature A Doctor  Bleep 1234  Review | 12 | | | | | | | | | | |
| Additional instructions Dose increased 7/1/15 | 16 | | | | | | | | | | |
| | 18 | | | | | | | | | | |
| | 22 | | | | | | | | | | |

**ONCE ONLY PRESCRIPTIONS**

| Date | Time to be given | DRUG | Dose | Route | Prescriber Signature | Bleep | Administration Date given | Time given | Given by |
|---|---|---|---|---|---|---|---|---|---|
| 1/1/15 | 10:00 | PHENYTOIN | 1.5 g | IV | A Doctor | 1234 | 1/1/15 | 10:15 | AN |
| | | | | | | | | | |

**OXYGEN**

| Target SpO₂ | ○ 94–98% ○ 88–92% |
|---|---|
| Mode of delivery | ○ Continuous ○ As required |
| Starting device | |
| Initials | Bleep | Date |

### What should I consider when deciding what to prescribe?

Phenytoin now has a limited role in the management of epilepsy because of the availability of newer drugs that are generally better tolerated. However, it retains a place in the management of status epilepticus (seizures that are unremitting or recur without complete inter-ictal recovery; see Case 6). The concentration of phenytoin in the blood has a reasonably good relationship with anti-epileptic efficacy. However, its therapeutic index is narrow (i.e. there is little

margin of safety between the dose required for therapeutic effect and the dose that may be toxic). For these reasons, it is important that the plasma concentration of phenytoin is measured to guide its dosage adjustment (therapeutic drug monitoring, TDM).

### Understanding phenytoin concentration monitoring

In the context of status epilepticus, you should first take a sample for phenytoin concentration measurement about an hour after administration of the IV loading dose. This is to ensure that a therapeutic concentration has been achieved, as was the case for Mr Raffiq. If maintenance therapy is then prescribed (which may be IV or oral, depending on the circumstances), you should take the next sample once *steady state* has been achieved. Steady state means that the rate of drug administration equals the rate of drug elimination; in other words, that the serum concentration has plateaued (other than for concentration oscillations associated with administration of individual doses). Measuring the phenytoin concentration before steady state is reached is likely to be misleading and should generally be avoided unless toxicity is suspected.

A good general rule is that steady state is achieved after the patient has been taking a stable dose for 5 half-lives of the drug. In the case of phenytoin this is more complicated because the half-life is not constant. Nevertheless, most authorities would recommend not sampling until the patient has been on a stable dosage for at least 5 days. It is best if the sample is taken just before a dose (i.e. a trough level; see Case 26), but because phenytoin has a long half-life and its absorption is slow, this is not crucial. In Mr Raffiq's case, the latest concentration appears to have been appropriately taken, so can be used to guide dosage adjustment.

### Understanding phenytoin dosage adjustment

At low serum phenytoin concentrations, the rate at which phenytoin is eliminated from the body increases in proportion to its serum concentration, such that its half-life is stable (first-order kinetics). However, as the phenytoin concentration approaches the therapeutic range, the body's capacity to eliminate it becomes saturated. Now, the rate of phenytoin elimination is fixed: it does not increase as the serum concentration rises (zero-order kinetics). This means that the half-life will *lengthen* in proportion to the serum concentration. If you increase the dose further, not only will more phenytoin be entering the body, but its half-life within the body increases. The practical implication of this is that phenytoin dosage changes can have a more dramatic effect on the serum concentration than you might expect. You should therefore only make small adjustments to the phenytoin dosage, unless working under specialist advice.

### Special circumstances

When interpreting a phenytoin level, you should also check the patient's serum albumin concentration. This is because, under usual conditions, about 90% of the circulating phenytoin is bound to albumin. Only the unbound 10% is pharmacologically active, and yet, when you send a sample for phenytoin concentration it will usually be the 'total' concentration (i.e. bound [inactive] plus free [active] phenytoin) that is measured and reported.

If the amount of albumin in the blood is reduced (as in, for example, liver disease or critical illness), the total phenytoin concentration will fall, because there is less phenytoin bound to albumin. However, the concentration of *free* phenytoin may remain constant. This means that the target range is no longer appropriate: the patient may have a therapeutic or toxic concentration of free phenytoin, despite the total serum phenytoin concentration being below the target range.

A similar effect occurs in renal failure, which changes the affinity with which phenytoin binds to albumin. Consequently, you should also check the renal profile when interpreting a serum phenytoin concentration: if there is renal impairment (high serum creatinine concentration or low eGFR), there may be more free (active) phenytoin than would be suggested by the total phenytoin level.

Mr Raffiq's renal function and serum albumin concentration are within normal limits. Had they not been, you would ideally request measurement of the *free* phenytoin concentration. As this facility is not widely available, an alternative is to apply a mathematical correction to the total concentration to take account of renal function and albumin concentration (see Further reading). Some hospital laboratories apply this correction automatically – check the report carefully and seek advice if in any doubt.

### How do I write the prescription?

As the current phenytoin dosage seems to yield a serum phenytoin concentration that is lower than what we are seeking to achieve (the upper half of the target range, i.e. 15–20 μg/mL), the dosage should be increased. This is usually done by stopping the existing prescription and re-prescribing the drug at the new dosage. This has been illustrated on the model chart, with an increase of the daily dose from 300 to 350 mg. The increment of 50 mg has been selected as it is the smallest dosage change that can be made without having to cut tablets or switch to a different formulation (capsules or syrup). A lower increment (25 mg) would be preferable in patients who are elderly, have a low serum albumin concentration or impaired renal function.

Mr Raffiq should now be monitored clinically (both for seizure frequency and signs of phenytoin toxicity, e.g. ataxia, nystagmus) and a further measurement of the serum phenytoin concentration should be performed after about 5 days at the new dosage. An earlier measurement could be made if features of toxicity supervene, but will otherwise just confuse matters.

Note that the formulation (tablets) has been specified in the phenytoin prescription. There is little evidence to suggest clinically significant difference between formulations (e.g. different brands; tablets, capsules or syrup). However, because of the drug's narrow therapeutic index, many specialists nevertheless recommend keeping patients on the same formulation.

### Further reading

Medical Pharmacology at a Glance. Chapter 25: Antiepileptic drugs.

Prescribing at a Glance. Chapter 21: Therapeutic drug monitoring.

*For adjustment of serum phenytoin concentration due to hypoalbuminaemia or renal impairment, online calculators are available, two examples of which are given below. These are provided for educational purposes only and are not intended to be taken as a recommendation for use in clinical practice. Take care to ensure that you are working in the same units of measurement, and that you check all results carefully.*

MDCalc. Phenytoin/dilantin correction for albumin or renal failure. Available at: http://www.mdcalc.com/phenytoin-dilantin-correction-for-albumin-or-renal-failure/ (accessed 24 January 2014).

ClinCalc.com. Phenytoin correction calculator. Available at: http://clincalc.com/Phenytoin/Correction.aspx (accessed 24 January 2014).

**REGULAR PRESCRIPTIONS**

| Surname | Hospital number | Weight | Drug intolerances |
|---|---|---|---|
| EDWARDS | 100042 | | None known |
| First name | Date of birth | 95 kg | |
| GARETH | 14/01/1956 | | |

| | | Circle / enter times below ↓ | ⊠ Enter dates below | | | Month: January | | Year: 2015 | | | |
|---|---|---|---|---|---|---|---|---|---|---|---|
| | | | 05 | 06 | 07 | | | | | | |
| **DRUG** DALTEPARIN | | 06 | | | | | | | | | |
| | | 08 | | | | | | | | | |
| Dose 5000 units | Route SC | Freq Daily | Start date 3/1/15 | 12 | | | | | | | |
| Signature A Doctor | Bleep 1234 | Review Daily | | 16 | | | | | | | |
| | | | | ⑱ | AM | AM | AM | | | | |
| Additional instructions | | | | 22 | | | | | | | |
| **DRUG** FLUCLOXACILLIN | | 06 | | AM | AM | | | | | | |
| | | 08 | | | | | | | | | |
| Dose 1 g | Route IV | Freq 6 hourly | Start date 3/1/15 | ⑰ | AM | AM | AM | | | | |
| Signature A Doctor | Bleep 1234 | Review 10/1/15 | | 16 | | | | | | | |
| | | | | ⑱ | AM | AM | | | | | |
| Additional instructions Cellulitis/diabetic foot ulcer | | | | ✗ ⓪⓪ | AM | AM | | | | | |
| **DRUG** METFORMIN | | 06 | | | | | | | | | |
| | | ⑧ | | AM | AM | | | | | | |
| Dose 1 g | Route Oral | Freq Twice daily | Start date 3/1/15 | 12 | | | | | | | |
| Signature A Doctor | Bleep 1234 | Review | | 16 | | | | | | | |
| | | | | ⑱ | AM | AM | | | | | |
| Additional instructions | | | | 22 | | | | | | | |
| **DRUG** ASPIRIN | | 06 | | | | | | | | | |
| | | ⑧ | | AM | AM | | | | | | |
| Dose 75 mg | Route Oral | Freq Daily | Start date 3/1/15 | 12 | | | | | | | |
| Signature A Doctor | Bleep 1234 | Review | | 16 | | | | | | | |
| | | | | 18 | | | | | | | |
| Additional instructions | | | | 22 | | | | | | | |

**Table 42.2** Examples of commonly used insulin preparations. Timings refer to subcutaneous *not* intravenous administration.

| Duration of action | Speed of onset (time to peak activity) | Examples (proprietary names) |
|---|---|---|
| Short | Short (2–4 hours) | Soluble insulin (Actrapid®, Insuman® Rapid) |
| | Rapid (30–90 min) | Insulin aspart (Novorapid®) Insulin lispro (Humalog®) Insulin glulisine (Apidra®) |
| Intermediate | Slow (4–10 hours) | Isophane (NPH) insulin (Humulin I®, Insulatard®, Insuman® Basal) |
| Long | Slow (variable peak) | Insulin glargine (Lantus®) Insulin detemir (Levemir®) |
| Biphasic | n/a | Novomix® 30 (insulin aspart/ insulin aspart protamine) Humalog® Mix25 or Mix50 (insulin lispro/insulin lispro protamine) |

## What should I consider when deciding what to prescribe?

Prescribing daily subcutaneous insulin for inpatients with diabetes mellitus is a common and often daunting task for junior doctors and non-medical prescribers, as the plethora of different insulin formulations and regimens can be overwhelming. However, by familiarising yourself with some of the more common therapeutic strategies and frequently used insulins, you can begin to grasp how to manage this regularly encountered prescribing problem. Why not shadow a diabetes ward round or diabetes nurse specialist to gain some experience of insulin prescribing?

The first thing to be aware of is that there are no hard and fast rules for prescribing insulin as every patient is different. In addition, acute illness alters appetite and food intake *and* increases insulin resistance, thereby changing the body's requirements. This can lead to erratic blood glucose measurements that can be difficult to predict and control. As well as modifying insulin therapy to control blood glucose concentrations, it is important to establish and treat the cause of altered insulin requirements (cellulitis for Mr Edwards).

When you are faced with having to alter an insulin prescription, we suggest you ask yourself the following questions.

### What insulin preparation does the patient usually take and how does it work?

The different insulin preparations can be classified in several ways: e.g., their duration of action, the speed at which they take effect or the way in which they are manufactured or sourced. The BNF groups insulins into three categories (based broadly on their *duration* of action): short-, intermediate- or long-acting. This is a helpful starting point, but we would recommend that you are also conscious of the *speed* at which insulins with a short duration of action take effect: a little confusingly this can be described as *short* (e.g. the soluble insulin Actrapid®; see Case 30) or *rapid* (e.g. insulin aspart, Novorapid®). Insulins with intermediate or long duration of action are generally felt to have a slower onset of effect. Insulin preparations may be monophasic, containing one insulin formulation with a single duration of action, or biphasic, containing two insulin formulations with different durations of action. Table 42.2 provides examples of some of the more commonly used insulins and indicates their duration and speed of action.

Insulins with a short duration of action are generally given with meals, to control increases in blood glucose associated with food intake. Insulins with an intermediate duration of action are given once or twice a day and insulins with a long duration of action are given just once a day. The combination of insulins used by patients will depend on individual circumstances. For people with type 2 diabetes, current guidelines recommend patients who require insulin for adequate glycaemic control should be prescribed a once or twice daily dose of an intermediate (NPH) acting insulin.

However, for patients with a particularly high $HbA_{1c}$ (>75 mmol/mol), like Mr Edwards, a once or twice daily biphasic preparation should be considered. Long-acting insulin preparations can be useful for patients who cannot tolerate multiple injections, for those who require carers to inject insulin or to avoid hypoglycaemic episodes that may be occurring through current therapy.

Mr Edwards uses Humalog® Mix25, a biphasic insulin, which contains a mixture of 25% short-acting insulin lispro and 75% intermediate-acting insulin lispro protamine. The intermediate-acting portion of this preparation is created by the addition of a protamine group to the short-acting insulin, which delays insulin absorption from the injection site. He injects this twice a day, just before breakfast and just before dinner. This provides him with basal insulin cover throughout a 24-hour period, as well as providing a boost of short-acting insulin to cover meals (with the exception of lunch). The proportion of short- and intermediate-acting insulins in biphasic preparations is defined by the number after the preparation name, e.g. Novomix® 30 contains 30% short- and 70% intermediate-acting insulin; Humalog® Mix50 contains 50% short- and 50% intermediate-acting insulin.

We would encourage you to reflect on the similarities between the different names of insulin preparations (e.g. Humalog® and Humalog® Mix; Novorapid® and Novomix®); a mistake as simple as writing the wrong last few letters or numbers on an insulin prescription can have dangerous consequences for your patient, such as hypoglycaemia. You must make sure that the insulin you prescribe is the correct preparation. Familiarising yourself with some of the more commonly used insulin preparations will help you do this.

| Name | | Hospital number | Date of birth | Intolerances |
|---|---|---|---|---|
| Gareth Edwards | | 100042 | 14/01/1956 | None known |

**INSULIN PRESCRIPTIONS**

| DATE | | TIME | 0600 | 1200 | 1800 | 2200 |
|---|---|---|---|---|---|---|
| 5/1/15 | INSULIN | Blood glucose concentration: | 12.1 | 14.9 | 13.6 | 13.8 |
| | | 1. HUMALOG | 23 units | x | 23 units | z |
| | | 2. | | | | |
| Prescriber: | A Doctor | | Initials AD | Initials | Initials AD | Initials |
| Administered by: | A Nurse | | Initials AN | Initials | Initials AN | Initials |
| 6/1/15 | INSULIN | | 0600 | 1200 | 1800 | 2200 |
| | | Blood glucose concentration: | 7.9 | 13.2 | 14.7 | 8.4 |
| | | 1. HUMALOG | 23 units | x | 23 units | x |
| | | 2. | | | | |
| Prescriber: | A Doctor | | Initials AD | Initials | Initials AD | Initials |
| Administered by: | A Nurse | | Initials AN | Initials | Initials AN | Initials |
| 7/1/15 | INSULIN | | 0600 | 1200 | 1800 | 2200 |
| | | Blood glucose concentration: | 8.6 | 13.5 | | |
| | | 1. HUMALOG MIX 25 | 23 units | x | 23 units | x |
| | | 2. | | | | |
| Prescriber: | A Doctor | | Initials AD | Initials | Initials AD | Initials |
| Administered by: | A Nurse | | Initials AN | Initials | Initials | Initials |
| 8/1/15 | INSULIN | | 0600 | 1200 | 1800 | 2200 |
| | | Blood glucose concentration: | | | | |
| | | 1. HUMALOG MIX 25 | 25 units | x | 25 units | x |
| | | 2. | | | | |
| Prescriber: | A Doctor | | Initials AD | Initials | Initials AD | Initials |
| Administered by: | | | Initials | Initials | Initials | Initials |
| 9/1/15 | INSULIN | | 0600 | 1200 | 1800 | 2200 |
| | | Blood glucose concentration: | | | | |
| | | 1. HUMALOG MIX 25 | 25 units | x | | |
| | | 2. | | | | |
| Prescriber: | A Doctor | | Initials | Initials | Initials | Initials |
| Administered by: | | | Initials | Initials | Initials | Initials |

### What blood glucose concentrations should I aim for?

Glucose control for hospital inpatients is important, as high blood glucose concentrations can be associated with adverse outcomes. In an outpatient setting, the aim of therapy is to maintain pre-meal glucose levels at 4–7 mmol/L, adjusting insulin doses about once a week. However, we now know that aiming for the same tight glucose control in hospital inpatients can be harmful as it can lead to accidental hypoglycaemia, which is associated with an increased risk of death. Glucose targets are therefore more liberal in hospital: local guidelines are likely to differ and should always be consulted. As a rough guide, therapy for most patients should aim for a blood glucose concentration of 5–10 mmol/L.

### How does blood glucose concentration relate to insulin dose?

Insulin dose adjustments should never be based on a single glucose measurement. When prescribing insulin you should review blood glucose measurements over the preceding 48–72 hours and look for patterns, e.g. are there particular times in the day when blood glucose concentrations are particularly high? The other maxim to remember is that 'current glucose levels tend to reflect the preceding insulin dose'. For example, consistently high glucose concentrations measured before lunch reflect insufficient insulin administration in the morning.

### How much should I change the insulin dose by?

The dose changes required will vary between patients and their insulin regimen. Table 42.3 suggests a scheme for altering twice daily biphasic insulin treatment, such as that used by Mr Edwards. It is slightly more cautious than the dose adjustments recommended by manufacturers of similar preparations, to take into account the special circumstances of his hospital admission. It is not possible to offer precise guidance on how to adjust the doses for all of the different types of insulin regimens as much depends on the individual patient and their situation (e.g. intercurrent infection, change in diet during illness) as well as their total insulin requirements. The following are a few 'top tips' to follow when changing an insulin dose:

1 'Do no harm': avoid hypoglycaemia and significant fluctations in glucose concentration by:
   ○ Never adjusting by more than 10% of the total daily dose

**Table 42.3** Suggested adjustments for twice daily biphasic insulin regimen. Adjust morning dose according to the glucose concentrations before lunch and evening meal. Adjust the evening dose according to the glucose concentrations before bed and breakfast

| Glucose concentration | Dose adjustment |
|---|---|
| <5 mmol/L | Reduce dose by 4 units |
| 5–10 mmol/L | No change to dose |
| 10–15 mmol/L | Increase dose by 2 units |
| 15–20 mmol/L | Increase dose by 4 units |
| >20 mmol/L | Seek senior help. Consider increasing dose by 6 units |

- Anticipating your patient's dietary changes, e.g. before and after surgery

**2** Try to make only one change at a time:
- In patients using basal-bolus insulin regimens, avoid changing both the long- and short-acting insulins at the same time

**3** Give your changes time to have an impact:
- Make sure you wait at least 24 hours before making another change

**4** Remember that the current blood glucose concentration reflects the previous insulin dose administered:
- Do not change the breakfast insulin dose to fix a high pre-breakfast glucose concentration.

### What does the patient think?

Patients with diabetes are often experts in their own insulin management. They will often be competent to change their own insulin doses to meet changing requirements and can therefore be an invaluable source of advice about what works for them. You should always talk to your patient about any adjustments you think should be made to their insulin regimen, particularly as many patients will be self-administering their insulin while in hospital.

### How do I write the prescription?

Insulin is usually prescribed on a separate or supplementary drug chart, the design of which varies between hospitals so you should familiarise yourself with the local prescribing policy. Blood glucose is usually recorded on the same chart. Frequency of blood glucose measurements will vary depending on the insulin regimen that the patient uses. When you are writing insulin prescriptions, you should use proprietary names as activity, dosing and administration may vary between preparations. Remember that 'units' *must* be written in full. If the insulin prescription chart in your hospital allows for prescriptions at several times of the day, clearly indicate with a dose where insulin should be given and a cross where it should not. Discuss changes with the patient and inform nursing staff of your prescription.

Mr Edward's blood sugar has been high since he came into hospital. You can see when looking at the prescription chart that his evening insulin dose was increased on the first day. This has had a good effect at managing his bedtime and early morning blood glucose concentration; however, his glucose concentration remains above 10 mmol/L during the day. You should therefore have altered his morning insulin dose, increasing it by 2 units.

You should also have prescribed Humalog® Mix25 rather than the ambiguous Humalog® that has been prescribed before. Without the addition of a Mix25, there is a danger that Mix50 could be given erroneously and, as this would contain a greater proportion of the rapidly active component than Mr Edwards is used to, it could lead to hypoglycaemia.

We recommend that you write prescriptions for the next 24–48 hours so that trends can be seen from any changes that are made and to avoid a situation where nursing staff cannot give insulin at the correct time because you have forgotten or been too busy to prescribe it.

### Further reading

NICE guideline CG66 (partially updated by CG87): The management of type 2 diabetes. Available at: http://www.nice.org.uk/CG66 (accessed 24 January 2014).

Medical Pharmacology at a Glance. Chapter 36: Antidiabetic agents.

Prescribing at a Glance. Chapters 33 & 34: Using drugs for the endocrine system.

## What should I consider when deciding what to prescribe?

### Adverse effects of smoking

Mr Hines smokes 30 cigarettes daily. Tobacco smoke increases inflammation, oxidative stress and thrombosis. These pathological processes drive the development of atherosclerosis and may precipitate acute arterial occlusion, leading to, for example, acute coronary syndrome (ACS). If Mr Hines is able to stop smoking now, this will reduce his risk of further adverse cardiovascular events and prolong his life. It will also reduce his risk of other smoking-related diseases including cancers (e.g. lung, mouth and throat, bladder), peripheral and cerebrovascular disease and chronic obstructive pulmonary disease.

### Smoking cessation for hospital inpatients

Hospital admission provides an opportunity for smoking review and cessation advice.

*Ask.* You should ask all patients if they smoke and document their tobacco use.

For those who smoke, you should:

*Advise.* You should ask them if they have considered giving up smoking and clearly advise them to do so. It is helpful to link their current condition to the potential benefits of smoking cessation. For example, for Mr Hines, you could advise him that stopping smoking will reduce the risk of further heart attacks.

*Assist.* As hospitals are non-smoking buildings, many inpatients undergo enforced smoking cessation. You should offer them nicotine replacement therapy (NRT) to reduce the discomfort of nicotine withdrawal. Long-term success of smoking cessation requires support and behavioural modification. Before discharge you should offer referral to a local smoking cessation service and, if accepted, make the appointment before they leave hospital.

### Mr Hines

Mr Hines is aware of his need to stop smoking and has asked for help. You should therefore prescribe NRT. Before writing the prescription you should consider the following.

*Choice of treatment.* NRT comes in many formulations including lozenges, chewing gum, oral spray, inhalator and patches. The choice of formulation depends on patient preference, degree of nicotine dependence and likely withdrawal reaction. Mr Hines is a heavy smoker who became generally irritable and cranky last time he tried to stop smoking and also experiences an intermittent strong urge to smoke. A suitable regimen for Mr Hines would therefore include a prolonged-release nic-

| Surname HINES | Hospital number 100043 | Weight 101 kg | Drug intolerances None known |
|---|---|---|---|
| First name MALCOLM | Date of birth 26/05/1961 | | |

**REGULAR PRESCRIPTIONS**

Month: January    Year: 2015

| | Circle / enter times below | 6 | 7 |
|---|---|---|---|
| DRUG ASPIRIN | 06 | | |
| | 08 | | *AM* |
| Dose 75 mg / Route Oral / Freq Daily / Start date 6/1/15 | 12 | | |
| Signature A Doctor / Bleep 1234 / Review | 16 | | |
| | 18 | | |
| Additional instructions | 22 | | |
| DRUG ATORVASTATIN | 06 | | |
| | 08 | | *AM* |
| Dose 40 mg / Route Oral / Freq Daily / Start date 6/1/15 | 12 | | |
| Signature A Doctor / Bleep 1234 / Review | 16 | | |
| | 18 | | |
| Additional instructions | 22 | | |
| DRUG CLOPIDOGREL | 06 | | |
| | 08 | | *AM* |
| Dose 75 mg / Route Oral / Freq Daily / Start date 6/1/15 | 12 | | |
| Signature A Doctor / Bleep 1234 / Review | 16 | | |
| | 18 | | |
| Additional instructions | 22 | | |
| DRUG FONDAPARINUX | 06 | | |
| | 08 | | *AM* |
| Dose 2.5 mg / Route S/C / Freq Daily / Start date 6/1/15 | 12 | | |
| Signature A Doctor / Bleep 1234 / Review 48 h | 16 | | |
| | 18 | | |
| Additional instructions | 22 | | |
| DRUG METOPROLOL | 06 | | |
| | 08 | | *AM* |
| Dose 12.5 mg / Route Oral / Freq 8-hrly / Start date 6/1/15 | 12 | | |
| Signature A Doctor / Bleep 1234 / Review | 16 | *AM* | |
| | 18 | | |
| Additional instructions | 22 | *AM* | |
| DRUG NICOTINE PATCH | 06 | | |
| | 08 | | |
| Dose 25 mg / Route Topical / Freq Daily / Start date 7/1/15 | 12 | | |
| Signature A Doctor / Bleep 1234 / Review | 16 | | |
| | 18 | | |
| Additional instructions Apply on waking, remove at night | 22 | | |

**ONCE ONLY PRESCRIPTIONS**

| Date | Time to be given | DRUG | Dose | Route | Prescriber Signature | Prescriber Bleep | Administration Date given | Administration Time given | Administration Given by |
|---|---|---|---|---|---|---|---|---|---|
| 6/1/15 | 12:00 | ASPIRIN | 300 mg | Oral | AD | 1234 | 14/9 | 12:00 | AN |
| 6/1/15 | 12:00 | CLOPIDOGREL | 300 mg | Oral | AD | 1234 | 14/9 | 12:00 | AN |
| 7/1/15 | 11:00 | NICOTINE PATCH | 25 mg | Topical | AD | 1234 | | | |

**OXYGEN**

| Target SpO₂ | ☑ 94–98% | ○ 88–92% |
|---|---|---|
| Mode of delivery | ☑ Continuous | ○ As required |
| Starting device | Face mask | |
| Initials AD | Bleep 1234 | Date 6/1/15 |

**AS REQUIRED MEDICATION**

| DRUG NICOTINE LOZENGE | Date | | |
|---|---|---|---|
| | Time | | |
| Dose 1 mg / Route Oral / Max freq hourly / Start date 7/1/15 | Dose | | |
| | Route | | |
| Signature A Doctor / Bleep 1234 / Review | Given | | |
| | Check | | |
| Additional instructions Maximum 15 lozenges daily | | | |

otine patch to address the background irritability and cravings, with an immediate-release preparation (e.g. lozenge, chewing gum, spray) available for when the urge to smoke strikes.

*Cautions and contraindications.* Nicotine infrequently causes palpitations and rarely causes atrial fibrillation. Therefore it should be used with caution in patients who are haemodynamically unstable due to severe arrhythmias, ACS or cerebrovascular event. Mr Hines has had an ACS, but is haemodynamically stable and in sinus rhythm. It is almost always considered safer to take NRT than to smoke tobacco. Mr Hines can therefore receive NRT.

*Potential interactions.* Nicotine does not interact with any of the other drugs that Mr Hines is taking. You should remember that cigarette smoke induces cytochrome P450 liver enzymes, increasing the metabolism of theophylline and some anti-psychotics. Patients taking these drugs should be monitored if they stop smoking to minimise the risk of toxicity.

## Other pharmacological support for smoking cessation

In addition to NRT, bupropion, originally an antidepressant, and varenicline, a selective nicotine-receptor partial agonist, have also been proven to help people stop smoking. NICE guidance states that these pharmacological therapies should normally only be used as part of an abstinent-contingent programme. This means that the drugs should only be prescribed where the patient makes a commitment to stop smoking on or before a particular date. All three treatments work best in combination with support, such as that provided by an NHS stop smoking service. Mr Hines should be encouraged to access smoking cessation support after discharge, where he can have further discussions on whether NRT, bupropion or varenicline would be the most suitable pharmacotherapy to support his smoking cessation attempt.

## Chart review

Mr Hines's present treatment is appropriate for his diagnosis of non-ST elevation ACS, although the addition of an ACE inhibitor (e.g. ramipril at an initial dose of 1.25 mg 12-hourly) would be desirable. There is no space for this on the drug chart provided. In real life, if you run out of space on one drug chart, you would need to add a second drug chart (clearly annotating the charts '1 of 2' and '2 of 2' as appropriate) to prescribe additional drugs. Note that fondaparinux is an anti-coagulant agent, so he does not require additional prophylaxis against venous thromboembolism at the moment.

## How do I write the prescription?
### Nicotine patch

Nicotine patch strengths describe the amount of nicotine they will release in 16 or 24 hours. Nicotine patches are available in sets of high/medium/low strengths, with the exact dose combination varying according to brand, being 15/10/5 mg (Nicorette®), 25/15/10 mg (Nicorette®) or 21/14/7 mg (Nicotinelle®, NiQuitin®). Your choice of dosage for hospital inpatients will depend on the brand stocked in your hospital.

You should start patients who smoke 10 or more cigarettes per day on a high-strength patch and patients who smoke fewer than 10 cigarettes per day on a medium-strength patch. As the smoking cessation attempt progresses, the strength of the nicotine patch is gradually reduced to stop at around 12 weeks, with speed of withdrawal tailored to the individual patient.

As Mr Hines smokes 30 cigarettes per day, he has been offered a high-strength patch. He should apply the patch on waking to a dry non-hairy area of skin on his hip, trunk or upper arm and hold it in place for 10–20 seconds to make sure it sticks. He should use a different area of skin for the patch each day to reduce the risk of skin reactions. As nicotine causes insomnia, he should be advised to remove the patch at night. However, patients who have severe cravings on waking can use a 24-hour nicotine patch.

### Immediate-release nicotine

As Mr Hines is very dependent on nicotine he may need both prolonged- and immediate-release nicotine replacement for successful control of withdrawal symptoms. In the model prescription, we have elected to prescribe immediate-release nicotine as a lozenge. We have chosen a low strength, 1 mg lozenge (1.5, 2 and 4 mg strengths are also available) to use in combination with the patch. We have exercised relative caution because of his recent ACS. However, the situation should be kept under review and the lozenge strength could be increased if the NRT prescribed does not control his withdrawal and he does not experience problematic side effects with the low-strength lozenge.

### Further reading

Medical Pharmacology at a Glance. Chapter 31: Drug misuse and dependence.

## What should I consider when deciding what to prescribe?

Mrs Dennis is a 90-year-old woman who has been admitted following a fall, which was probably due to postural hypotension. She normally takes seven regular medications. Since being admitted to hospital the number of medications she is taking has increased to 13. She is being treated for musculoskeletal pain with paracetamol, codeine phosphate and diclofenac; for constipation with senna; and she has been receiving night sedation on a regular basis.

## Polypharmacy

You should recognise the potential problems of poly-pharmacy in Mrs Dennis's case. Loosely, this term means the use of numerous medicines in an individual patient. There are various stricter definitions for poly-pharmacy, but in the context of prescribing practice we find the most useful definition is simply the state in which more drugs are being taken than are clinically indicated. Polypharmacy is most common in the elderly; people who have multiple chronic co-morbidities; those who use over-the-counter medications; and those who receive prescriptions from multiple care providers. It can sometimes result from the practice of prescribing new drugs in an attempt to treat the side effects of others: the 'vicious cycle of prescribing'. The risks of polypharmacy include adverse drug reactions (ADRs), drug–drug interactions and non-adherence – and these risks increase with the number of drugs prescribed.

## Prescribing for the elderly

Ageing changes the way the body absorbs, distributes, metabolises and eliminates drugs (pharmacokinetics) and the way drugs affect the body (pharmacodynamics). The clinical significance of this on prescribing depends on the drug used: e.g. CNS sensitivity is increased to hypnotics such as benzodiazepines, meaning lower doses are needed to achieve a desired effect, and toxicity may occur at 'standard' doses.

When reviewing any patient's medications you should make sure there is a clear indication for each drug and that the correct drug, at the correct dose, has been prescribed. This is particularly important in the elderly and in the context of multiple prescriptions. While it is not appropriate to stop long-term prognostic medications (e.g. those taken for the prevention of cardiovascular disease) simply on the basis of a patient's age, it is reasonable to take the patient's likely life expectancy into account when assessing the relative benefits and risks of treatment. For example, the potential benefits of a medicine when taken over a number of years may not sufficiently outweigh the day-to-day side effects experienced by an individual patient.

Adverse effects associated with polypharmacy of particular concern in elderly patients like Mrs Dennis include constipation, depression and falls (with the associated risk of injury). When reviewing an elderly patient who has fallen, it is useful to look out for a few specific classes of drug that are associated with an increased risk of falls: hypnotics (e.g. benzodiazepines), antihypertensives, laxatives, diuretics and drugs with an anticholinergic effect.

Finally, you need to check for potential interactions between drugs and, where a potentially hazardous drug combination arises, consider the risks and benefits of the drugs individually and in combination.

### Applying this understanding to Mrs Dennis's case
*Rationalising new medication*

Mrs Dennis is on a combination of analgesics for her right hip pain following her fall, but her pain has improved and the intensity

| Surname DENNIS | Hospital number 100044 | Weight 56 kg | Drug intolerances None known |
|---|---|---|---|
| First name RACHEL | Date of birth 09/03/1924 | | |

**REGULAR PRESCRIPTIONS**  DRUG CHART 1 OF 2

Month: January  Year: 2015

| DRUG DALTEPARIN | Circle / enter times below | 5 | 6 | 7 | | | | |
|---|---|---|---|---|---|---|---|---|
| Dose 5000 units | Route SC | Freq Once daily | Start date 5/1/15 | 06 08 12 | | | | |
| Signature A Doctor | Bleep 1234 | Review | | 16 | | | | |
| | | | | (18) | AM | AM | | |
| Additional instructions VTE prophylaxis | | | | 22 | | | | |
| DRUG ASPIRIN | | | | 06 | | | | |
| Dose 75 mg | Route Oral | Freq Once daily | Start date 5/1/15 | (08) 12 | AM | AM | AM | |
| Signature A Doctor | Bleep 1234 | Review | | 16 18 | | | | |
| Additional instructions | | | | 22 | | | | |
| DRUG CLOPIDOGREL | | | | 06 | | | | |
| Dose 75 mg | Route Oral | Freq Once daily | Start date 5/1/15 | (08) 12 | AM | AM | AM | STOP 7/1/15 |
| Signature A Doctor | Bleep 1234 | Review | | 16 18 | | | | A Doctor 1234 |
| Additional instructions | | | | 22 | | | | |
| DRUG RAMIPRIL | | | | 06 | | | | |
| Dose 5 mg | Route Oral | Freq Once daily | Start date 5/1/15 | (08) 12 | AM | AM | AM | STOP 7/1/15 |
| Signature A Doctor | Bleep 1234 | Review | | 16 18 | | | | A Doctor 1234 |
| Additional instructions | | | | 22 | | | | |
| DRUG BISOPROLOL | | | | 06 | | | | |
| Dose 2.5 mg | Route Oral | Freq Once daily | Start date 5/1/15 | (08) 12 | AM | AM | AM | |
| Signature A Doctor | Bleep 1234 | Review | | 16 18 | | | | |
| Additional instructions | | | | 22 | | | | |
| DRUG ATORVASTATIN | | | | 06 | | | | |
| Dose 40 mg | Route Oral | Freq Once daily | Start date 5/1/15 | 08 12 | | | | |
| Signature A Doctor | Bleep 1234 | Review | | 16 18 | | | | |
| Additional instructions | | | | (22) | AM | AM | | |

## Drug Chart

| Surname: DENNIS | Hospital number: 100046 | Weight | Drug intolerances |
|---|---|---|---|
| First name: RACHEL | Date of birth: 09/03/1924 | 56 kg | None known |

**Month: January    Year: 2015**

Enter dates below: 5, 6, 7

**PARACETAMOL**
Dose: 1 gram | Route: Oral | Freq: 6-hrly | Start date: 5/1/15
Signature: A Doctor | Bleep: 1234

- 06: AM AM AM
- 12: AM AM
- 18: AM AM
- 24: AM AM

**CODEINE PHOSPHATE**
Dose: 30 mg | Route: Oral | Freq: 6-hrly | Start date: 5/1/15
Signature: A Doctor | Bleep: 1234
STOP 7/1/15 — A Doctor 1234

- 06: AM AM AM
- 12: AM AM
- 18: AM AM
- 24: AM AM

**SENNA**
Dose: Two tablets | Route: Oral | Freq: Once daily | Start date: 5/1/15
Signature: A Doctor | Bleep: 1234

- 22: AM AM

**FOLIC ACID**
Dose: 5 mg | Route: Oral | Freq: Once daily | Start date: 5/1/15
Signature: A Doctor | Bleep: 1234
STOP 7/1/15 — A Doctor 1234

- 08: AM AM AM

**LEVOTHYROXINE**
Dose: 100 micrograms | Route: Oral | Freq: Once daily | Start date: 5/1/15
Signature: A Doctor | Bleep: 1234

- 08: AM AM AM

**DICLOFENAC**
Dose: 50 mg | Route: Oral | Freq: 8-hrly | Start date: 5/1/15
Signature: A Doctor | Bleep: 1234
STOP 7/1/15 — A Doctor 1234

- 06: AM AM AM
- 14: AM AM
- 22: AM AM

| Date | Time to be given | DRUG | Dose | Route | Prescriber Signature | Bleep | Date given | Time given | Given by |
|---|---|---|---|---|---|---|---|---|---|
| | | | | | | | | | |

**OXYGEN**

Target SpO₂: ○ 94–98% ○ 88–92%
Mode of delivery: ○ Continuous ○ As required
Starting device:
Initials | Bleep | Date

**AS REQUIRED MEDICATION**

**TEMAZEPAM**
Dose: 10 mg | Route: Oral | Max: Once daily | Start date: 5/1/15
Signature: A Doctor | Bleep: 1234
Additional instructions: For night sedation
STOP 7/1/15 — A Doctor 1234

| Date | 5/1 | 6/1 |
|---|---|---|
| Time | 2330 | 2200 |
| Dose | 10 mg | 10 mg |
| Route | Oral | Oral |
| Given | AM | AM |
| Check | AM | AM |

**CODEINE PHOSPHATE**
Dose: 30 mg | Route: Oral | Max: 4-6 hourly | Start date: 7/1/15
Signature: A Doctor | Bleep: 1234
Additional instructions: For breakthrough hip pain

---

of her analgesic treatment can probably now be reduced. The priority should be to stop her diclofenac. This is because it could worsen her existing renal impairment and increases her risk of gastrointestinal bleeding and cardiovascular events. It would be reasonable to continue paracetamol regularly, but switch the codeine phosphate to the as required section of the drug chart for breakthrough pain. Her constipation is likely to be related to the regular codeine phosphate, so it is hoped that reducing the frequency of administration will reduce her need for regular laxatives.

Mrs Dennis has been receiving night sedation as an inpatient. Hypnotics, including short-acting benzodiazepines, can increase the risk of falls, particularly in the elderly. They should not be prescribed routinely to inpatients. When taken over the longer term there is a risk of inducing a state of dependence.

### Rationalising existing medication

You should stop her folic acid. Mrs Dennis takes folic acid for a folate-deficiency megaloblastic anaemia. Normally, a 4-month period of treatment is sufficient to replenish the body's stores and correct the anaemia. In this case we can see Mrs Dennis is replete of folate from her recent blood tests and is no longer anaemic.

You should stop her clopidogrel. Mrs Dennis had a myocardial infarction 18 months ago requiring insertion of a drug-eluting stent. Clopidogrel should generally only be continued for 1 year for this indication. In this case the clopidogrel has been prescribed in error resulting from the use of an outdated discharge summary as the reference source. Lifelong aspirin treatment is generally advocated following myocardial infarction and stent insertion, but even this should be judged on a case-by-case basis, taking account of its adverse effects and tolerability for the individual patient.

Mrs Dennis initially presented with a fall, and had symptoms and signs of postural hypotension. You should withhold ramipril as she continues to have features of postural hypotension. Although there is evidence to support anti-hypertensive treatment in the very elderly, aggressive blood pressure-lowering treatment should not be pursued at the expense of causing more immediate adverse effects such as falls.

### Participants in the decision-making process

All the risk–benefit analyses mentioned above, and the decisions on which medications to stop or continue, should be undertaken in partnership with the patient and, as appropriate, those close to them. Moreover, you should ideally consult with her GP regarding changes to her long-term medication. The GP may have considerably more knowledge of the patient's history and past treatment than you do, and will have to deal with the ramifications of any treatment decisions you make.

## How do I write the prescription?

When stopping medications you should cross through both the prescription and administration sections clearly, but you should still be able to read the original prescription. Sign and date the change, and make a note in the patient's medical records of why the drugs have been stopped and whether they need to be restarted at a later date.

To summarise the actions taken in this case:

- Codeine phosphate has been stopped in the regular section of the drug chart and re-prescribed in the as required section
- Diclofenac has been stopped as it increases her risk of acute kidney injury
- Temazepam has been stopped as the indication for its use is not well justified and may put Mrs Dennis at increased risk of falls
- Folic acid has been stopped as her folate stores are replete and she is no longer anaemic

- Clopidogrel has been stopped as it is not indicated for more than 12 months after a myocardial infarction
- Ramipril has been stopped because of her symptoms of postural hypotension. It may be appropriate later to reintroduce it at lower dose with close monitoring of her symptoms and postural blood pressure.

Mrs Dennis has two drug charts. It is not uncommon for patients on multiple medications to require more than one drug chart to prescribe all their current medications. Make sure when reviewing multiple drug charts there is no accidental duplication of prescriptions and do not forget to review the as required section of the drug chart for duplications, particularly of analgesic drugs.

### Further reading

Medical Pharmacology at a Glance. Chapter 4: Drug metabolism.
Prescribing at a Glance. Chapter 17: Prescribing in the elderly.

---

## 45 | A 54-year-old woman with a peptic ulcer

### What should I consider when deciding what to prescribe?

Mrs McKinnon is now well following hospital admission for a bleeding duodenal ulcer. When planning her discharge medication you need to determine whether she needs on-going treatment for her duodenal ulcer to ensure healing and prevent recurrence. You also need to consider whether prior medicines for her hypertension should be restarted and whether there could be interactions between old and new therapies. It is essential that all changes in medication are communicated clearly to Mrs McKinnon and her GP.

### Consider new diagnoses

Mrs McKinnon was found to have a duodenal ulcer causing haematemesis. She was treated with adrenaline at endoscopy to achieve haemostasis, followed by a 72-hour infusion of omeprazole to reduce the risk of rebleeding. Prior to discharge you need to consider whether any additional treatment is required to promote ulcer healing and reduce the risk of recurrence. As she was found to have *Helicobacter pylori* infection on CLO test, you should prescribe an *H. pylori* eradication regimen.

### New medicines to start

*H. pylori* eradication regimens usually include a proton pump inhibitor (PPI) with two antibiotics, chosen from amoxicillin, clarithromycin and metronidazole. A range of regimens have been proven to be effective in diverse clinical trials. The regimens may involve different doses and frequency of administration of the component drugs to those you would normally use in other indications. Therefore, you should look them up in the British National Formulary (BNF) in the section that deals specifically with *H. pylori* eradication. Choice of

### DISCHARGE SUMMARY

| Surname MCKINNON | Hospital number 100045 | Date of admission 04/01/2015 | Ward 2B |
|---|---|---|---|
| First name SHEILA | Date of birth 03/03/1960 | Date of discharge 07/01/2015 | Consultant PETERS |
| Address 47 Any Street Anytown AT1 2BC | Drug intolerances Erythromycin causes itching and a rash | General practitioner name and address Dr Albert Boather Boather Medical Practice Anytown AT1 5DE | |

**Principal diagnosis**
Upper gastrointestinal bleed secondary to *H. pylori*-associated duodenal ulcer

**Other diagnoses and summary of management**
Mrs McKinnon was admitted with haematemesis and malaena. Red cells were transfused and she underwent urgent upper gastrointestinal endoscopy. A duodenal ulcer was identified as the source of bleeding and bleeding was controlled with adrenaline. The CLO test was positive, so an *H. pylori* eradication regimen has been prescribed. Comorbidity: hypertension (no changes to treatment).

### Medicines to take away

| DRUG | DOSE | FREQ | ROUTE | DURATION | GP TO CONTINUE | COMMENTS |
|---|---|---|---|---|---|---|
| AMLODIPINE | 5 mg | Daily | ORAL | Long-term | Y | |
| RAMIPRIL | 5 mg | Daily | ORAL | Long-term | Y | |
| OMEPRAZOLE | 20 mg | 12-hrly | ORAL | 4 weeks | Y | ~~Complicated ulcer. Will~~ need repeat prescription to complete 4-week ~~course~~ |
| AMOXICILLIN | 500 mg | 8-hrly | ORAL | 7 days | N | *H. pylori* eradication |
| METRONIDAZOLE | 400 mg | 8-hrly | ORAL | 7 days | N | *H. pylori* eradication |
| | | | | | | |
| | | | | | | |
| | | | | | | |

| Print name A DOCTOR | Grade F1 | Bleep 1234 | Signature A Doctor | Date 7/1/2015 |
|---|---|---|---|---|

regimen may depend on local prescribing policy. In Mrs McKinnon's case you should choose a regimen that does *not* include clarithromycin as she is allergic to erythromycin, a macrolide antibiotic in the same class.

### New medicines to stop
She has not required the anti-emetic drug cyclizine for 3 days. This can now be stopped.

### Anything else?
As Mrs McKinnon has had a large bleed you should consider whether she needs any iron to allow her to replenish her red blood cells. At present she has no symptoms of anaemia and her haemoglobin concentration is in the normal range, so this is not necessary. The lifespan of transfused red cells is less than that of native red cells, so you might suggest to her that if she develops fatigue or shortness of breath in coming weeks she should see her GP to check she has not become anaemic.

## Prior medication
### To continue
Mrs McKinnon was taking amlodipine 5 mg daily and ramipril 5 mg daily as long-term treatment for hypertension. These were stopped at admission, presumably because of hypotension and hypovolaemia secondary to her haematemesis. Her gastrointestinal bleeding has now stopped, her blood pressure is rising and her renal function and potassium are normal. You should therefore now restart both medicines. It is often a good idea to restart existing medicines around 24 hours before hospital discharge to make sure they are still tolerated in the context of recovery from an acute illness. In Mrs McKinnon's case you do not need to delay her discharge while these drugs restart.

### To stop / interactions
There are no identified clinically significant interactions between new and prior therapy and no prior medications that need to be stopped.

## Communication
### Patient
You should advise Mrs McKinnon that her new medicines are to clear an infection that is causing her ulcer and that it is important that she completes the 1-week course of treatment. You should explain the difference between the antibiotics, which she needs to take for 1 week, and the acid-suppressing medicine (PPI), which she should take for 4 weeks in total. As most discharge medicines are provided as a 14-day supply, she will need to get more of the acid suppressant from her GP before it runs out. You should mention possible side effects of medicines, particularly gastrointestinal symptoms such as sickness, loose stool and abdominal cramps. You should advise her not to drink alcohol while taking the metronidazole as she may experience an extremely unpleasant reaction involving flushing, throbbing headache and vomiting (a disulfiram-like reaction). She should also avoid any cough/cold medicines or mouthwash that contains alcohol, as these will have the same effect. While you are on the topic you could remind her of the safe daily limit for alcohol consumption (2–3 units for a woman) and ask if she has considered stopping smoking.

It is important to remind her that she should take her blood pressure treatment as usual from this morning and see her GP for her usual review and repeat prescriptions.

### GP
A good discharge summary concisely explaining events in hospital and changes in treatment is essential. This is invariably combined with the discharge prescription.

## Writing a discharge prescription
This case illustrates the process of writing a discharge prescription, commonly referred to on the wards as the TTA (to take away) or TTO (to take out). This is a very important task which is commonly undertaken by foundation doctors. We illustrate the process on paper, but it is much the same for electronic discharge summaries, which are increasingly the norm.

The principles of writing a discharge prescription are no different from any other form of prescription writing, although a couple of points require particular emphasis:
- Specifying the duration of therapy, as the GP needs to know whether they are expected to take on responsibility for providing repeat prescriptions
- Highlighting changes that have been made to the patient's previous medication regimen (particularly medicines that were stopped), so that the GP knows that any differences are intentional rather than being due to oversights.

Your prescription will be reviewed by a pharmacist, who will ensure that the patient has at least a 14-day supply of medicines to take away.

Often, dealing with the discharge prescription is the rate-limiting step between the decision to discharge a patient and them actually leaving the hospital. It is therefore very important both to the patient and to the smooth running of the hospital that you deal with discharge prescriptions as expeditiously as possible. It may be helpful to write them *in anticipation* of the patient going home in the next 1–2 days. However, if you do this, you must be especially careful to ensure any last-minute changes to their drug chart or treatment plan have been reflected in the discharge prescription.

### How do I write the prescription?
#### H. pylori eradication regimen
The eradication regimen shown in the model prescription was chosen to avoid clarithromycin, as Mrs McKinnon is allergic to erythromycin. She therefore needs to receive amoxicillin and metronidazole, which are only recommended in combination with omeprazole or lansoprazole. She has tolerated intravenous omeprazole for the past 72 hours and so oral omeprazole is a reasonable substitute, although lansoprazole would also be an acceptable choice.

Triple therapy (PPI and two antibiotics) is usually for 1 week and this will eradicate *H. pylori* and bring about ulcer healing in approximately 85% of cases. As Mrs McKinnon has had a significant bleed from her ulcer, BNF advice is to continue the PPI for 3 more weeks after completing the eradication regimen.

The regimen has therefore been prescribed as described in the BNF with recommended doses, administration frequency and duration of treatment. In accordance with good antibiotic prescribing principles, the indications for antibiotic use have been given.

### Anti-hypertensive medication
Amlodipine and ramipril have been prescribed on the discharge prescription. With her blood pressure now rising she should ideally restart these sooner rather than later. Therefore, you would also

prescribe them on the inpatient prescription chart and ask the nursing staff to administer doses this morning.

## Other

As required prescriptions should generally be stopped once they are no longer needed. You should not therefore prescribe cyclizine on the discharge prescription.

## Further reading

Medical Pharmacology at a Glance. Chapter 12: Drugs acting on the gastrointestinal tract I: peptic ulcer.

Prescribing at a Glance. Chapter 19: How to write a drug prescription.

National Institute for Health and Clinical Excellence (2004). Dyspepsia: Managing dyspepsia in adults in primary care. Clinical guidline CG17. Available: http://www.nice.org.uk/nicemedia/live/10950/29460/29460.pdf (accessed 24 January 2014). NB update in progress, no scheduled publication date.

---

## 46 | A 64-year-old woman with chronic kidney disease

## What should I consider when deciding what to prescribe?

### General principles

CKD is defined by impaired renal function (estimated glomerular filtration rate (eGFR) $<60\,mL/min/1.73\,m^2$) or another renal abnormality (e.g. proteinuria) that persists for 3 months or more. The general principles of management of CKD are similar to those for acute kidney injury (AKI; see Case 31), with one addition, highlighted below in bold:

- Maintain appropriate fluid balance
- Review the patient's medicines for safety in renal impairment
- Identify and treat reversible causes
- Identify and treat complications
- Seek specialist advice
- **Slow the rate of CKD progression.**

### Putting these into practice

#### Maintain appropriate fluid balance

The best way of managing fluid balance in CKD is by modifying dietary sodium intake (recall that sodium is the principal determinant of extracellular fluid volume). In view of her oedema, you should advise her to limit her dietary sodium intake. In some cases, diuresis (with a loop diuretic) is also needed, but this should not be started without first trying non-pharmacological therapy.

| Surname MORRIS | Hospital number 100046 | Weight 82 kg | Drug intolerances None known |
| First name JANET | Date of birth 16/01/1950 | | |

**REGULAR PRESCRIPTIONS**

Month: **January**  Year: **2015**

| DRUG ATORVASTATIN | | | | Dose 10 mg / Route ORAL / Freq Daily / Start date 6/1/15 | Signature A Doctor / Bleep 1234 / Review | Additional instructions |
| DRUG METFORMIN | Dose 1 g / Route ORAL / Twice daily / Start date 6/1/15 | Signature A Doctor / Bleep 1234 / Review | Additional instructions With meals | STOPPED 7/1/15 due to renal impairment A Doctor 1234 |
| DRUG HEPARIN | Dose 5000 units / Route SC / Freq 12-hrly / Start date 6/1/15 | Signature A Doctor / Bleep 1234 / Review | Additional instructions Used instead of LMHW due to CKD |
| DRUG RAMIPRIL | Dose 1.25 mg / Route ORAL / Freq Daily / Start date 7/1/15 | Signature A Doctor / Bleep 1234 / Review | Additional instructions First dose at bedtime |

#### Medication review

Review all her medications, including those not prescribed (especially over-the-counter non-steroidal anti-inflammatory drugs, which she should be advised to avoid). The BNF recommends that metformin should be stopped if the eGFR is $<30\,mL/min/1.73\,m^2$, as in this case. Insulin requirements may fall in renal impairment; equally, they may rise after stopping metformin. However, you cannot make any adjustments to her insulin doses without knowing her daily blood glucose concentration profile, so ensure this is monitored closely (four times a day would be adequate). Atorvastatin is eliminated by hepatic metabolism then excretion of the metabolites in faeces, so its dosage is not affected by renal impair-

ment (in the BNF, this is implied by the absence of a 'renal impairment' paragraph in the atorvastatin monograph).

#### Identify and treat reversible causes

Appropriate investigations have been performed to identify potential reversible causes (particularly nephrotoxic drugs and urinary tract obstruction), and none have been found.

#### Identify and treat complications

The potential complications of CKD are similar to those of AKI, and may be recalled with reference to the SWEAT mnemonic (see

| Name | Hospital number | Date of birth | Intolerances |
|---|---|---|---|
| Janet MORRIS | 100046 | 16/01/1950 | None known |

**INSULIN PRESCRIPTIONS**

| DATE | | TIME | 0600 | 1200 | 1800 | 2200 |
|---|---|---|---|---|---|---|
| 6/1/15 | | Blood glucose concentration: | | | 6.1 | 6.7 |
| | INSULIN | 1. NOVOMIX 30 | x | x | 18 units | x |
| | | 2. | | | | |
| Prescriber: | A Doctor | | Initials | Initials | Initials AD | Initials |
| Administered by: | A Nurse | | Initials | Initials | Initials AN | Initials |
| 7/1/15 | | Blood glucose concentration: | 7.1 | 6.3 | | |
| | INSULIN | 1. NOVOMIX 30 | 24 units | x | 18 units | x |
| | | 2. | | | | |
| Prescriber: | A Doctor | | Initials AD | Initials | Initials AD | Initials |
| Administered by: | A Nurse | | Initials AN | Initials | Initials | Initials |
| 8/1/15 | | Blood glucose concentration: | | | | |
| | INSULIN | 1. NOVOMIX 30 | 24 units | x | | |
| | | 2. | | | | |
| Prescriber: | A Doctor | | Initials AD | Initials | Initials | Initials |
| Administered by: | | | Initials | Initials | Initials | Initials |
| | | Blood glucose concentration: | | | | |
| | INSULIN | 1. | | | | |
| | | 2. | | | | |
| Prescriber: | | | Initials | Initials | Initials | Initials |
| Administered by: | | | Initials | Initials | Initials | Initials |
| | | Blood glucose concentration: | | | | |
| | INSULIN | 1. | | | | |
| | | 2. | | | | |
| Prescriber: | | | Initials | Initials | Initials | Initials |
| Administered by: | | | Initials | Initials | Initials | Initials |

Case 31). Mrs Morris does not appear to have any major complications of kidney disease (pulmonary oedema, hyperkalaemia, acidosis, uraemic complications) at present.

In CKD, you also need also to consider two hormonally mediated complications (think: 'SWEAT and hormones'):

- *Anaemia.* The kidneys are responsible for producing erythropoietin (EPO) – the hormone that regulates the production of red blood cells. Mrs Morris has a mild normochromic normocytic anaemia, typical of that commonly found in CKD. However, the decision to start EPO is one that should be taken by a specialist. A useful thing that you can do at this stage is to request iron studies (serum ferritin, transferrin saturation, total iron binding capacity), as patients should have normal iron stores before being treated with EPO.
- *Renal bone disease.* The kidneys perform the final step in the pathway that makes calcitriol (the most active form of vitamin D). In addition, they are responsible for excreting phosphate. It is therefore common to find hyperphosphataemia in patients with CKD, as is evident in Mrs Morris's case. The combined effects of vitamin D deficiency and hyperphosphataemia (stimulating parathyroid hormone secretion) can produce a range of bone changes. In addition to dietary changes, she may require treatment with a phosphate binder (such as calcium carbonate) and supplementary vitamin D (which may be provided in a combined preparation with calcium carbonate), but this is best dealt with in the specialist clinic.

### Specialist advice

Patients with CKD should be referred to a nephrologist if their eGFR is $<30\,mL/min/1.73\,m^2$ or is falling rapidly. They should also be referred if the diagnosis is uncertain, unusual or in doubt (e.g. if there is unexplained haematuria or heavy proteinuria); if they have uncontrolled hypertension despite appropriate therapy; or if renal artery stenosis is suspected. Patients with urinary tract obstruction must be referred urgently to a urological surgeon.

### Slow the rate of CKD progression

Compensatory changes that occur in CKD include enlargement of remaining functional glomeruli, and increased blood pressure both systemically and within the glomeruli. The aim of these changes is to increase glomerular filtration. This may be useful over the short term, but in the longer term it probably contributes to renal damage.

All patients with CKD require careful management of hypertension. However, a particularly important group of patients is those with detectable protein in their urine. The protein may sometimes be detected on routine dipstick testing (proteinuria), but often is only found on laboratory measurement of the urine albumin : creatinine ratio (ACR). Protein in the urine provides a clue that the glomeruli are being 'stressed' by high pressures, and that they may benefit from having this treated.

The best way to relieve high pressures within the glomeruli is with an angiotensin converting enzyme (ACE) inhibitor or angiotensin receptor blocker (ARB). Recall that angiotensin II is a general vasoconstrictor, but that its vasoconstrictor effect is particularly pronounced on the arteriole that takes blood out of the glomerulus (the efferent arteriole). Therefore, blocking the effect of angiotensin II releases pressure in the glomerulus by allowing blood to flow out of it more easily. As a side effect, this reduces the amount of fluid that filters into the nephron. You will observe this though the slight rise in serum creatinine concentration (and fall in the eGFR) that typically occurs on starting an ACE inhibitor/ARB. However, provided the changes are within certain limits of acceptability, they may be tolerated – because in the longer term, the rate of progression will be lower.

The indications for starting an ACE inhibitor/ARB in CKD are:

- *Diabetic:* urine ACR >2.5 (men) or >3.5 (women)
- *Non-diabetic:* urine ACR $\geq 30$ mg/mmol with hypertension.

Mrs Morris is diabetic and has an ACR of 18.3 mg/mmol, so she should be offered treatment with an ACE inhibitor or ARB. ACEIs are usually preferred in the first instance, as they are less expensive and the data supporting their use are more extensive. However, some patients cannot tolerate ACE inhibitors due to cough, and in such cases an ARB should be offered.

## How do I write the prescription?

Stop Mrs Morris's metformin treatment by clearly crossing through the prescription. Sign and date this, and record the decision and its reason in the notes. You should also ensure this is clearly communicated to the patient's GP via the discharge summary, so that he knows it is not just an omission. You should not adjust the insulin at this stage.

You should start an ACE inhibitor. Which one will depend mainly on the local formulary choice and your own familiarity. Ramipril is the most commonly used ACE inhibitor in the UK: it should be prescribed at an initial dosage of 1.25 mg/day, and she should be advised to take the first dose just before bed. You should make arrangements for her renal function and electrolytes to be checked in the next 1–2 weeks. The ACE inhibitor should be stopped if the serum creatinine concentration rises by more than 30%, the serum potassium concentration exceeds 6.0 mmol/L, or the eGFR falls by more than 25%. Changes of less than this should be monitored to ensure they do not progress further, but the ACE inhibitor may be continued in the meantime.

Over the subsequent weeks the dose of the ACE inhibitor should be titrated up to the maximum tolerated dose (up to 10 mg/day in the case of ramipril), again with monitoring of electrolytes and renal function. Make sure this is all clearly documented on the discharge summary. The NICE guidelines on CKD (see Further reading) provide details on the level of blood pressure control needed.

## Further reading

National Institute for Health and Clinical Excellence. Early identification and management of chronic kidney disease in adults in primary and secondary care. Clinical guideline CG73 (2008). Available: http://guidance.nice.org.uk/CG73 (accessed 24 January 2014).

Prescribing at a Glance. Chapter 15: Prescribing in renal disease.

---

# 47    A 66-year-old man with palpitations

## What should I consider when deciding what to prescribe?

Mr Edwards is a 66-year-old man with symptoms (palpitations, nausea) and signs (bradycardia, premature ventricular complexes) of digoxin toxicity. Digoxin toxicity is likely to have occurred due to reduced renal clearance of digoxin, caused by acute kidney injury, and to have been exacerbated by hypokalaemia due to gastrointestinal electrolyte losses. Although high plasma concentrations of digoxin do not always indicate toxicity, the likelihood of toxicity increases as the digoxin plasma concentration increases. Hypokalaemia in particular can predispose to digoxin toxicity, even when digoxin concentration is within the therapeutic range. Other risk factors for digoxin toxicity include, hypomagnesaemia, hypercalcaemia and drug interactions, e.g. with amiodarone and calcium channel blockers (which increase the plasma concentration of digoxin), and diuretics (if hypokalaemia occurs).

Your priorities in this case are to provide initial supportive care, correct the hypokalaemia and manage his digoxin toxicity.

## Supportive care

You should first take an ABCDE approach to Mr Edwards' acute deterioration and in particular organise for him to be placed on a cardiac monitor as he is at risk of developing a life-threatening arrhythmia such as a ventricular tachycardia.

You should also make an assessment of Mr Edwards fluid balance. His diarrhoea has stopped and his acute kidney injury appears to be improving (creatinine 144 from 184 μmol/L) but clinically he still appears to be dehydrated (dry mucous membranes, prolonged capillary refill). You need to continue to replace his existing fluid deficit. As he is nauseated, this is best done with intravenous fluids. Because of his gastrointestinal losses you will need to replace both water and electrolytes. Sodium chloride with additional potassium chloride is the best choice here (see Case 19). His overall estimated fluid balance is negative (−1040 mL). You therefore need to prescribe maintenance fluids (approximately 2.4 L over 24 hours) and replace his deficit (approximately 1 L over 24 hours): a total of 3.4 L over 24 hours. This is roughly equivalent to 1 L over 6 hours, and 3 further litres over 8 hours each.

## Correction of hypokalaemia

Mr Edwards has had diarrhoea and so is likely to have lost a lot of potassium as well as fluid and other electrolytes. You need to replace his potassium deficit and also account for any additional

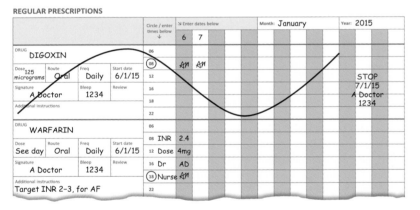

## ONCE ONLY PRESCRIPTIONS

| Date | Time to be given | DRUG | Dose | Route | Prescriber Signature | Prescriber Bleep | Administration Date given | Administration Time given | Administration Given by |
|------|------|------|------|-------|------|------|------|------|------|
|  |  |  |  |  |  |  |  |  |  |
|  |  |  |  |  |  |  |  |  |  |
|  |  |  |  |  |  |  |  |  |  |

### OXYGEN

| | |
|---|---|
| Target SpO₂ | ○ 94–98%  ○ 88–92% |
| Mode of delivery | ○ Continuous  ○ As required |
| Starting device | |
| Initials | Bleep | Date |

## AS REQUIRED MEDICATION

**DRUG** SALBUTAMOL

| | | | | | Date | |
|---|---|---|---|---|---|---|
| | | | | | Time | |
| Dose 1–2 puffs | Route INH | Max freq Every 15 minutes | Start date 6/1/15 | | Dose | |
| | | | | | Route | |
| Signature A Doctor | | Bleep 1234 | Review | | Given | |
| | | | | | Check | |

Additional instructions: 100 micrograms per puff

**DRUG** METOCLOPRAMIDE

| | | | | | Date | |
|---|---|---|---|---|---|---|
| | | | | | Time | |
| Dose 10 mg | Route IV | Max freq 8-hrly | Start date 7/1/15 | | Dose | |
| | | | | | Route | |
| Signature A Doctor | | Bleep 1234 | Review | | Given | |
| | | | | | Check | |

Additional instructions:

**DRUG**

| | | | | | Date | |
|---|---|---|---|---|---|---|
| | | | | | Time | |
| Dose | Route | Max freq | Start date | | Dose | |
| | | | | | Route | |
| Signature | Bleep | Review | | | Given | |
| | | | | | Check | |

Additional instructions:

**DRUG**

| | | | | | Date | |
|---|---|---|---|---|---|---|
| | | | | | Time | |
| Dose | Route | Max freq | Start date | | Dose | |
| | | | | | Route | |
| Signature | Bleep | Review | | | Given | |
| | | | | | Check | |

Additional instructions:

## INFUSION PRESCRIPTIONS

| Date | Time | Fluid | Vol | Drug | Dose | Rate | Doctor initials | Nurse initials | Batch no | Start time | Stop time |
|------|------|-------|-----|------|------|------|------|------|------|------|------|
| 6/1/15 | 14:00 | 5% GLUCOSE | 1 L | POTASSIUM CHLORIDE | 20 mmol | 125 mL/hr | AD | AN | 1001 | 14:00 | 22:00 |
| 6/1/15 | 22:00 | 0.9% SODIUM CHLORIDE | 1 L | POTASSIUM CHLORIDE | 20 mmol | 125 mL/hr | AD | AN | 2001 | 22:00 | 06:00 |
| 7/1/15 | 06:00 | 5% GLUCOSE | 1 L | POTASSIUM CHLORIDE | 20 mmol | 125 mL/hr | AD | AN | 1002 | 06:00 | 14:00 |
| 7/1/15 | 14:00 | 0.9% SODIUM CHLORIDE | 1 L | POTASSIUM CHLORIDE | 40 mmol | 166 mL/hr | AD | | | | |

on-going losses (see Case 19). This is particularly important in view of Mr Edwards's digoxin toxicity, as the hypokalaemia places him at high risk of arrhythmias. You therefore need to restore his plasma potassium to safe concentrations as quickly as possible. Intravenous administration is the most appropriate route in this instance. As potassium infusion can also cause dangerous arrhythmias, in a general ward setting potassium should be infused at a rate no faster than 20 mmol/hour.

### Treatment of digoxin toxicity

In treating digoxin toxicity you should consider correct any relevant electrolyte disturbances, minimise the risk of drug interactions, stop or reduce the dose of digoxin (at least in the short term) and consider using a specific antidote if indicated. Digoxin has a long half-life, around 30–40 hours, and this can be increased to around 4 days in the context of renal impairment (as digoxin is predominantly excreted by the kidneys).

In cases of serious overdose you may need to give the specific antidote: digoxin-specific antibody fragments (DigiFab®), administered intravenously. Digoxin-specific antibody fragments bind to digoxin in the blood, preventing it from interacting with cardiac cells, allowing it to be safely excreted by the kidneys.

In general, the antidote is indicated where there are life-threatening complications of digoxin toxicity that do not respond to other measures. Specific indications for the administration of digoxin-specific antibody fragments are as follow:

- Severe digoxin toxicity with haemodynamic compromise
- Ventricular arrhythmias
- Digoxin toxicity with hyperkalaemia
- Acute ingestion of >4 mg in a child (or 0.1 mg/kg) or >10 mg in an adult
- Serum digoxin concentration ≥10 µg/L 4–6 hours post dose
- Serum digoxin concentration ≥15 µg/L at any time.

Always consult a cardiologist and toxicologist (in the UK, via the National Poisons Information Service) in all cases of severe digoxin toxicity.

### Mr Edwards

Aside from correcting Mr Edwards' hypokalaemia, which in itself may correct his symptoms and abnormal ECG changes, you should stop his digoxin prescription. Digoxin binding therapy is not indicated.

### Continuing usual treatment

Mr Edwards's should continue his warfarin as charted, as prescribed according to his INR. The decision to restart digoxin, or an alternative agent for atrial fibrillation management, will depend on his clinical condition, resolution of ECG changes and correction of electrolyte abnormalities and renal function.

### How do I write the prescription?
### Potassium replacement

Potassium is available as an oral or intravenous preparation. In this context, the intravenous route is preferred. However, given his co-existing renal impairment his fluid balance and potassium levels will need careful monitoring.

0.9% sodium chloride 1 L with potassium chloride 20 or 40 mmol should be prescribed in the infusions section of the drug chart. This comes as a pre-mixed solution. The rate of infusion should deliver no more than 20 mmol of potassium in an hour, and we have already established the ideal rate to replace his fluid losses is 166 mL/hour. The serum potassium concentration should be rechecked following the infusion or if there are any further abnormalities on the cardiac monitor, and the rate of potassium replacement adjusted accordingly.

### Stopping digoxin

Digoxin should be stopped for the time being. This should be signed and dated, and you should make a note of why it was stopped in the medical notes.

### Further reading

Medical Pharmacology at a Glance. Chapters 17: Antiarrhythmic drugs; Chapter 18: Drugs used in heart failure.
Prescribing at a Glance. Chapters 26–28: Using drugs for the cardiovascular system.

## What should I consider when deciding what to prescribe?

Mr Hawkins is a 70-year-old man who has had a ST-elevation ACS requiring percutaneous coronary intervention with a drug-eluting stent. He is currently making a good recovery. However, around one in five patients with this condition will be readmitted to hospital with cardiac disease within a year of their initial cardiac event. There is therefore an important role for secondary prevention in reducing recurrent ischaemic events.

## Secondary prophylaxis

All patients who have had an ST-elevation or non-ST-elevation ACS should be offered long-term treatment with aspirin, an ACE inhibitor, a beta blocker and a statin to reduce their risk of recurrent coronary events, cardiac complications and death.

Successful insertion of a coronary artery stent can effectively restore coronary flow, as illustrated in Mr Hawkins's case. However, patency of the vessel can subsequently be lost through gradual narrowing due to cellular proliferation (*restenosis*) or abrupt narrowing due to the formation of clot (*stent thrombosis*). Patients with restenosis typically present with increasingly severe angina, which occurs within 9 months in 20–30% of cases in which a bare-metal stent has been inserted. Drug-eluting stents were developed in an attempt to prevent this. They are associated with lower rates of restenosis due to the anti-proliferative agents (e.g. sirolimus or paclitaxel) that are released locally to prevent cellular proliferation around the stent.

Anti-proliferative drugs from drug-eluting stents delay the formation of an endothelial layer over the atherogenic stent material and so the period over which there is risk of stent thrombosis is longer than for bare-metal stents. Stent thrombosis is a very serious complication that invariably results in ST-elevation ACS, which sadly is often fatal. Dual antiplatelet therapy (with aspirin and a P2Y12 receptor blocker such as clopidogrel or ticagrelor) effectively reduces the risk of this complication. Aspirin should be continued lifelong as, in addition to helping to prevent stent thrombosis, it reduces risk of recurrent coronary events and death. The addition of a second antiplatelet drug such as clopidogrel or ticagrelor is important for the period during which there is a risk of stent thrombosis. After insertion of a drug-eluting stent, this is about 12 months, as has been recommended by Mr Hawkins's cardiologist. Mr Hawkins should be advised about the risks of discontinuing this prematurely, as the implications of stent thrombosis are severe.

An ACE inhibitor (or angiotensin receptor blocker, if an ACE inhibitor is not tolerated) should be started as soon as possible following diagnosis of an ACS, and continued indefinitely, particularly in patients with signs of left-sided heart failure. ACE inhibitors reduce mortality, ACS, heart failure and stroke in patients with previous cardiovascular disease. This occurs through multiple mechanisms including favourable effects on left ventricular remodelling, vasodilatation with improved coronary blood flow, and neurohormonal effects. You should prescribe an ACE inhibitor licensed for use following ACS, as guided by the BNF. Here we have chosen to prescribe ramipril.

A beta blocker should be introduced as soon as the patient is sufficiently stable to tolerate its negative inotropic and chronotropic effects. Studies have shown that this reduces the risk of recurrent ACS. Usual practice is to commence this within 24 hours of admission if possible, and then increase it to the maximum tolerated dose over a period of weeks to achieve a heart rate of 50–60 beats/min. There are many beta blockers licensed for use following an ACS. They reduce the risk of death by around 20%

| Surname | Hospital number | Weight | Drug intolerances |
|---|---|---|---|
| HAWKINS | 100048 | 80 kg | None known |
| First name | Date of birth | | |
| BEN | 25/11/1944 | | |

**REGULAR PRESCRIPTIONS**  **DRUG CHART 1 OF 2**

| | Circle / enter times below | Enter dates below — Month: January  Year: 2015 | | | | | | | | |
|---|---|---|---|---|---|---|---|---|---|---|
| | | 6 | 7 | | | | | | | |
| **DRUG** ASPIRIN | 06 | | | | | | | | | |
| | 08 | | AM | | | | | | | |
| Dose 75 mg / Route Oral / Freq Daily / Start date 6/1/15 | 12 | | | | | | | | | |
| Signature A Doctor / Bleep 1234 / Review | 16 | | | | | | | | | |
| | 18 | | | | | | | | | |
| Additional instructions ACS, lifelong | 22 | | | | | | | | | |
| **DRUG** CLOPIDOGREL | 06 | | | | | | | | | |
| | 08 | | AM | | | | | | | |
| Dose 75 mg / Route Oral / Freq Daily / Start date 6/1/15 | 12 | | | | | | | | | |
| Signature A Doctor / Bleep 1234 / Review | 16 | | | | | | | | | |
| | 18 | | | | | | | | | |
| Additional instructions ACS, for 12 months | 22 | | | | | | | | | |
| **DRUG** FONDAPARINUX | 06 | | | | | | | | | |
| | 08 | | | | | | | | | |
| Dose 2.5 mg / Route SC / Freq Daily / Start date 6/1/15 | 12 | | | | | | | | | |
| Signature A Doctor / Bleep 1234 / Review | 16 | | | | | | | | | |
| | 18 | | | | | | | | | |
| Additional instructions ACS, until discharge | 22 | | | | | | | | | |
| **DRUG** LANSOPRAZOLE | 06 | | | | | | | | | |
| | 08 | | AM | | | | | | | |
| Dose 30 mg / Route Oral / Freq Daily / Start date 6/1/15 | 12 | | | | | | | | | |
| Signature A Doctor / Bleep 1234 / Review | 16 | | | | | | | | | |
| | 18 | | | | | | | | | |
| Additional instructions | 22 | | | | | | | | | |
| **DRUG** METOPROLOL | 06 | | | | | | | | | |
| | 08 | | | | | | | | | |
| Dose 12.5 mg / Route Oral / Freq 8-hrly / Start date 7/1/15 | 12 | | | | | | | | | |
| Signature A Doctor / Bleep 1234 / Review | 16 | | | | | | | | | |
| | 18 | | | | | | | | | |
| Additional instructions Do not give if HR<50. Increase dose to max. tolerated | 22 | | | | | | | | | |
| **DRUG** RAMIPRIL | 06 | | | | | | | | | |
| | 08 | | | | | | | | | |
| Dose 2.5 mg / Route Oral / Freq Twice daily / Start date 7/1/15 | 12 | | | | | | | | | |
| Signature A Doctor / Bleep 1234 / Review | 16 | | | | | | | | | |
| | 18 | | | | | | | | | |
| Additional instructions | 22 | | | | | | | | | |

| Surname<br>HAWKINS | Hospital number<br>100048 | Weight<br>80 kg | Drug intolerances<br>None known |
|---|---|---|---|
| First name<br>BEN | Date of birth<br>25/11/1944 | | |

**REGULAR PRESCRIPTIONS**

| | Circle / enter times below ↓ | ⬐ Enter dates below | Month: January | | | | Year: 2015 | | |
|---|---|---|---|---|---|---|---|---|---|

| DRUG EPLERENONE | 06 | | | | | | | | |
|---|---|---|---|---|---|---|---|---|---|
| | (08) | | | | | | | | |
| Dose 25 mg | Route Oral | Freq Daily | Start date 7/1/15 | 12 | | | | | |
| | | | | 16 | | | | | |
| Signature A Doctor | Bleep 1234 | Review | | 18 | | | | | |
| Additional instructions | | | | 22 | | | | | |

| DRUG ATORVASTATIN | 06 | | | | | | | | |
|---|---|---|---|---|---|---|---|---|---|
| | 08 | | | | | | | | |
| Dose 40 mg | Route Oral | Freq Daily | Start date 7/1/15 | 12 | | | | | |
| | | | | 16 | | | | | |
| Signature A Doctor | Bleep 1234 | Review | | 18 | | | | | |
| Additional instructions | | | | (22) | | | | | |

**ONCE ONLY PRESCRIPTIONS**

| | | | | | Prescriber | | Administration | | | OXYGEN |
|---|---|---|---|---|---|---|---|---|---|---|
| Date | Time to be given | DRUG | Dose | Route | Signature | Bleep | Date given | Time given | Given by | Target SpO₂ ✓ 94–98% ○ 88–92% |
| 6/1/15 | 18:00 | ASPIRIN | 300 mg | Oral | AD | 1234 | 6/1/15 | 1800 | AN | Mode of delivery ○ Continuous ✓ As required |
| 6/1/15 | 18:00 | CLOPIDOGREL | 300 mg | Oral | AD | 1234 | 6/1/15 | 1800 | AN | Starting device Nasal cannula |
| 6/1/15 | 18:00 | FONDAPARINUX | 2.5 mg | SC | AD | 1234 | 6/1/15 | 1800 | AN | Initials AD  Bleep 1234  Date 6/1/15 |

**AS REQUIRED MEDICATION**

| DRUG GLYCERYL TRINITRATE | | | | Date | 6/1 | | | |
|---|---|---|---|---|---|---|---|---|
| | | | | Time | 18:00 | | | |
| Dose 400 micrograms | Route SL | Max freq | Start date 6/1/15 | Dose | 400mcg | | | |
| | | | | Route | SL | | | |
| Signature A Doctor | Bleep 1234 | Review | | Given | AN | | | |
| | | | | Check | AD | | | |
| Additional instructions<br>For chest pain, call doctor if repeated doses required | | | | | | | | |

| DRUG MORPHINE | | | | Date | 6/1 | | | |
|---|---|---|---|---|---|---|---|---|
| | | | | Time | 18:00 | | | |
| Dose 5 mg | Route IV | Max freq 4-hrly | Start date 6/1/15 | Dose | 5 mg | | | |
| | | | | Route | IV | | | |
| Signature A Doctor | Bleep 1234 | Review | | Given | AN | | | |
| | | | | Check | AD | | | |
| Additional instructions | | | | | | | | |

| DRUG METOCLOPRAMIDE | | | | Date | 6/1 | | | |
|---|---|---|---|---|---|---|---|---|
| | | | | Time | 18:00 | | | |
| Dose 10 mg | Route IV | Max freq 8-hrly | Start date 6/1/15 | Dose | 10 mg | | | |
| | | | | Route | IV | | | |
| Signature A Doctor | Bleep 1234 | Review | | Given | AN | | | |
| | | | | Check | AD | | | |
| Additional instructions | | | | | | | | |

and the risk of recurrent infarction by around 25%. Beta blockers reduce heart rate and contractility. These effects reduce myocardial oxygen demand and increase the duration of diastole, which improves coronary perfusion. In patients with a recent acute coronary event, metoprolol is a reasonable choice as it has a short half-life and can be stopped quickly if side effects develop (e.g. worsening heart failure, atrioventricular block).

Statins, which are HMG-CoA reductase inhibitors with a lipid-lowering effect, should be considered in all patients following an ACS irrespective of their initial cholesterol levels. They reduce the risk of recurrent ACS and can reduce mortality by 20% over 2 years. The evidence is strongest for high-dose atorvastatin or pravastatin following an myocardial infarction (MI).

## Aldosterone antagonists for heart failure

The aldosterone antagonist eplerenone should be considered in patients with heart failure resulting from left ventricular systolic dysfunction. In patients with severe left ventricular impairment (ejection fraction ≤35%) following ACS, eplerenone can reduce mortality by around 15%. This is thought to occur through improved ventricular remodelling and modulation of other pathophysiological mechanisms following an ACS. You should check renal function and the serum potassium concentration before starting treatment as aldosterone antagonists can cause renal impairment and hyperkalaemia. Spironolactone is an alternative aldosterone antagonist for severe heart failure, but does not have the same level of evidence to support its early use after an MI.

## Managing other cardiovascular risk factors

*Smoking.* Patients who smoke should be offered advice and support to help them quit (see Case 43).

*Diabetes mellitus.* Good control of blood glucose is important for both short- and long-term outcomes following ACS. In the short term, hyperglycaemia is an independent risk factor for adverse outcomes and death during recovery from ACS. In the long term, good blood glucose control may help to prevent further macrovascular disease (such as MI and stroke), and you should check Mr Hawkins's glycosylated haemoglobin (HbA₁c) level to assess his diabetic control and whether his treatment needs adjusting.

*Fondaparinux,* a factor Xa inhibitor that prevents thrombin formation and thereby reduces further clot formation, can be continued until his discharge tomorrow.

## How do I write the prescription?
### Beta blocker

Metoprolol should be started at a low dose of 12.5 mg 8-hourly orally. This can be titrated up to a maximum dose of 100 mg 8-hourly in order to achieve a heart rate of 50–60 beats/min. If tolerated, this can later be switched to a longer acting beta blocker, such as bisoprolol or a modified-release metoprolol formulation, to reduce tablet burden.

### ACE inhibitor

Ramipril should be started at a low dose of 1.25 or 2.5 mg twice daily. This should be gradually increased to the maximum tolerated dose (maximum dose 10 mg daily, usually administered in divided doses to minimise post dose hypotension).

### Aldosterone antagonist

Eplerenone should be prescribed regularly at a low dose of 25 mg daily, given orally. This dose should be increased to 50 mg after 1 month.

### Statin

Atorvastatin has been prescribed at a dose of 40 mg daily. The intention would be to titrate this up to 80 mg daily (the maximum dose) before discharge, in keeping with the evidence base supporting its use after MI.

## Existing medications

Aspirin and clopidogrel are already charted and the intended duration of therapy is already stated in the additional instructions box, which should also be added to the discharge summary to advise Mr Hawkins's GP.

## Further reading

Medical Pharmacology at a Glance. Chapter 15: Drugs used in hypertension; Chapter 16: Drugs used in angina; Chapter 19: Drugs used to affect blood coagulation; Chapter 20: Lipid-lowering drugs.

Prescribing at a Glance. Chapters 27 & 28: Using drugs for the cardiovascular system.

NICE clinical guideline 172. MI: secondary prevention. 2013. Available at: http://www.nice.org.uk/nicemedia/live/14302/65691/65691.pdf (accessed 19 January 2014).

---

## 49 A 49-year-old woman with chronic liver disease complaining of pain

### What should I consider when deciding what to prescribe?

Angela Morrison has been admitted with decompensated chronic liver disease and now requires analgesia for an arm injury. When selecting analgesia and reviewing her treatment you should consider whether her liver disease will reduce drug metabolism, which could for example increase the risk of side effects. You should reflect on whether any of her medications could worsen hepatic impairment or its complications. It is also a good opportunity to ensure that her liver disease and any complications are adequately treated.

### Assessing severity of chronic liver disease

It is difficult to estimate the likely effect of chronic liver disease on hepatic drug metabolism as there is no one simple parameter that encapsulates hepatic function (unlike chronic kidney disease which can be described by eGFR). Useful indicators of poor hepatic function are albumin, clotting and bilirubin, which describe synthetic and excretory functions, and the presence of hepatic complications, including ascites and hepatic encephalopathy. The Child–Pugh score uses these parameters to determine prognosis in patients with liver disease. This score may also have some utility in directing prescribing (Table 49.2).

This score was initially used to evaluate surgical risk as good (grade A, 5–6 points), moderate (grade B, 7–9 points) or poor (grade C, 10–15 points). A higher Child–Pugh score indicates increased need for caution when prescribing drugs metabolised by the liver.

### Angela Morrison

Mrs Morrison has a low albumin, raised INR and elevated bilirubin, indicating poor liver function. The finding that her liver enzymes (ALT, ALP, GGT) are only mildly elevated is misleading in determining the severity of her liver disease. This is because a large proportion of her hepatic tissue has been replaced by fibrosis, reducing the amount available to release these enzymes. Mrs Morrison's liver disease is complicated by portal hypertension with oesophageal varices, ascites and mild hepatic encephalopathy (inattention, irritability and mild confusion). Taken together, poor liver function and complications indicate that Mrs Morrison has

| Surname MORRISON | Hospital number 100049 | Weight | Drug intolerances |
|---|---|---|---|
| First name ANGELA | Date of birth 13/12/1965 | 55 kg | None known |

**REGULAR PRESCRIPTIONS**

| | Circle / enter times below ↓ | Month: January | | | | Year: 2015 | |
|---|---|---|---|---|---|---|---|
| | | 5 | 6 | 7 | | | |
| DRUG FUROSEMIDE — Dose 40 mg — Route Oral — Freq Daily — Start date 5/1/15 — Signature A Doctor — Bleep 1234 — Review — Additional instructions | 06 / (08) / 12 / 16 / 18 / 22 | | An (at 08) | An (at 08) | | | |
| DRUG PROPRANOLOL — Dose 20 mg — Route Oral — Freq 12-hrly — Start date 5/1/15 — Signature A Doctor — Bleep 1234 — Review — Additional instructions | 06 / (08) / 12 / 16 / (18) / 22 | An (at 18) | An (at 08), An (at 18) | An (at 08) | | | |
| DRUG SPIRONOLACTONE — Dose 100 mg — Route Oral — Freq Daily — Start date 5/1/15 — Signature A Doctor — Bleep 1234 — Review — Additional instructions | 06 / (08) / 12 / 16 / 18 / 22 | | An (at 08) | An (at 08) | | | |
| DRUG THIAMINE — Dose 100 mg — Route Oral — Freq Daily — Start date 5/1/15 — Signature A Doctor — Bleep 1234 — Review — Additional instructions | 06 / (08) / 12 / 16 / 18 / 22 | | An (at 08) | An (at 08) | | | |
| DRUG MENADIOL SODIUM PHOSPHATE — Dose 10 mg — Route Oral — Freq Daily — Start date 7/1/15 — Signature A Doctor — Bleep 1234 — Review 3 days — Additional instructions (vitamin K) | 06 / (08) / 12 / 16 / 18 / 22 | | | | | | |
| DRUG LACTULOSE — Dose 20 ml — Route Oral — Freq 3 times daily — Start date 7/1/15 — Signature A Doctor — Bleep 1234 — Review — Additional instructions | (06) / 08 / (12) / 16 / 18 / (22) | | | | | | |

severe hepatic impairment. Considerable caution should therefore be taken when prescribing medication for her. You can make this judgement without the complexities of the Child–Pugh score. However, her Child–Pugh score of 13 backs up your clinical assessment.

| Date | Time to be given | DRUG | Dose | Route | Prescriber | | Administration | | | OXYGEN | | |
|---|---|---|---|---|---|---|---|---|---|---|---|---|
| | | | | | Signature | Bleep | Date given | Time given | Given by | | | |

OXYGEN

| Target SpO₂ | ○ 94–98% |
| | ○ 88–92% |
| Mode of delivery | ○ Continuous |
| | ○ As required |
| Starting device | |

| Initials | Bleep | Date |
|---|---|---|
| | | |

**AS REQUIRED MEDICATION**

DRUG **TEMAZEPAM**

| Dose 10 mg | Route Oral | Max freq Daily | Start date 5/1/15 |
| Signature A Doctor | Bleep 1234 | Review | |

| Date | 5/1 | 6/1 |
| Time | 2200 | 2200 |
| Dose | 10mg | 10mg |
| Route | Oral | Oral |
| Given | AM | AM |
| Check | | |

Stopped 7/1/15
A Doctor 1234

Additional instructions

DRUG **PARACETAMOL**

| Dose 500mg-1g | Route Oral | Max freq 8-hrly | Start date 7/1/15 |
| Signature A doctor | Bleep 1234 | Review | |

| Date | |
| Time | |
| Dose | |
| Route | |
| Given | |
| Check | |

Additional instructions
Max 3 g per day

---

**Table 49.2** Child–Pugh score. Published Child–Pugh scores vary slightly in the exact levels of each parameters used as a cut off. Many online calculators can be found with a simple online search (Pugh et al. 1973)

| | 1 point | 2 points | 3 points |
|---|---|---|---|
| Albumin (g/L) | >35 | 28–35 | <28 |
| Bilirubin (µmol/L) | <34 | 34–50 | >50 |
| INR | <1.7 | 1.7–2.3 | >2.3 |
| Ascites | None | Mild | Moderate to severe |
| Hepatic encephalopathy | None | Grade 1 and 2 | Grade 3 and 4 |

### Prescribing for patients with liver disease

General principles you should follow when prescribing for patients with severe liver disease:

1 Prescribe as few drugs as possible
2 For individual drugs check in the BNF for any special considerations when prescribing for patients with hepatic impairment
3 For drugs metabolised by the liver or with potential to exacerbate liver disease or complications, choose an alternative drug (e.g. one excreted by the kidney) or reduce the dose
4 Monitor patients carefully for response and side effects
5 When starting new drugs, always consider setting a stop date.

### Prescribing for Angela Morrison

*Analgesia*

Paracetamol can be used safely for pain relief in patients with liver disease. However, dose reduction may be required. Paracetamol is metabolised in the liver to the toxic metabolite *N*-acetyl-*p*-benzoquinone imine (NAPQI), which is inactivated and excreted by conjugation with glutathione. Intracellular glutathione stores are depleted by malnutrition, alcohol and in people with liver disease. Paracetamol may therefore be hepatotoxic at the usual 'normal' maximum dose (1 g every 6 hours) in people who are underweight (<50 kg), poorly nourished or who have severe liver disease. Although Mrs Morrison weighs 55 kg, do not forget that

she has several litres of ascites, masking an even lower body weight. As she has severe liver disease and is probably malnourished, you should reduce the daily maximum paracetamol dose allowed when prescribing this for her.

Non-steroidal anti-inflammatory drugs (NSAIDs) are contraindicated in severe liver disease as they increase the risk of gastrointestinal bleeding, worsen sodium and water retention and may precipitate renal failure.

Opioid analgesics may precipitate coma in patients with hepatic impairment due to accumulation of the drug or direct or indirect worsening of hepatic encephalopathy. They should only be used with considerable caution. Most opioid analgesics are metabolised by the liver and so may accumulate when liver function is impaired. Opioids slow intestinal transit and cause constipation, which increases gastrointestinal absorption of nitrogenous compounds that cause or exacerbate hepatic encephalopathy. Furthermore, opioids and other sedative drugs, including benzodiazepines, antidepressants and antipsychotics, can directly worsen encephalopathy through their central nervous system effects. If paracetamol does not control Mrs Morrison's pain you could consider prescribing a moderate opioid analgesic such as dihydrocodeine. However, you should use a low dose (e.g. 15 mg not 30 mg), avoid regular administration or combination with paracetamol (i.e. not co-dydramol) and co-prescribe lactulose to prevent constipation. Stronger opioids should only be prescribed with specialist advice and support.

*Other issues*

*Clotting.* Mrs Morrison has a raised INR, purpura and bruising where she has injured her shoulder. You could prescribe menadiol sodium phosphate (oral vitamin K), which may improve her coagulation. Her impaired coagulation and previous variceal bleed are contraindications to pharmacological VTE prophylaxis, although anti-embolism stockings could be considered.

*Encephalopathy.* Mrs Morrison has some disorientation, inattention and irritability, consistent with grade 1 or 2 hepatic encephalopathy. You should address this by cancelling the prescription for benzodiazepines and prescribing lactulose to increase intestinal transit and reduce intestinal absorption of nitrogenous compounds.

### How do I write the prescription?
### Analgesia

You should prescribe paracetamol on the as required side of the chart so that Mrs Morrison only takes it when needed. On the model prescription, 500 mg to 1 g is prescribed 8-hourly to a maximum of 3 g/day. This is lower than the usual adult dose of 1 g 6-hourly, maximum 4 g/day.

It would not be unreasonable for you to have written up a low dose of dihydrocodeine (15 mg) either as a once only or as required (e.g. max 12-hourly) medication. However, we have chosen not to do this as a routine on the model prescription, but to wait to prescribe opioids only if paracetamol is ineffective and they are really needed.

## Oral vitamin K

You should consider prescribing the oral form of vitamin K, using its non-proprietary name of menadiol sodium phosphate. On the model prescription, this has been prescribed at a dose of 10 mg daily for 3 days. You should reserve higher doses, intravenous administration and/or clotting factor infusion for patients with coagulopathy who are bleeding.

## Lactulose

On the model prescription the lactulose dose of 20 mL three times daily is slightly higher than the usual initial dose recommended for constipation (15 mL twice daily). The aim of treatment is for Mrs Morrison to achieve at least two loose stools per day as a treatment for hepatic encephalopathy, and you should increase the dose until this is achieved.

## Night sedation

This has been crossed off to prevent worsening of encephalopathy.

## Further reading

Medical Pharmacology at a Glance. Chapter 29: Opioid analgesics.
Prescribing at a Glance. Chapter 14: Prescribing in liver disease.
Pugh RN, Murray-Lyon IM, Dawson JL, Pietroni MC, Williams R. Transection of the oesophagus for bleeding oesophageal varices. Br J Surg 1973;60:646–9.

---

# 50 An 89-year-old man approaching the end of life

## What do I need to consider when reviewing therapy?

It is common for dying patients not to be able to tolerate their usual medicines. Moreover, the risk–benefit balance of medicines is likely to change: those that may have been valuable when the patient was active and had a life expectancy of several years may just cause unnecessary discomfort as they approach the end of life. So, when caring for a dying patient, an important task is to review all their medicines and stop those that are no longer appropriate.

## Medication review

In Mr Smith's case, it is no longer appropriate to administer a statin. Statins are valuable as long-term prognostic medicines in appropriately selected patients, but will offer no benefit for a patient who is imminently dying. In addition, Mr Smith is now unlikely to be able to tolerate his inhaler. Attempting to administer it will cause distress without providing any meaningful benefit. By contrast, analgesic and anti-emetic medicines remain valuable. There is no reason to suspect that his pain will have subsided, and indeed, his tachypnoea might be a consequence of pain. It is therefore important to find an alternative route of delivery for these medicines as he is no longer able take them orally. Of the various parenteral routes available, subcutaneous administration is usually preferred in palliative care. Subcutaneous injections are relatively painless (unlike intramuscular injections) and they do not require an intravenous cannula. If multiple injections are likely to be required, a continuous subcutaneous infusion (CSCI) can be used, as has been advised in Mr Smith's case. This is often called simply a syringe driver.

## Medicines to include in the subcutaneous infusion

You should only include medicines that are important to maintain or improve the patient's comfort. This will

| Surname | Hospital number | Weight | Drug intolerances |
|---|---|---|---|
| SMITH | 100050 | | None known |
| First name | Date of birth | 64 kg | |
| TERRY | 27/01/1925 | | |

**REGULAR PRESCRIPTIONS**

Month: January    Year: 2013

Enter dates below: 4 5 6 7

| DRUG HALOPERIDOL | | | |
|---|---|---|---|
| Dose 1.5 mg | Route ORAL | Freq Nightly | Start date 4/1/13 |
| Signature A Doctor | | Bleep 1234 | Review |
| Additional instructions | | | |

STOP 7/1/13 A Doctor 1234
22: AM AM AM

| DRUG MST CONTINUS | | | |
|---|---|---|---|
| Dose 30 mg | Route ORAL | Freq 12-hrly | Start date 4/1/13 |
| Signature A Doctor | | Bleep 1234 | Review |
| Additional instructions Morphine sulfate m/r | | | |

06: AM AM Unable to take
STOP 7/1/13 A Doctor 1234
18: AM AM AM

| DRUG SENNA | | | |
|---|---|---|---|
| Dose 15 mg | Route ORAL | Freq Nightly | Start date 4/1/13 |
| Signature A Doctor | | Bleep 1234 | Review |
| Additional instructions | | | |

STOP 7/1/13 A Doctor 1234
22: AM AM AM

| DRUG SIMVASTATIN | | | |
|---|---|---|---|
| Dose 40 mg | Route ORAL | Freq Nightly | Start date 4/1/13 |
| Signature A Doctor | | Bleep 1234 | Review |
| Additional instructions | | | |

STOP 7/1/13 A Doctor 1234
22: AM AM AM

| DRUG SYMBICORT 400/12 | | | |
|---|---|---|---|
| Dose 2 puffs | Route INH | Freq 12-hrly | Start date 4/1/13 |
| Signature A Doctor | | Bleep 1234 | Review |
| Additional instructions | | | |

06: AM AM Unable to take
STOP 7/1/13 A Doctor 1234
18: AM AM Unable to take

| DRUG | | | |
|---|---|---|---|
| Dose | Route | Freq | Start date |
| Signature | Bleep | Review | |
| Additional instructions | | | |

## ONCE ONLY PRESCRIPTIONS

| Date | Time to be given | DRUG | Dose | Route | Prescriber | | Administration | | | |
|------|------|------|------|------|------|------|------|------|------|------|
| | | | | | Signature | Bleep | Date given | Time given | Given by | |
| | | | | | | | | | | |
| | | | | | | | | | | |
| | | | | | | | | | | |

### OXYGEN

| Target SpO₂ | ○ 94–98% ○ 88–92% |
|------|------|
| Mode of delivery | ○ Continuous ○ As required |
| Starting device | |

| Initials | Bleep | Date |
|------|------|------|
| | | |

## AS REQUIRED MEDICATION

**DRUG** ORAMORPH

| Dose 10 mg | Route ORAL | Max freq 2-hrly | Start date 4/1/13 |
|------|------|------|------|
| Signature A Doctor | Bleep 1234 | Review | |

Additional instructions
Morphine sulfate oral solution (immediate release). For breakthrough pain.

| Date | 4/1 | 5/1 | 5/1 | 6/1 | | |
|------|------|------|------|------|------|------|
| Time | 1900 | 1000 | 2200 | 1800 | | STOP |
| Dose | 10 mg | 10 mg | 10 mg | 10 mg | | 7/1/13 |
| Route | ORAL | ORAL | ORAL | ORAL | | A Doctor |
| Given | AM | AM | AM | AM | | 1234 |
| Check | AM | AM | AM | AM | | |

**DRUG** MORPHINE

| Dose 5 mg | Route SC | Max freq 2-hrly | Start date 7/1/13 |
|------|------|------|------|
| Signature A Doctor | Bleep 1234 | Review | |

Additional instructions
For breakthrough pain. Call if more frequent administration required.

| Date | | | | | | |
| Time | | | | | | |
| Dose | | | | | | |
| Route | | | | | | |
| Given | | | | | | |
| Check | | | | | | |

**DRUG** MIDAZOLAM

| Dose 2.5–5 mg | Route SC | Max freq 2-hrly | Start date 7/1/13 |
|------|------|------|------|
| Signature A Doctor | Bleep | Review | |

Additional instructions
For agitation. Call if more frequent administration required.

| Date | | | | | | |
| Time | | | | | | |
| Dose | | | | | | |
| Route | | | | | | |
| Given | | | | | | |
| Check | | | | | | |

**DRUG**

| Dose | Route | Max freq | Start date |
|------|------|------|------|
| Signature | Bleep | Review | |

Additional instructions

| Date | | | | | | |
| Time | | | | | | |
| Dose | | | | | | |
| Route | | | | | | |
| Given | | | | | | |
| Check | | | | | | |

## INFUSION PRESCRIPTIONS

| Date | Time | Fluid | Vol | Drug | Dose | Rate | Doctor initials | Nurse initials | Batch no | Start time | Stop time |
|------|------|------|------|------|------|------|------|------|------|------|------|
| Continuous subcutaneous infusion (CSCI) | Date 7/1/13 Time 14:00 | | | MORPHINE HALOPERIDOL | 30 mg 1.5 mg | Make up to 18 ml with water for injection and administer via McKinley T34 syringe pump (0.75 mL/h) | AD | | | | |
| | | | | | | | | | | | |
| | | | | | | | | | | | |

---

usually comprise an opioid analgesic (morphine, diamorphine or, occasionally, fentanyl or alfentanil) and an anti-emetic (low-dose haloperidol is often a good choice for drug-induced nausea). In selected cases, it may also include an anxiolytic drug for agitation (e.g. midazolam), or an anti-secretory drug (e.g. hyoscine butylbromide) for severe and distressing respiratory secretions. Not all drugs can be given by subcutaneous infusion, and some drugs cannot be co-administered in the same infusion due to chemical incompatibility. You should seek advice from a palliative medicine specialist in most cases in which you contemplate starting a CSCI, and in all cases in which you have any doubt over medication choice and compatibility.

### Converting between routes of administration

When changing between routes of administration, it is usually necessary to change the dose of the drug. This is because most drugs are not completely absorbed from the gut (i.e. their bioavailability is less than complete), but are more completely absorbed from subcutaneous tissue. For example, in chronic use, about one-third of an oral dose of morphine sulfate is absorbed, whereas about 80% of a subcutaneously administered dose will be absorbed.

For this reason, when converting from oral to subcutaneous administration, divide the *total daily dosage* by two (some would argue that it is safer to divide by three). In Mr Smith's case, as he usually takes 60 mg/day morphine (two doses of MST Continus 30 mg), the dose that should be prescribed for subcutaneous infusion is 30 mg.

Approximately 75% of an oral dose of haloperidol is absorbed. When dealing with low doses (<5 mg/day) it is not usually necessary to make an adjustment when switching to subcutaneous administration.

### Other considerations

You should ensure adequate provisions are made for breakthrough symptoms – in this case, breakthrough pain. A good rule of thumb is that the dose of opioid required for breakthrough analgesia is about one-sixth of the total daily dose of regular analgesia. So, in this case, the existing prescription for Oramorph® (morphine sulfate immediate release) 10 mg is appropriate. This should be converted for subcutaneous administration as described above (divide by two), but this time morphine sulfate (not Oramorph®) should be prescribed for administration by subcutaneous injection.

It is also a good idea to prescribe other 'rescue' drugs that may be needed in the care of a dying patient. Some symptoms (particularly agitation) can arise quite abruptly, and may be distressing for the patient and those close to him. If nothing has been prescribed pre-emptively, the resulting delays in treatment add to this distress.

Prescriptions for fluids are not usually required when caring for a patient expected to die imminently – good mouth care is usually more important – but this should always be determined on a case-by-case basis. Likewise, oxygen is rarely indicated. If the patient is breathless, it is better to treat this non-pharmacologically (e.g. with a fan) or, if necessary, with an opioid.

You should be aware that many drugs administered by subcutaneous infusion are not licensed for use in this way. The use of drugs outside the terms of their license ('off-label') is allowed, but places some extra responsibility on the prescriber. Normally, you should explain to the patient why you are recommending use of a medicine in a way that has not been formally approved, and seek their consent to prescribe it. In palliative care, however, attempting to do this may not be practical, and may cause distress. In such cases it may be preferable not to draw attention to the licence status.

### How do I write the prescription?

Stop all unnecessary medicines in the usual way by clearly crossing through the prescription and signing and dating this. In the model prescription, all of Mr Smith's existing medicines have been stopped. His regular oral morphine regimen has been represcribed as a subcutaneous infusion, and his prescription for oral breakthrough analgesia has been represcribed for subcutaneous injection. A prescription for midazolam 2.5–5 mg SC has also been written in the as required section, in case it is needed for agitation arising in the last stages of his life.

There are various forms of syringe pumps, each of which has slightly different requirements for how the infusion should be prepared. Likewise, hospitals have different policies for how the prescription should be written: whether it should be on the standard infusions chart, a sticker affixed to the chart or a separate prescription altogether. You should familiarise yourself with the syringe driver policy for the hospital in which you work.

In this case, we illustrate an approach using a sticker affixed to the prescription chart. The details of the prescription are tailored to one commonly used syringe pump (the McKinley T34 device). The drugs to be given in the infusion (over 24 hours) are morphine sulfate 30 mg (half the dose administered orally) and haloperidol 1.5 mg (no dosage adjustment). Water for injection is usually the preferred diluent.

Note that when prescribing oral morphine preparations it is good practice to use brand names (e.g. MST Continus, Oramorph) to avoid confusion between immediate- and modified-release preparations. This is not necessary when prescribing opioids for injection, when non-proprietary names (e.g. morphine) should be used.

### Further reading
Watson M, Lucas C, Hoy A, Back I, Armstrong P (eds). Palliative care adult network guidelines plus. http://book.pallcare.info/ (accessed 7 November 2013).

National Institute for Health and Clinical Excellence. Opioids in palliative care (CG140). 2012. http://www.nice.org.uk/CG140 (accessed 24 January 2014).

# Appendix 1 Antibiotic guidelines

## SUGGESTED EMPIRICAL ANTIBIOTIC CHOICE FOR COMMON INFECTIONS IN ADULT PATIENTS

| | INFECTION | FIRST-LINE ANTIBIOTIC | ALTERNATIVE ANTIBIOTIC IF UNABLE TO USE FIRST CHOICE |
|---|---|---|---|
| GASTROINTESTINAL SYSTEM | Gastroenteritis | Antibiotic not usually indicated | Antibiotic not usually indicated |
| | Clostridium difficile infection<br>Oral. Suggested duration of treatment 10–14 days | Metronidazole | Vancomycin |
| RESPIRATORY | Acute exacerbations of chronic obstructive pulmonary disease<br>Oral. Suggested duration of treatment 5 days | Amoxicillin or doxycycline | Clarithromycin |
| | Community-acquired pneumonia mild<br>Oral. Suggested duration of treatment 7 days | Amoxicillin | Doxycycline or clarithromycin |
| | Community-acquired pneumonia moderate<br>Oral or IV. Suggested duration of treatment 7 days | Amoxicillin + clarithromycin | Doxycycline |
| | Community-acquired pneumonia severe<br>IV. Suggested duration of treatment 7–10 days | Benzylpenicillin + clarithromycin | Seek microbiology advice |
| | Hospital-acquired pneumonia<br>Oral or IV. Suggested duration of treatment 7 days | Co-amoxiclav | Seek microbiology advice |
| CENTRAL NERVOUS SYSTEM | Meningitis<br>IV. Suggested duration of treatment at least 10 days | Cefotaxime | Seek microbiology advice |
| URINARY TRACT | Acute pyelonephritis<br>IV. Suggested duration of treatment 10–14 days | Co-amoxiclav | Ciprofloxacin |
| | Uncomplicated urinary tract infection<br>Oral. Suggested duration of treatment 3–7 days | Trimethoprim or nitrofurantoin | Amoxicillin |
| SKIN | Cellulitis<br>Oral or IV. Suggested duration of treatment 7–14 days | Flucloxacillin | Clarithromycin |
| EYE | Purulent conjunctivitis<br>Topical. Suggest continue until 48 hours after healing | Chloramphenicol | Seek microbiology advice |

*Prescribing Scenarios at a Glance*, First Edition. Emma Baker, Daniel Burrage, Dagan Lonsdale, and Andrew Hitchings.

# Appendix 2 Case summaries

| Case no | Title | Brief case summary | Level |
|---|---|---|---|
| | *Section 1: The acute take* | | |
| 1 | An 82-year-old woman who requires venous thromboembolism prophylaxis | Prescribing thromboprophylaxis for a patient following surgical treatment for a fractured tibia | 1 |
| 2 | A 104-year-old woman with respiratory failure | Prescribing oxygen for a patient at risk of carbon dioxide retention | 1 |
| 3 | A 64-year-old man with severe acute abdominal pain | Prescribing and administration of intravenous morphine for severe acute abdominal pain | 2 |
| 4 | A 55-year-old woman with atrial fibrillation | Initial management of acute atrial fibrillation, including rate control and reduction of thromboembolic risk | 2 |
| 5 | A 32-year-old man with community-acquired pneumonia | Prescribing appropriate admission medication for a patient with community-acquired pneumonia | 2 |
| 6 | A 45-year-old woman with status epilepticus | Prescribing admission treatment for a patient presenting in status epilepticus | 2 |
| 7 | A 27-year-old woman with suspected bacterial meningitis | Prescribing appropriate admission medication for a patient with suspected bacterial meningitis | 2 |
| 8 | A 31-year-old woman with paracetamol overdose | Interpreting a paracetamol level and prescribing acetylcysteine for a significant paracetamol overdose | 3 |
| 9 | A 59-year-old man with acute pulmonary oedema | Initial emergency management of acute pulmonary oedema in a patient with a background of ischaemic heart disease and chronic heart failure | 3 |
| 10 | A 24-year-old woman with acute asthma | Initial management of a patient with an acute severe asthma exacerbation | 3 |
| 11 | A 57-year-old man who has suddenly deteriorated | Immediate management of suspected anaphylaxis, in which potential triggers include co-amoxiclav and gelatin | 3 |
| 12 | An 84-year-old man taking warfarin who has a headache | Reversal of over-anticoagulation in a patient taking warfarin who develops a subdural haematoma following a minor head injury | 3 |
| 13 | A 66-year-old man with acute coronary syndrome | Initial emergency management of acute coronary syndrome in a patient with multiple cardiovascular risk factors | 4 |
| 14 | A 67-year-old man with an exacerbation of COPD | Prescribing admission medication for a patient with a COPD exacerbation, taking into account current medication and comorbidities | 4 |
| | *Section 2: On call in the hospital* | | |
| 15 | A 91-year-old man with hypoglycaemia | Treatment of severe hypoglycaemia with IV glucose | 1 |
| 16 | A 60-year-old woman requesting night sedation | Prescribing a hypnotic–anxiolytic drug the night before elective surgery | 1 |
| 17 | A 62-year-old man with suspected opioid toxicity | Prescribing naloxone for suspected opioid toxicity due to morphine sulfate in the context of renal impairment | 1 |
| 18 | A 58-year-old man who has low blood pressure | Review of medications in a postoperative patient with postural hypotension | 1 |
| 19 | A 44-year-old woman who is 'nil by mouth' | Prescribing intravenous fluid therapy to cover maintenance requirements | 2 |
| 20 | A 59-year-old man with circulatory compromise | Prescribing a fluid challenge for a patient with reduced effective circulating volume due to sepsis | 2 |
| 21 | A 15-month-old girl with gastroenteritis | Prescribing intravenous fluids for a dehydrated but haemodynamically stable child | 2 |
| 22 | A 5-year-old boy with a painful right arm | Prescribing analgesia for a 5-year-old boy with postoperative pain | 2 |
| 23 | A 12-hour-old boy with signs of sepsis | Prescribing intravenous antibiotics for a neonate with suspected neonatal sepsis | 2 |
| 24 | A 60-year-old man who has developed a hot joint | Managing acute gout (starting an NSAID and stopping a potential precipitant) | 2 |

*Prescribing Scenarios at a Glance*, First Edition. Emma Baker, Daniel Burrage, Dagan Lonsdale, and Andrew Hitchings.

**164**   © 2014 John Wiley & Sons, Ltd. Published 2014 by John Wiley & Sons, Ltd. Companion website: www.ataglanceseries.com/prescribingscenarios

| Case no | Title | Brief case summary | Level |
|---|---|---|---|
| 25 | A 65-year-old man with hypokalaemia | Prescribing intravenous potassium replacement for hypokalaemia | 2 |
| 26 | A 69-year-old woman being treated with gentamicin | Interpreting a gentamicin concentration to determine whether a dose should be administered | 2 |
| 27 | A 69-year-old man anti-coagulated with warfarin | Dose adjustment of warfarin in the context of a high INR | 2 |
| 28 | A 28-year-old woman with nausea | Prescribing an anti-emetic drug for postoperative nausea | 2 |
| 29 | A 29-year-old man who is in pain following an operation | Prescribing postoperative analgesia | 3 |
| 30 | A 49-year-old man due to undergo surgery | Initiating a variable rate intravenous insulin infusion for a patient with diabetes due to undergo surgery | 3 |
| 31 | A 79-year-old woman with acute kidney injury | Prescription chart review for a patient with acute kidney injury | 3 |
| 32 | An 85-year-old woman with hospital-acquired pneumonia | Managing a patient found to have hospital-acquired pneumonia, including antibiotic prescription | 3 |
| 33 | A 47-year-old man who has developed an abnormal liver profile | Reviewing medication in a patient on multiple drugs for acute and chronic illness who develops an abnormal liver profile | 4 |
| 34 | An 83-year-old man who develops diarrhoea | Reviewing treatment for a patient in hospital who develops diarrhoea with a likely diagnosis of *Clostridium difficile* infection | 4 |
| 35 | An 88-year-old man with hyperkalaemia | Prescribing urgent treatment for severe hyperkalaemia, including calcium gluconate and insulin–glucose | 4 |
| 36 | A 69-year-old woman with acute alcohol withdrawal | Management of a hospital inpatient with acute alcohol withdrawal | 4 |

*Section 3: Routine inpatient review*

| Case no | Title | Brief case summary | Level |
|---|---|---|---|
| 37 | A 69-year-old woman with constipation | Prescribing a laxative for a patient with constipation | 1 |
| 38 | A 71-year-old man who has developed a tremor | Reviewing and stopping medication for a patient with drug-induced parkinsonism | 2 |
| 39 | An 81-year-old woman at risk of fragility fractures | Prescribing secondary prevention following an osteoporotic fracture in a post-menopausal woman | 2 |
| 40 | A 23-year-old pregnant woman with pulmonary embolism | Prescribe anti-coagulation for a patient with pulmonary embolism in the third trimester of pregnancy | 2 |
| 41 | A 31-year-old man with increased seizure frequency | Interpreting and acting on serum phenytoin concentration data to guide dosage adjustment | 2 |
| 42 | A 58-year-old man with diabetes mellitus treated with insulin | Prescribing subcutaneous insulin for a hospital inpatient with diabetes mellitus | 2 |
| 43 | A 53-year-old man who wants to stop smoking | Prescribing medication to support a smoking cessation attempt in a patient who has recently had an acute coronary syndrome | 2 |
| 44 | A 90-year-old woman on numerous medications | Reviewing and rationalising medications in an elderly patient with polypharmacy | 2 |
| 45 | A 54-year-old woman with a peptic ulcer | Prescribing discharge medication for a patient found to have a duodenal ulcer as a cause of haematemesis | 3 |
| 46 | A 64-year-old woman with chronic kidney disease | Global assessment of a patient with newly diagnosed CKD with particular attention to medication review and initiation of ACE inhibitor | 3 |
| 47 | A 66-year-old man with palpitations | Management of a patient with digoxin toxicity secondary to renal impairment and hypokalaemia | 3 |
| 48 | A 70-year-old man with ST-elevation acute coronary syndrome | Prescribing medication for secondary prevention following a non-ST-elevation acute coronary syndrome | 3 |
| 49 | A 49-year-old woman with chronic liver disease complaining of pain | Choosing an analgesic and reviewing treatment for a patient with decompensated chronic liver disease | 4 |
| 50 | An 89-year-old man approaching the end of life | Reviewing the medication regimen of a dying patient and writing a continuous subcutaneous infusion ('syringe driver') prescription | 4 |

# Index

Note:
Items that are the main subject of cases/clinical scenarios are denoted by **bold** page locators, with those pages referring to scenario referred to simply by number and those pages referring to the model chart and explanation having a suffix **A**. Page numbers in *italics* refer to figures and tables. Index entries relating to information from within the scenarios, model charts or explanations are in normal type.